INTRODUCTION TO ANATOMY AND PHYSIOLOGY FOR HEALTHCARE STUDENTS

This book provides a highly accessible introduction to anatomy and physiology. Written for students studying the subject for the first time, it covers the human body from the atomic and cellular levels through to all the major systems and includes chapters on blood, immunity and homeostasis.

Logically presented, the chapters build on each other and are designed to develop the reader's knowledge and understanding of the human body. By the end of each chapter, the reader will understand and be able to explain how the structures and systems described are organised and contribute to the maintenance of health. Describing how illness and disease undermine the body's ability to maintain homeostasis, this text helps readers to predict and account for the consequences when this occurs.

Complete with self-test questions, full-colour illustrations and a comprehensive glossary, this book is an essential read for all nursing and healthcare students in both further and higher education.

David Sturgeon is a Senior Lecturer in Nursing at Canterbury Christ Church University, UK.

INTRODUCTION TO ANATOMY AND PHYSIOLOGY FOR HEALTHCARE STUDENTS

DAVID STURGEON

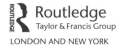

Routledge
Taylor & Francis Group

LONDON AND NEW YORK

FIGURES

TABLES

ACRONYMS AND CHEMICAL SYMBOLS

ACE	angiotensin-converting enzyme	**COPD**	chronic obstructive pulmonary disease
ACh	acetylcholine		
ACTH	adrenocorticotropic hormone	**cP**	centipoise
ADH	antidiuretic hormone	**CPR**	cardio-pulmonary resuscitation
AF	atrial fibrillation	**CRH**	corticotropin-releasing hormone
AIDS	acquired immune deficiency syndrome	**CSF**	cerebrospinal fluid
		CVC	cardiovascular centre
ANH	atrial natriuretic hormone	**DCT**	distal convoluted tubule
ANS	autonomic nervous system	**DEXA**	dual energy X-ray absorptiometry
ATP	adenosine triphosphate	**DNA**	deoxyribonucleic acid
AV	atrio ventricular	**ECG**	electrocardiogram
BCG	bacillus calmette-guérin	**EDV**	end-diastolic volume
BMI	body mass index	**EF**	ejection fraction
BMR	basal metabolic rate	**EPO**	erythropoietin
BP	blood pressure	**ER**	endoplasmic reticulum
2,3-BPG	2,3-biphosphoglycerate	**ESV**	end systolic volume
°C	centigrade	**Fe**	iron
Ca	calcium	**FSH**	follicle-stimulating hormone
Ca^{++}	calcium ion	**ft**	feet
CCK	cholecystokinin	**g**	gram/s
C$_6$H$_{12}$O$_6$	glucose	**GFR**	glomerular filtration rate
Cl	chlorine	**GH**	growth hormone
Cl$^-$	chlorine ion	**GHIH**	growth hormone inhibiting hormone
cm	centimetre/s		
cm^2	centimetre/s squared	**GHRH**	growth hormone releasing hormone
CNS	central nervous system		
CO	cardiac output	**GnRH**	gonadotropin-releasing hormone
CO$_2$	carbon dioxide	**H**	hydrogen

H^+	hydrogen ion	MS	multiple sclerosis
Hb	haemoglobin	mV	millivolts
HbCO	carboxyhaemoglobin	N	nitrogen
$HbCO_2$	carbaminohaemoglobin	Na	sodium
HbO_2	oxyhaemoglobin	Na^+	sodium ion
hCG	human chorionic gonadotropin	NaCl	sodium chloride
HCl	hydrochloric acid	NK (cell)	natural killer
HCO^{3-}	bicarbonate	nmol	nanomole/s
H_2CO_3	carbonic acid	NO	nitrous oxide
HIV	human immunodeficiency virus	O_2	oxygen
H_2O	water	PCO_2	partial pressure carbon dioxide
HR	heart rate	PCT	proximal convoluted tubule
Ig	immunoglobulin	pH	power/potential of hydrogen
IGF	insulin-like growth factors	PIH	prolactin-inhibiting hormone
IV	intravenous	PO_2	partial pressure oxygen
K	potassium	PNS	parasympathetic nervous system
K^+	potassium ion	PP	pulse pressure
kg	kilogram/s	PWS	Prader-Willi syndrome
kPa	kilopascal/s	Rh	Rhesus
l	litre/s	RNA	ribonucleic acid
LATS	long-acting thyroid stimulants	SA	sino-atrial
l/d	litres daily	SCN	suprachiasmatic nucleus
LH	luteinising hormone	SD	standard deviation
m	metre/s	SNS	sympathetic nervous system
m^2	metre/s squared	STEMI	ST elevation myocardial infarction
MALT	mucosa-associated lymphoid tissue	STT	spinothalmic tract
MAP	mean arterial pressure	SV	stroke volume
MI	myocardial infarction	TPR	total peripheral resistance
ml	millilitre/s	TRH	thyroid-releasing hormone
mm	millimetre/s	tRNA	transfer ribonucleic acid
mmHg	millimetres of mercury	TSH	thyroid-stimulating hormone
mmol	millimole/s	UTI	urinary tract infection
MMR	measles mumps rubella	UV	ultraviolet
MND	motor neuron disease	VF	ventricular fibrillation
mRNA	messenger ribonucleic acid	VT	ventricular tachycardia

ACKNOWLEDGEMENTS

I would like to acknowledge my colleagues Gill Pocock, Barbara Worster, Debbie King, Martin Bailey, Steve O'Connor and Karen Daniels for their personal and professional support. In particular, I would like to thank Gill whose advice has been invaluable during the writing of this book. All errors and inaccuracies are entirely my own.

I would also like to thank the team at Taylor and Francis for their patience and professionalism at all times.

Finally, I would like to thank Louise, Sofia, Ezra and Flynn for putting up with my crankiness during the writing of this book (and generally).

INTRODUCTION

This book is not intended to be an exhaustive or definitive account of human anatomy and physiology. There are many weightier texts available that discuss this topic in more detail and at greater length. What this book does provide is an accessible introduction to how the body works for healthcare students and other 'curious' individuals. It can be read cover to cover or used on a chapter-to-chapter basis as a reference guide to the different systems of the body. You may want to skip sections that are not relevant to your course or not appropriate to your level of study. However, I would encourage you to read it from beginning to end if possible for a number of reasons. Firstly, it is important to understand how the body is organised in terms of structural sophistication (i.e. from atom to organism). Just because something is small doesn't mean it is unimportant: quite the opposite, in many cases. The expression 'look after the pennies and the pounds will look after themselves' could just as easily apply to the smallest functional unit of the body – the cell. Unfortunately, the phrase 'ensure cellular health and the organ systems will continue to benefit from homeostatic regulation' is not very catchy and may put some people off reading further. Nonetheless, it is useful to have some understanding of the microscopic anatomy of the body in order to appreciate how many of the larger structures work. It is no coincidence that the tiny structures contained within the cell are known as organelles (tiny organs) and many of the activities they undertake (e.g. metabolism, digestion and excretion) are comparable with similar processes undertaken by the larger organs and systems of the body. The two are, of course, intricately connected and, for this reason, it is important to understand how the different organs and organ systems rely upon one another.

One of the difficulties when writing an anatomy and physiology book (at any level) is deciding the order in which to present the information, since everything is interconnected. For example, in order to understand the role of the heart you need to understand how oxygen is carried in the blood. However, in order to understand this, you need to know a little bit about the lungs and the respiratory system. At the same time, the heart and lungs both respond to chemical messengers (hormones) secreted by the endocrine system, as well as electrical signals (action potentials) generated by the nervous system! So which one first? Hopefully, as you progress through the book this 'interconnectedness' will become increasingly apparent. The final reason I would encourage you to read the entire book is that the chapters contain useful nuggets of information about washing-up liquid, the physiology of *Star Wars* (and other films), parasites and mind control, the difference between blackheads and whiteheads, how to get rid of skunk smell, which part of the brain is called the 'tough mother', poo-sausage research (really), blood type and personality in Japan, and other useful information.

People often find the study of anatomy and physiology challenging because there is so much unfamiliar vocabulary used to describe the different parts of the body and the activities they undertake. Even the terms 'anatomy' and 'physiology' are potentially bewildering. Most people are aware that they refer to the human body in some way or other but what is the difference? Put simply, anatomy refers to the structure of the human body or 'where everything is' in relation to the rest of the body. Physiology, on the other hand, refers to how these structures actually work. Many of the terms used to describe the different parts of the body (anatomy) and the processes that occur there (physiology) are derived from Greek, Latin or – infuriatingly – both at the same time. However, once you start to familiarise yourself with this vocabulary (and realise that it isn't as intimidating as it first appears) you quickly start to recognise how different phrases are put together to explain related concepts. For example, pathophysiology simply refers to the processes that occur when the body is diseased or injured (patho + physiology = disease + how it works). You can dress this up as much as you like but the essential concept is quite straightforward. Hopefully, this book will make clear that you already know an awful lot about the way in which the body functions in health and illness, as well as provide insights and explanations for processes that you may not have previously considered or known about. Please refer to the glossary at the back of the book to help with any vocabulary you can't remember or don't understand and use the 'Test yourself' sections to revise key knowledge (answers are provided).

Another reason people tend not to read anatomy and physiology books is because they can be extremely boring (I say this with confidence since I have read many good ones and many bad ones). Obviously, boring is a relative concept. What is boring for me (golf) may be very interesting for you. However, the human body *is* really interesting, you just don't know it yet! For example, as you are reading this text, your body's defences are battling away to destroy the potentially dangerous microorganisms introduced onto the pages of this book (or tablet if you are reading an electronic copy). Of course I am exaggerating; there was no need for me to introduce microorganisms onto the surface of the book/tablet since whoever touched it before you has already done so. However, don't panic, your body possesses an incredibly sophisticated immune system that (in health at least) is more than capable of destroying the large number of pathogenic (patho + genic = disease + forming) microorganisms that you have already come into contact with today and during the course of your life so far. The world is full of them but your body is working tirelessly to ensure that it continues to function in well-defined, healthy parameters. Consequently, it is essential to understand how the body operates in health in order to understand what happens when things go wrong. Sometimes, it is simply that we are unable to produce a particular substance (there is a deficit). For example, type 1 diabetes occurs when the beta cells of the pancreas are unable to produce enough of the hormone (chemical messenger) insulin. Without insulin we struggle to provide the cells of the body with glucose which they require to produce energy. If you understand how this process works in health it is very easy to understand what the consequences will be if it does not happen.

Finally, although the book is structured in terms of normal anatomy and physiology there are frequent references to disease and altered health states throughout since it helps to contextualise the particular body system from a healthcare perspective. It also serves to illustrate the inevitable consequences when something goes wrong. Reference to disease and illness in this book is certainly not complete, it is simply intended to aid understanding and demonstrate why it is important to know some of this information in practice. I am frequently asked by students: 'Do I need to know this?' My answer is almost always 'Yes' but I find they are far more likely to believe me (and, if I'm lucky, remember what I've said) if I can provide a tangible example of how the information applies to real-life healthcare situations. This is difficult to do all the time since some disease processes are simply too complicated to explain without a great deal of underpinning knowledge. However, I have tried to provide examples when the opportunity allows. I also apologise in advance for my frequent use of analogy and reference to films and characters that seem (to me) to demonstrate a particular point.

Contents

CHAPTER 1

ATOMS, ELEMENTS AND COMPOUNDS

STARTING SMALL

When thinking about how the human body works most of us tend to consider the familiar structures of the heart, lungs, kidneys, etc. We faintly remember from school that the heart is a muscular pump, the lungs allow us to breathe and the kidneys produce urine (but how any of this actually happens is a distant memory). Whilst these and other organs are self-evidently of great importance for our health, we should not overlook the much smaller and equally important structures that collectively make up these well-known parts of the human body. For example, the smallest functional unit of the body is the cell and it is estimated that the average adult possesses about 30 trillion (30,000,000,000,000) of these. However, even these microscopic units are composed of even smaller structures that are constantly engaged in the breakdown and production of chemicals and compounds necessary to maintain cellular and overall health. I know what you are thinking – 'this already sounds boring' – but hopefully I can convince you that the small as well as the big is worth knowing about and even quite interesting. In order to understand how the body works we first need to look at the simplest level of organisational structure – the atom. The way in which these fickle and impulsive particles bond and dis-associate with one another enables the body to function in the manner that it does. I am perhaps being a little unfair to all atoms since some of them possess relatively calm and settled dispositions. However, it is also fair to say that many have personality disorders that rival the average Big Brother contestant and some are extremely (and usefully) unstable.

ATOMS

The word atom is derived from an idea first formulated by the ancient Greek philosopher Democritus over 2,000 years ago. Democritus believed that everything was made from indivisible, imperishable and unchanging particles which he called *atamos*. A remarkable and insightful deduction for someone with no modern scientific equipment at his disposal. Today, atoms are often described as the smallest unit of matter that can exist in a stable form. They are made up of a number of smaller subatomic (literally 'below' or 'less than' atomic) particles that behave in a much more unpredictable fashion. However, for the purposes of this book, we are only interested in three of these particles: protons, neutrons and electrons. Each atom has a central core called a nucleus which contains varying numbers of protons and neutrons. The nucleus is surrounded by one or more energy layers called a shell which contains the electrons (Figure 1.1). Protons are positively charged particles, neutrons have no charge (they are neutral) and electrons are negatively charged. This is important since, under 'normal' circumstances, the number of protons in the atom's nucleus is equal to the number of electrons in the atom's outer shell (or shells).

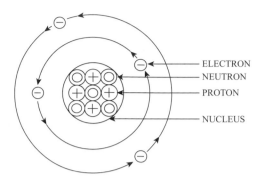

Figure 1.1   Basic structure of an atom.

This ensures that the atom remains electrically neutral since the positive charge of the proton is cancelled out by the negative charge of the electron. It doesn't matter how many neutrons there are in the nucleus of the atom (in terms of electrical charge) since they are always neutral.

ELEMENTS

Do you remember the periodic table of elements from school? Every physics and chemistry classroom had one of these impressively large charts on the wall somewhere. Each of the elements represented on the periodic table is composed of atoms of the same type (Figure 1.2). That is to say, each element is composed of either a single atom or a number of atoms of the same type. For example, an atom of hydrogen (chemical symbol H) represents the element hydrogen. If we add another hydrogen atom (H_2) it remains the element hydrogen but can also be described as a molecule of hydrogen. The term molecule can be confusing since it is applied when two or more atoms form chemical bonds with each other. However, in the case of a molecule, it doesn't matter if the atoms are the same or different from each other (unlike a compound which refers to the combination of two or more DIFFERENT atoms). I chose hydrogen as an example simply because it is the first element of the periodic table and has the atomic number 1. Did you ever wonder why hydrogen receives this pre-eminent position in the league table of elements? Why should hydrogen be number 1 when gold (Au) is languishing at number 79 and platinum (Pt) is only doing slightly better at 78? The answer is very simple and relates to the number of protons contained in the atom's nucleus. Hydrogen has the atomic number 1

The relative atomic mass of an element whose isotopic composition is variable is shown in parenthesis.
*Elements marked with * are those which do not occur naturally on earth.*

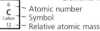

6 — Atomic number
C — Symbol
12 — Relative atomic mass

Figure 1.2 Periodic table of elements. Ninety-nine percent of the human body is composed of those highlighted in orange.

because it has one proton in its nucleus. Gold has the atomic number 79 because it has 79 protons in its nucleus. Oxygen (O) has the atomic number 8 because, you guessed it, it has eight protons in its nucleus. The fundamental difference between lead (Pb, atomic number 82) and gold (Au, atomic number 79) is the number of protons in the nucleus. However, as any good alchemist will tell you, it turns out to be incredibly tricky converting one into the other.

NEUTRONS

Neutrons are also found in the nucleus . . . but what do they actually do? We know that the number of neutrons in the nucleus does not affect the electrical charge of the atom since they are always uncharged particles. They do, however, help to determine the mass number of the atom. Mass simply means how much matter a solid, liquid or gas contains. You are probably thinking: 'Isn't that the same as weight?' Well, yes and no. For example, the mass of a small gold bar may be 2 kilograms (a unit of weight). Mass *is* commonly measured by how much something weighs but, crucially, weight can change depending on where you happen to be at the time. Mass, on the other hand, will always remain the same. For example, if we weighed the same gold bar on the moon, it would weigh less than it does on earth but still have the same mass. Following this argument to its logical conclusion: if you wish to lose weight, without going on a diet, simply move to the moon or other low-gravity environment. Anyway, what has this got to do with neutrons? The atomic mass number is the total of the number of protons and the number of neutrons in the nucleus of the atom. Helium, for example, has two protons and two neutrons in its nucleus. Consequently, it has an atomic number of 2 and an atomic mass number of 4. Just to confuse matters, not all atoms of an element have the same number of neutrons in their nucleus. We refer to these atoms as isotopes since they have a different atomic mass. Atomic weight (or relative atomic mass) is slightly different. It is calculated by taking an average (mean) of the relative atomic mass numbers of all the isotopes for a particular element. However, I feel this is getting unnecessarily complicated. The bottom line is that protons + neutrons = the mass number of the atom.

STABLE OR UNSTABLE?

The final constituent of the atom is the electron. These, as you remember, are negatively charged particles that whip around the nucleus of the atom in shells of varying size. The first or innermost shell can house a maximum of two electrons. The second shell can accommodate a maximum of eight electrons. The third shell is a little more complicated, and the first 20 elements (hydrogen to calcium) possess outer/third shells that hold a maximum of eight electrons. After this, the outer/third shell electron numbers become more variable and iron, for example, has 14 electrons in its third shell (2, 8, 14, 2) whilst copper (and all elements following it) have 18. Anyway, the point is this: elements are much like us in that they are constantly searching for harmony and inner peace in their lives. In order to achieve this seemingly impossible goal all they have to do is completely fill their outer electron shell. To put it another way, atoms with an incomplete outer shell are said to be chemically active since they are looking to combine (or bond) with another atom's electrons. Those that have already achieved this Nirvana-like state of completeness (e.g. those with a full outer electron shell) are referred to as chemically inactive or stable. The best example of this phenomenon is provided by the first two elements of the periodic table: hydrogen (H) and helium (He). Hydrogen has one proton in its nucleus and one electron in its first (and only) shell. It has one spare space, therefore, and is constantly on the look-out for an electron to fill this yawning gap in its life. Hydrogen is definitely an unstable (or chemically active) atom. If you don't believe me just consider the hydrogen bomb. Helium, on the other hand, has two protons in its nucleus and two electrons in its first (and only) shell. In contrast to hydrogen, therefore, helium is a very easy-going atom and forms one of a very exclusive group of elements who can boast a complete outer electron shell. These elements are known as the noble (or inert) gases and occupy the right-hand column of the periodic table (atomic numbers: 2, 10, 18, 36, 54, 86). Run 15,000 volts of electricity through neon whilst in a sealed glass tube and it just glows a pretty colour (irritatingly smug). Another good example of the difference in the personality between hydrogen and helium is, and I am slightly embarrassed to say this, airships. Let me explain before you throw this book away in exasperation. On 6 May 1937, the German airship *Hindenburg* burst into flames whilst attempting to land in New Jersey, killing 36 passengers and crew. What has this got to do with hydrogen, you may well ask? Well, unstable hydrogen was the gas used to lift this enormous aircraft off the ground. Inert (and non-flammable) Helium was also available but United States law prohibited the export of the gas to Germany (and other countries) since it feared that it would be used for military purposes. Ironically, the worst-ever airship disaster involved the helium-filled USS *Akron* four years earlier – it crashed in a storm (also in New Jersey).

COMPOUNDS

Another extremely unstable element (and highly flammable gas) is oxygen. Yes, good old oxygen is not as well balanced as we give it credit for. Oxygen has eight protons in its nucleus and eight electrons in its two shells (Figure 1.3). This leaves two available spaces that oxygen is restlessly looking to fill. Just like hydrogen then, oxygen suffers from a profound inadequacy complex that often leads to anti-social and volatile behaviour. As mentioned above, oxygen (in sufficient concentration) reacts rather aggressively when exposed to a naked flame. One of the common misconceptions about the earth's atmosphere is that it is composed entirely of oxygen. If we consider this proposition for a second it doesn't take long to formulate an experiment to disprove it: if I light a match, will the entire world explode? No. In fact, only 21% of the atmosphere is oxygen (78% is nitrogen) which, fortunately for cigarette smokers and everyone else, is insufficient to pose a threat when lighting a match. However, oxygen is self-evidently a chemically active element and it is not too fussy how it fills its spare electron capacity. Oxygen's most enduring and lasting relationship (you might even say the love of its life) is with that other highly strung element – hydrogen. Actually, it is more of a *ménage à trois* since it involves one oxygen atom and two hydrogen atoms. Since hydrogen has one electron and one space in its electron shell, and oxygen has six electrons and two spaces in its outer electron shell, it is possible for oxygen to bond with two hydrogen atoms simultaneously and for all three to achieve a complete outer shell (Figure 1.4). When two different elements combine to form a new molecule it is known as a compound. In this case, the elements hydrogen and oxygen combine to form the compound H_2O or water – the most important compound of them all for organic life.

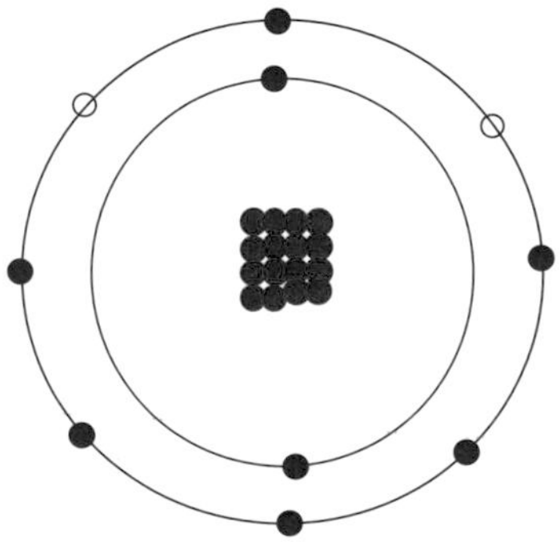

Figure 1.3 Oxygen atom with two empty spaces in outer electron shell.

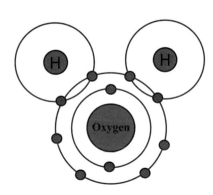

Figure 1.4 Water (H_2O) compound.

COVALENT AND HYDROGEN BONDING

The way in which the two atoms of hydrogen and one atom of oxygen combine is called covalent bonding. The term valence simply refers to the number of electrons in an atom's outer shell that are available for bonding. Hydrogen has a valance of 1^+ since it has one electron available for bonding. Although oxygen has six electrons in its outer shell it is usually said to have a valence of 2^- since it has two available spaces (from a total of eight) for bonding. In simple terms, therefore, a covalent bond means that the atoms share valence. The force of attraction is strong in these bonds and they are very difficult to separate once combined. Since the average adult consists of about 40 litres of water this is rather fortunate since it prevents us from unexpectedly disintegrating into chemical soup. But what keeps the individual H_2O molecules together and makes them so . . . watery? Well, the answer is hydrogen bonding. We already know that in a discrete H_2O molecule there are two hydrogen atoms (with positive valence) and one oxygen atom (with negative valence). Because the bonding electrons are shared unequally by the oxygen and hydrogen atoms (think of oxygen as Micky Mouse's head and the two hydrogen atoms as his comically oversized ears) a partial negative charge forms at the oxygen end of the water molecule (Micky's chin) and a partial positive charge forms at the hydrogen end (Micky's ears). Since the hydrogen and oxygen atoms carry opposite charges, nearby water molecules are attracted to each other like tiny little magnets (Figure 1.5). Consequently, despite the fact that hydrogen bonds are weaker than other types of atomic bond, they allow water molecules to 'stick' together. When water becomes ice, the molecules become frozen in place and begin to arrange themselves into a solid grid or lattice-like structure. This rigid and buoyant form of water is highly desirable when floating in a glass of gin, but highly undesirable when floating in the North Atlantic directly in front of an 'unsinkable' ocean liner. Conversely, if we heat water to boiling

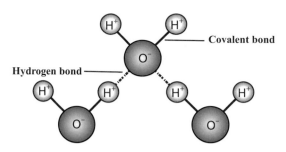

Figure 1.5 Covalent and hydrogen bonding.

point, some molecules attain enough kinetic (motion) energy to temporarily escape from the liquid as steam. Amazingly almost every element can exist as a solid, a liquid and a gas – it is just a question of finding the right temperature.

IONIC BONDING

The next type of bond that can occur between atoms is called an ionic bond. An ion is an electrically charged atom that is formed when an atom gains or loses an electron. In normal circumstances, atoms contain the same number of protons and electrons which ensures they are electrically neutral. In this case, however, the total number of electrons is not equal to the total number of protons, providing the atom with a positive or negative electrical charge. An ionic bond occurs when an electron is 'transferred' or 'donated' from one atom to another. This creates an attraction between the atom that has lost one or more electrons (known as a cation) and the atom that has gained one or more electrons (known as an anion). Since the cation has more protons than electrons it is positively charged; whilst the anion, which has more electrons than protons, is negatively charged. A good example of this process is provided by the slightly on/off relationship between sodium (Na) and chlorine (Cl) better known as salt (NaCl). Sodium has the atomic number 11 and has a total of 11 electrons (2 in the first shell, 8 in the second shell and 1 in the third shell). If sodium could only get rid of, or give away, this irritating single electron in its third shell it could achieve a complete outer shell (consisting of eight electrons) and become the stable element it had always dreamed of. Chlorine, on the other hand, has the atomic number 17 and has 2 electrons in the first shell, 8 electrons in the second shell and 7 electrons in the third shell – 1 short of perfection. If only chlorine could find or borrow an extra electron, it too could achieve its dream of becoming more like an easy-going noble gas. Just like a romantic comedy, therefore, the solution is right under the noses of our two mismatched but highly compatible protagonists. The sodium atom lends (or donates) an electron to the chlorine atom and they both benefit from their newly acquired stable state (Figure 1.6). OK, but how do they actually bond? In simple terms, they are held together by the strong electrostatic attraction between the positive and negative charges of each atom. This sounds complicated but is actually quite straightforward. The sodium atom has lost an electron and now has one more proton than electron. Consequently, it has a charge of 1$^+$ (a cation). The chlorine, on the other hand, has gained an electron and now has one more electron than proton. It has a charge of 1$^-$ (an anion). The attraction between the positive and negative charges pulls them towards one another and bonds them together (remember the 'tiny magnets' of hydrogen bonding). However, it is something of a marriage of convenience and you have to wonder if the commitment is really there. Although ionic compounds are often incredibly hard they also tend to be quite brittle (physically and emotionally). One of the most interesting properties of ionic compounds is that they can conduct electricity when dissolved in water (e.g. plasma). The water molecules pull the positive and negative ions apart and although this seems a cruel and tragic end to their fleeting and underdeveloped relationship, it does allow all sorts of important reactions to occur in the body.

IONS AND ELECTROLYTES

The term ion simply refers to a particle that has a positive or negative charge (cation or anion). Electrolytes are substances that separate (dissociate) into ions in solution and acquire the capacity to conduct electricity. For example, salt (NaCl) dissolves in water to produce positively charged sodium ions (Na$^+$) and negatively chloride ions (Cl$^-$). Other positively charged ions include potassium (K$^+$), calcium (Ca^{2+}) and magnesium (Mg^{2+}), whilst bicarbonate (HC0$_3^-$) and phosphate (PO$_4^{3-}$) are negatively charged. Ions are important since they provide the impetus for muscle and nerve functions, help to regulate fluid balance, maintain acid-alkaline balance (see below) and even trigger sour and salty tastes in the mouth. For example, both calcium (Ca^{2+}) and potassium (K$^+$) are important for normal muscular contraction including the cardiac muscle of the heart. In health, the body can excrete excess potassium ions via the kidneys (see Chapter 10). This is fortunate since so many delicious foods contain high levels of potassium including chocolate, yogurt, salmon, potatoes, beans, pistachios, almonds, avocados, sun-dried tomatoes, orange juice and of course bananas. In certain circumstances, however, potassium levels may become elevated (e.g. if the kidneys are not functioning properly) or depleted (e.g. after prolonged diarrhoea and vomiting). In normal circumstances, 98% the body's potassium is contained within the cells (intracellular) with only 2% outside the cell (extracellular). High levels of potassium in the blood (hyperkalaemia) can lead to an abnormal heart rate known as a cardiac arrhythmia (see Chapter 7). In extreme cases, this may result in cardiac arrest (where the heart stops altogether) and one of the 'ingredients' used to execute prisoners by lethal injection is potassium

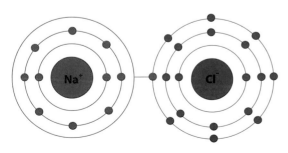

Figure 1.6 Ionic bonding of sodium chloride (Na$^+$Cl$^-$).

chloride. Low levels of potassium in the blood (hypokalaemia) may also prove dangerous and can result in muscle weakness, cramps, constipation and, in severe cases, respiratory depression.

DIFFUSION

Electrolytes are also extremely important for ensuring that water is distributed in the correct fluid compartments throughout the body (see below). As we know, electrolytes are substances that separate (dissociate) into ions in solution and acquire the capacity to conduct electricity. The term solution simply refers to what is formed when one substance is dissolved into another. In solution, all of the ingredients are uniformly distributed at a molecular level and no residue remains. For example, if we dissolve sugar in tea, the sugar changes physical state (from a solid to a liquid) and is equally distributed throughout the tea. The movement (or transport) of sugar in this way is an example of diffusion, whereby a substance moves from a high concentration to a low concentration. The sugar cube that has been dropped into the tea moves from a high concentration (around the cube) to a lower concentration (everywhere else) until it is equally distributed throughout (equilibrium is achieved). This is described as a passive process since it does not require energy to occur and is an important transport mechanism within the human body (think of glucose dissolved in blood plasma). However, although diffusion will take place of its own accord over a period of time, it is possible to influence the speed at which the reaction occurs. For example, diffusion rate is directly proportional to temperature: the higher the temperature, the faster the rate of diffusion. This is because raising temperature increases molecular activity. Returning to our cup of tea then, the hotter the water, the faster the rate at which the sugar will diffuse into the surrounding liquid. It is also possible to encourage this process by stirring the tea. Please feel free to casually remark to friends or family next time you are stirring sugar into your tea/coffee that you are actually attempting to agitate the molecules in the beverage to hasten the rate of diffusion (you will almost certainly receive a puzzled look). It is important to emphasise, however, that diffusion is not limited to the transport of substances in a liquid. It is also the process by which the gases oxygen (O_2) and carbon dioxide (CO_2) move from a high to a low concentration across the alveolar (air sac) membranes of the lung and elsewhere within the body (see Chapter 9). A more familiar example for those of you who have children (or similar small animals) is provided by farting. Imagine if you will, a typical family group sitting in close proximity to one another in a small, three-door hatchback (a Nissan Micra maybe). Towards the beginning of their journey the parents become increasingly aware of an unpleasant and unwelcome smell emanating from the back of the vehicle. After the usual recriminations and denials have taken place a window is opened and the smell begins to dissipate. If this is an occurrence that you are familiar with, or have recently been subjected to, consider how fortunate you have been to have experienced diffusion in action. The foul-smelling gas emanating from one of the children's bottoms is slowly but surely diffusing from a high concentration (in their pants) to a low concentration (everywhere else) until it is equally distributed throughout the car and all may 'enjoy' the pungent aroma of yesterday's dinner. Opening the window encourages diffusion to continue into the previously unadulterated air of the outside world.

OSMOSIS

Whilst all this talk of diffusion is quite interesting (and slightly gross) how does it relate to the way in which ions (and other solutes) help to ensure that water is distributed in the correct fluid compartment? Well, water also moves from a high concentration to a low concentration across a semi-permeable membrane. The term 'semi-permeable membrane' simply refers to a thin barrier that separates the water with few solutes dissolved in it, from the water with a higher concentration of solutes dissolved in it. Think of a teabag (it is permeable to water but the tea cannot escape). Imagine that we have two small reservoirs of tap water divided by a semi-permeable membrane. On the left side, we add a table spoon of salt (NaCl). We already know what will happen to this ionic compound when dissolved in water: the sodium chloride framework will disintegrate as the Na^+ and Cl^- ions become surrounded by water molecules. Anyway, the water on the left side is now less concentrated than that on the right because it is no longer normal tap water. The concentration of Na^+ and Cl^- ions is higher on the left BUT the concentration of water is lower compared to the tap water on the right. Consequently, water will diffuse from a high concentration on the right (tap water) to a low concentration on the left (tap water + NaCl) through the semi-permeable membrane that divides them. Water will stop diffusing only when the concentration on both sides is once again equal (by which time the water level on the left will be higher than that on the right). This process of water diffusion is known as osmosis and we will refer to it again and again regarding normal body function. In short, the quantity of ions (and other solutes) dissolved in water dissolved in water will have a profound effect on the osmotic concentration (osmolality) of that solution. If the osmotic concentration is too high, then the solute will attract water (until equilibrium is achieved). If the osmotic concentration is too low, water will be lost as it is attracted elsewhere. In either case, if this occurs in the human body, it can result in fluid overload or fluid depletion which may result in severe ill-health. This is one of reasons why we are (correctly) advised to limit our salt and sugar intake since they can affect the osmolality of our blood plasma, etc.

pH

Finally, some ions are very important for the regulation of acidity and alkalinity within the human body. This is also known as acid-base balance. But what are acids and bases? Well, an acid is simply a substance that releases hydrogen ions (H^+) when it disassociates in solution (typically water). The strength of an acid depends upon how completely the hydrogen ions disassociate in solution (e.g. how many H^+ are released). A base, on the other hand, is a substance that releases hydroxyl ions (OH^-) when dissolved in solution. It then accepts or 'soaks up' hydrogen ions resulting in a solution with more hydroxyl than hydrogen ions (an alkaline solution). Alkalinity is simply a measure of the capacity of a solution to neutralise or 'buffer' acids. Pure water is said to be neutral since it contains the same number of hydrogen and hydroxyl ions leading to a 1:1 ratio. The relative concentration of hydrogen to hydroxyl ions is represented by the pH scale. The p stands for power (or potential) and the H for hydrogen. Hence pH = the power of hydrogen. The pH scale usually runs from 1 to 14 and a change of 1 pH unit indicates a tenfold difference in actual hydrogen ion concentration. However, somewhat confusingly for non-mathematicians such as myself, the pH scale is expressed backwards and pH goes down as H^+ concentration goes up. That is to say, each whole pH value below 7 (the pH of pure water) is 10 times more acidic than the higher value, and each whole pH value above 7 is 10 times less acidic (or more alkali) than the one below it. For example, the pH of tomato juice is about 4 which is 10 times more acidic than a banana which has a pH of 5. Interestingly, milk has a pH of about 6.5 which seems to make a nonsense of my mother's advice to me as a child to drink milk to settle an acidic stomach. I would have been better off drinking water with a pH of 7. In fairness, milk is still significantly less acidic than stomach acid (hydrochloric acid/ HCl) which has a pH of between 1 and 3 (see Chapter 11). Alkali substances include sea water (pH 8), sodium bicarbonate (pH 9), toothpaste (pH 10 – which explains why it blanches your T-shirt when dribbled down the front) and ammonia (pH 12). The pH of human blood plasma is maintained within a very narrow range, 7.35–7.45, and is therefore ever-so-slightly alkaline. The body maintains this fine balance in two ways: hydrogen ions (H^+) are absorbed by other molecules in a process known as buffering and acid products are excreted from the body via the kidneys and lungs. Dysfunction of the body's buffer system can result in acidosis (as H^+ concentration increases and plasma pH falls) or alkalosis (as the H^+ concentration decreases and plasma pH rises). Either can result in severe ill-health and the extreme (potentially life-threatening) limits for plasma pH are considered to be below pH 6.8 and above pH 7.8.

METABOLISM

So far we have seen how the human body is made up of atoms, elements and compounds (some of which are bonded covalently and some of which are bonded ionically). But how does this actually relate to everyday life and how do they provide substance and form? The term metabolism refers to the many different biochemical processes that contribute to the distribution and breakdown of nutrients, the production of energy, the elimination of wastes and growth and development within the body. To put it another way, we are all dependent on the way atoms come together and break apart, and the body is involved in a constant cycle of catabolism and anabolism (see Chapter 11). Catabolism, or destructive metabolism, refers to breakdown of complex molecules into simple ones often resulting in the release of energy. For example, when you put a piece of bread in your mouth, an enzyme in your saliva (amylase) immediately begins to break down (catabolise) the carbohydrate from complex polysaccharide chains to simple monosaccharide chains (glucose). This is why, if you put a piece of bread in your mouth and resist the temptation to chew, it will soon begin to taste sweet (and very soggy). The amylase in your saliva quickly breaks apart the complex carbohydrate chains and converts them into simple sugars. Anabolism, on the other hand, refers to the process by which simple structures are transformed into more complex molecules. For example, at this very moment, the cells of your body are arranging simple amino acids (monomers) into complex chains (polymers) in order to produce proteins. In the following chapters we will see how this cycle of creative destruction is repeated over and over again in order to maintain health, growth and repair. However, putting to one side the

organisational complexity of the body for one moment, we are essentially comprised of a variety of combinations of four key elements: oxygen, carbon, hydrogen and nitrogen. It is true that we also consist of potassium, sodium, magnesium, iron, iodine and many other elements but all in very small quantities. Arguably the most important of these combinations, as mentioned earlier, is that of hydrogen and oxygen as H_2O.

FLUID COMPARTMENTS

An average human being contains about 40 litres of water accounting for 55–60% of their total body weight. In a new-born baby (neonate) this may be as high as 75% but will progressively decrease as the child matures. One of the reasons for this is that much of the new-born's skeleton consists of cartilage (see Chapter 4) which has very high water content (about 85%). There are many well-documented examples of babies and young children surviving falls from heights that would (or did) prove fatal to adults. Although on many occasions they were cushioned from the impact by other factors, the relative flexibility of their skeleton – and high water content overall – undoubtedly enhanced their chances of survival. In some fish (e.g. sharks and rays) cartilage is the only component of the skeleton and in 2012 a 2-foot leopard shark survived a significant fall onto a Californian golf course. Apparently, it was dropped by a bird (who had snatched it from the ocean some 5 miles away) and was returned alive to the Pacific in a bucket of salted water by a golf club employee. In humans, water is contained in three fluid compartments. About two-thirds (25 litres) is enclosed within the cells as intracellular fluid (Table 1.1). This can be a little hard to comprehend since cells are so small and individually at least they seem rather insignificant. However, when we consider that we each possess about 30 trillion (or thereabouts) it suddenly becomes more credible. The remaining fluid (about 15 litres) is contained outside the cells as extracellular fluid. About 12 litres of this is found around

TABLE 1.1 Fluid compartments

Total body fluid = 60% total body weight (40 litres of water)		
Intracellular fluid = 40% total body weight	Extracellular fluid = 20% total body weight	
Intracellular fluid = 25 litres of water	Interstitial fluid = 12 litres of water	Plasma = 3 litres of water

the cells in what is known as the interstitial space or compartment. Essentially this fluid bathes the cells and facilitates the delivery and removal of molecules and metabolic waste to and from the cells. The remaining 3 litres or so of fluid is found in the blood and lymphatic system as intravascular fluid (fluid in the vessels). The blood is said to consist of a cellular component (red blood cells, white blood cells, etc.) and a non-cellular matrix or plasma (see Chapter 5). It is this liquid plasma that allows blood to transport a variety of substances around the body and also provides an effective mechanism for maintaining a constant internal temperature (see Chapter 3). The balance between the different fluid compartments is very important for health and the body tries hard to maintain them in the approximate quantities outlined above. However, fluid can move between the blood vessel and the plasma membrane of the cell depending on the distribution of ions and plasma proteins in the fluid. That is to say, the osmotic concentration (osmolality) of fluid within the compartments will determine whether fluid is attracted towards it or whether it is attracted to water of a higher concentration.

FLUID BALANCE

A fluid that has the same concentration as another fluid is said to be isotonic (of equal tension). Within the body this means that the fluid on one side of a semi-permeable membrane (e.g. inside a cell) has the same osmolality as that on the other side. This ensures that fluid remains constant within the intracellular and extracellular compartments. For example, if we are dehydrated and require a transfusion of normal saline solution (0.9% NaCl) it is considered to be isotonic since it is a close

approximation to the osmolality of our blood in health. It is considered safe to transfuse, therefore, since it will not result in large-scale fluid shift from one compartment to another. A hypertonic (high tension) solution, on the other hand, has a high solute concentration and high osmotic pressure. Water is attracted towards it in order to dilute the solution. This can be useful in some circumstances and highly dangerous in others. For example, imagine you are sitting in a boat, adrift in the ocean, with nothing to eat or drink. If you drink the sea water (saline), the high concentration of NaCl will quickly alter the osmolality of your blood plasma and it will become relatively hypertonic compared to the fluid within your cells and interstitial compartment. Consequently, water from both of these compartments will be attracted towards the hypertonic blood plasma resulting in cellular dehydration (not good). Far from quenching your thirst, therefore, it will (for reasons explained in more detail in Chapter 10) make you even thirstier and almost certainly hasten your death at sea. Much better then to start-off drinking your own (or someone else's) urine since, initially at least, it will contain a more 'palatable' and safer mixture of water and dissolved substances. Finally, a solution that has very low solute concentration (few solutes dissolved in) is said to be hypotonic (low tension). For example, half-strength normal saline (0.45% NaCl) is hypotonic because the sodium chloride content is lower than the concentration in the blood plasma. In normal circumstances, therefore, it would be dangerous to transfuse a hypotonic fluid since it would be attracted to the relative hypertonicity of the fluid within the cells. This would cause them to swell, and perhaps even burst, as water passes through the cell membrane in order to equalise the concentrations. A good way to remember the difference between high and low osmolality is the expression: the higher the drier. When we are dry (e.g. dehydrated) our plasma osmolality is typically high or hypertonic. If, on the other hand, we have excess water in the vascular compartment (or elsewhere) our plasma osmolality will be low or hypotonic. In health, however, our body is constantly trying to achieve an isotonic or balanced state.

In the next chapter we will look at the smallest functional unit of the body, the cell, and how this tiny but complicated structure ensures health, growth and repair. We will also look again at the role of ions and explore other mechanisms of transport in and out of the cell. Hopefully, this chapter has got you thinking about how the small stuff underpins everything else. How something as seemingly insignificant as the concentration of salt or sugar in water can have a profound effect on health and well-being. Even as the body grows in organisational complexity, the way in which molecules bond and interact with one another remains crucial and any excess or deficit can prove harmful to health. We haven't quite finished with the small, therefore, and in the next chapter we need to look inside the nucleus of the cell at the way our genetic material is organised using only a few simple chemicals.

CHAPTER 1: TEST YOURSELF

Q. What are the three principle components (or particles) of an atom?
A. Protons, electrons and neutrons.

Q. What type of electrical charge does each of these particles possess (e.g. positive, negative or neutral)?
A. Protons have a positive charge, electrons have a negative charge and neutrons have no charge.

Q. What is the difference between an element and a compound?
A. An element is composed of either a single atom or a number of atoms of the same type. A compound is composed of a combination of two (or more) different atoms.

Q. What is the chlorine chloride, nitrogen, iron, calcium, water, carbon dioxide, sodium chloride and hydrochloric acid?
A. H, O_2, C, Cl, N, Fe, Ca, H_2O, CO_2 NaCl and HCl.

Q. What is the difference between covalent and ionic bonding?
A. Covalent bonding occurs when atoms share one or more electron. The force of attraction is strong in these bonds since both atoms complete their outer shell of electrons. Ionic bonding occurs when an electron is 'transferred' or 'donated' from one atom to another. This creates an attraction between the atom that has lost one or more electron (a positively charged cation) and the atom that has gained one or more electron (a negatively charged anion).

Q. What is an ion and what is an electrolyte?
A. An ion is an atom that has a positive or negative charge (cation or anion). Electrolytes are substances that separate (dissociate) into ions in solution and acquire the capacity to conduct electricity.

(Continued)

(Continued)

Q. What is the chemical symbol for the following ions: hydrogen, sodium, potassium, calcium and chloride?
A. H^+, Na^+, K^+, Ca^{++} and Cl^-.

Q. What is meant by the term diffusion?
A. Diffusion refers to the process where molecules (e.g. O_2) move from an area of high concentration to an area of low concentration (until equilibrium is achieved).

Q. What is meant by the term osmosis?
A. Osmosis refers to movement of water from a high concentration to an area of low concentration through a semi-permeable membrane.

Q. What does pH stand for?
A. Percentage of power of hydrogen (H^+).

Q. What is measured by the pH scale?
A. The pH scale measures acidity (low pH) and alkalinity (high pH) in relation to the concentration of H^+ in solution.

Q. Put the following into ascending order of pH (from most acidic to least): water, bicarbonate, hydrochloric acid, ammonia and urine.
A. Hydrochloric acid (pH 1–3), urine (pH 6), water (pH 7), bicarbonate (pH 9), ammonia (pH 11).

Q. What is the pH of blood plasma? Is it acid or alkaline?
A. 7.35–7.45 (slightly alkaline).

Q. What is the difference between anabolism and catabolism?
A. Anabolism is the phase of metabolism in which simple structures are transformed into complex molecules (e.g. amino acids into proteins). Catabolism refers to the breakdown of complex molecules into simple structures (e.g. protein into amino acids).

Q. How many litres of water does the average human being contain?
A. 40 litres.

Q. What are the three fluid compartments in the human body and roughly how much water do they contain?
A. Intracellular compartment (25 litres), interstitial compartment (12 litres), plasma compartment (3 litres).

Contents

THE CELL MEMBRANE

There are over 200 different types of cell in the human body including skins cells, bone cells, blood cells and nerve cells. They are essentially tiny parcels of chemicals enclosed by a thin plasma membrane and it is extraordinary to think that we all originated and developed from just one of these microscopic units. Following conception, cell multiplication takes place and cells with different structural specialisations develop (see Chapter 14). Human cells vary greatly in sophistication and function from relatively simple skin cells to highly specialised nerve cells (neurons). For the most part, human cells require three basic components: a cell membrane, cytoplasm (cyte + plasma = cell + water) and a nucleus. There are some notable exceptions that do not have a nucleus including red blood cells (erythrocytes). Although, in actual fact, they do have a nucleus but just for a very short period of time – it is ejected (extruded) as they mature. Anyway, let's not quibble. All cells need some form of plasma membrane in order to maintain structural integrity.

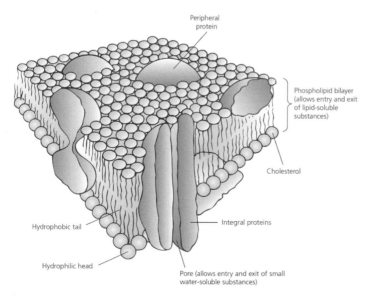

Peripheral protein

Phospholipid bilayer (allows entry and exit of lipid-soluble substances)

Cholesterol

Integral proteins

Hydrophobic tail

Hydrophilic head

Pore (allows entry and exit of small water-soluble substances)

Figure 2.1 Phospholipid bi-layer of the cell membrane.

Human cell membranes consist of two layers of phospholipids, sometimes referred to as a fatty bi-layer. This provides a barrier that ensures water and ions remain in the correct concentrations within the cell (cytoplasm) and outside the cell (interstitial fluid). It is able to do this because each lipid molecule contains a hydrophilic (water-loving) head and a hydrophobic (water-hating) tail (Figure 2.1). The bi-layer is arranged like a sandwich with the hydrophilic layers on the outer surfaces (the bread) and the tails on the inside (the butter). In other words, the hydrophilic head of the molecule is attracted to water whilst the hydrophobic tail is repelled. The same principle helps to explain how washing-up liquid works! If, like me, you do a lot of washing-up you will be well aware that fat does not dissolve in water. It either floats on top of the water, making crazy psychedelic patterns, or it stubbornly refuses to let go of whatever piece of crockery it has come into contact with. The hydrocarbon chains found in washing-up liquid also have hydrophilic and hydrophobic ends (they are said to be amphipathic). The hydrophobic ends attach themselves to the grease on the plate and surround it with their hydrophilic ends pointing outwards (towards the water). This makes the enclosed oil particles water-soluble and they can be washed away. Those of you who use dishwashers are missing out on this daily battle of wits. Anyway, in human cells, amphipathic phospholipid molecules are arranged in a continuous bi-layer and provide a highly impermeable barrier (which is fortunate for the cell since it is constantly exposed to water of some description).

ION CHANNELS

Embedded into the phospholipid bi-layer (the plasma membrane) are protein molecules known as ion channels. These facilitate the transport of ions and non-fat-soluble substances in and out of the cell. We have already observed in Chapter 1 that water is transported from a high concentration to a low concentration, across a semi-permeable membrane, depending on the relative osmolality of the two solutions. But how do these ions or solutes move between the intracellular and extracellular compartments? Firstly, ions are present in different concentrations in different fluid compartments. For example, sodium (Na^+) is the most abundant ion in the extracellular (outside the cell) fluid, whilst potassium (K^+) is the most abundant ion in the intracellular (inside the cell) fluid. Because they are present in such small concentrations in body fluids they are expressed in millimoles per litre (mmol/l). The concentration of sodium in extracellular fluid, therefore, is 135–145 mmol/l but only 10 mmol/l in intracellular fluid. The concentration of potassium, on the other hand, is 3.5–5 mmol/l in extracellular fluid and a whopping 140 mmol/l in intracellular fluid. Given the significant difference in the concentrations of both ions in different compartments it is not always necessary (or practical) for them to travel from a high to a low concentration and frequently they have to be transported in the opposite direction (e.g. against the gradient). Ion channels only allow ions of a certain size and/or electrical charge (e.g. cation or anion) to pass through the cell membrane. This is known as selective permeability. In many cases, movement of ions through the channel is governed by a 'gate' which is opened or closed in response to a chemical or electrical signal (Figure 2.2).

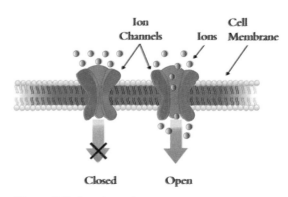

Figure 2.2 Ion channel.

ACTIVE TRANSPORT

When ions want to move from an area of low concentration to an area of high concentration they require energy to do so. Imagine that you are in a boat again but this time for fun (rather than faced with the dilemma of drinking sea water or your own urine). If you are travelling with the current, there is no need to expend energy paddling in the same direction – you simply go with the flow. If, on the other hand, you are travelling against the current you will need to expend a great deal of energy in order to make any progress at all (in fairness, that probably isn't much fun unless you really enjoy a challenge). The same applies to our ions. The energy required for an ion to be transported against the concentration gradient is provided by a chemical produced in the cells known as adenosine triphosphate or ATP (energy is stored in the covalent bonds between the phosphates). This process is called active transport since it requires the expenditure of chemical energy/ATP. Sodium and potassium also use ATP to move in and out of the cell in a form of active transport known as the sodium-potassium pump. In simple terms, three sodium ions from inside the cell bind to the ion channel (gate) whilst ATP provides the energy to open (or change the shape of) the channel. One phosphate group from the ATP (remember it was a *tri*phosphate) remains bound to the channel and the sodium is released into the interstitial compartment outside the cell. The new shape of the ion channel can now accommodate two potassium ions and when they bind to it, the phosphate group is released back into the cytoplasm of the cell. This, in turn, allows the channel to return to its original shape and the potassium ions are transported from outside to inside the cell. This process is repeated over and over again. However, the most important characteristic of this mechanism is that both sodium and potassium are transported from an area of low to an area of high concentration and this can only be achieved through the expenditure of chemical energy in the form of ATP (hence active transport).

CELL-EATING AND DRINKING

Another form of transport that requires the use of ATP is bulk transport or the movement of large (macro) molecules such as proteins and polysaccharides (long chain sugars) in and out of the cell. There are two types of bulk transport: endocytosis (into the cell) and exocytosis (out of the cell). The most common types of endocytosis are phagocytosis (cell-eating) and pinocytosis (cell-drinking) and both involve the cell membrane. Both of these processes put me in mind of the 1958 science fiction movie *The Blob*. In this movie, a giant amorphous 'blob' from outer space wreaks ponderous havoc on a small US town as it engulfs hapless victims into its gelatinous mass. During phagocytosis the cell membrane surrounds or engulfs a macromolecule from outside the cell and 'buds off' to form a food vacuole (cavity) or phagosome (devouring body). Once ingested in this way, the phagosome fuses with a small intracellular vesicle called a lysosome (separating or splitting body) whose enzymes digest the food particles contained within it. Pinocytosis is a similar process in which the cell membrane engulfs or drinks a small quantity of fluid by 'pinching' it and forming a vacuole around it. This process is non-selective and any solutes present within the fluid will also be 'drunk' in this way. Exocytosis, on the other hand, refers to the process by which waste products and other substances such as hormones are exported out of the cell by secretory vesicles (such as lysosomes) and deposited into the interstitial compartment outside the cell. Before we move on to look at some of the structures to be found inside the cell it is important to quickly mention that the cell membrane also contains a number of hormone receptors on its outer surface which will be discussed in Chapter 13.

CYTOPLASM

The second 'essential' component of a human cell is cytoplasm (essentially cell water). The liquid component of cytoplasm is known as cytosol and accounts for approximately 70% of the total volume of a typical human cell. We have already observed that the intracellular compartment contains approximately 25 litres of fluid (about 40% of our body weight) so it is no surprise that much of the cell comprises this watery substance. The cytoplasm helps maintain the structural integrity of the cell and provides a medium for transport and the many chemical reactions that take place within the cell. Cytoplasm also contains a high percentage of solutes and ions, chief amongst which, as we know, is potassium (K+). The final 'vital' component of a human cell (except when it's a red blood cell) is the nucleus.

THE NUCLEUS AND DNA

The nucleus contains the cell's genetic material, deoxyribonucleic acid (DNA), which it uses to control cellular activity. DNA is essentially *information* and is sometimes compared to a blueprint since it contains the instructions necessary to control the cell and, in most cases, the organism as a whole. Just like a builder uses an architectural blueprint to build a house, therefore, DNA is used to ensure that an organism is constructed and functions correctly. Unless you have an identical twin, no other human has your exact DNA code (unless you believe in parallel universes). As you can imagine, you require an awful lot of information to build and maintain a human being. If, like me, you have ever picked up a car manual and then quickly put it down again (thoroughly intimidated after a few pages) spare a thought for the people currently working on the Human Genome Project. These clever folk are attempting to map the sequence of chemical base pairs which make up human DNA in order to identify the totality of human genetic information. DNA exists as tightly wound packages called chromosomes. If we were to unravel a chromosome and look at the DNA strand at extremely high magnification, we would see the DNA double helix (Figure 2.3). This is the unique twisted-ladder structure that makes DNA unlike any other molecule.

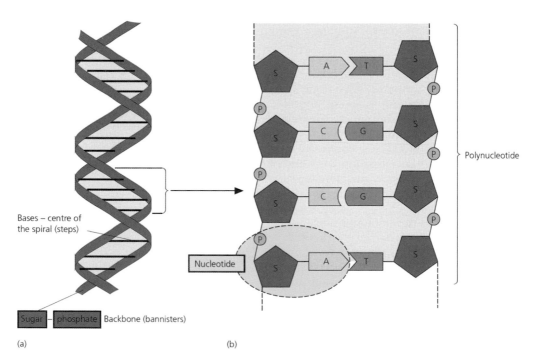

Figure 2.3 (a) DNA double helix. (b) DNA components: S = sugar (deoxyribose), P = phosphate, A = Adenine, C = Cytosine, G = Guanine, T = Thymine.

It was only confirmed in 1953 when James Watson and Francis Crick published the results of their research in *Nature* magazine (based upon the findings of Maurice Wilkins and Rosalind Franklin's X-ray studies). Watson and Crick's modelling of the double helix served to explain how DNA replicates and has enabled numerous advances in our understanding of the transmission of genetic information and disease. The discovery of DNA is also notable in that (according to Crick) it was first announced in a pub (The Eagle in Cambridge).

GENETIC INFORMATION

The sides or strands of the DNA double helix 'ladder' are composed of alternating sugars (deoxyribose) and phosphates. The 'rungs' between the strands, on the other hand, are made up of paired nucleotides or bases: adenine (A), thymine (T), cytosine (C) and guanine (G). The key to understanding this molecule is that these four bases bond together in a very precise fashion: adenine only bonds with thymine (A-T) and cytosine only bonds with guanine (C-G). The DNA code is then 'read' as a three-letter phrase (codon) that make up much longer sequences (on each side of the strand) called genes. You may be thinking that this seems a rather unlikely way to store huge amounts of sophisticated information. However, if we consider that computers can encode and store massive amounts of data simply using two binary digits (0 and 1) it seems quite generous. Other forms of communication that transmit information using limited means include Morse code (on/off tones) and Braille (six dot positions). The easiest way to conceptualise DNA, therefore, is to think of the bases as letters in an alphabet. By putting them together in sequences it becomes possible to form words or phrases. These words are then stored or collected as genes which represent a book of information. Genes (or books) are arranged along the length of each chromosome in a comparable fashion to books on a shelf. Finally, there are 46 chromosomes in the nucleus of a typical human cell which represents the stored information from these

many shelves in a similar fashion to a great library of knowledge. This may be a little simplistic but it helps to conceptualise the cumulative organisation of information from simple bases to human blueprint.

MUTATION

From time to time, normal cells are transformed into cancer cells when their DNA mutates (undergoes a change that causes unusual characteristics to develop). A neoplasm or 'new growth' results from a series of mutations that occur to genes involved in controlling cell growth. This may result in uncontrolled cellular proliferation (rapid multiplication) and the exaggeration of some normal cellular activities. In simple terms, therefore, cancer cells are good cells gone bad. They no longer follow the same 'rules' as normal cells and can produce their own growth signals, ignore anti-growth signals, invade other tissue, replicate an unlimited number of times and evade programmed cell death (apoptosis). The mutated cells develop a degree of autonomy and grow at a rate that is uncoordinated with the needs of the host. A cinematic example of the way in which some cancer cells behave can be found in the *Matrix* trilogy of films. The character Agent Smith (played by Hugo Weaving) replicates himself over and over again until he threatens to destroy the system that created him in a similar fashion to some aggressive cancers and microorganisms (see Chapter 6).

GENETIC DIVERSITY

Each species has a different number of chromosomes in their cells and it is sobering to learn that, genetically at least, we are less diverse than dogs. Dogs have a whopping 78 chromosomes compared to humans 46. However, if you consider the enormous variability of characteristics that dogs exhibit it doesn't seem quite as improbable. For example, compare an Afghan hound with a chihuahua or a Saint Bernard with a Pomeranian. Practicalities allowing, they can successfully produce crossed offspring that are still 'dogs' and are themselves able to reproduce. There are many comically named examples of crossed species including the labradoodle (Labrador/poodle cross), the chihuachshund (chihuahua/dachshund cross) and the cockapoo (cocker spaniel/poodle cross). Humans demonstrate some notable physical variations (such as differences in height, hair colour/ texture, eye colour/ shape and of course skin colour) but none of these mark us out as particularly different. However, it would be wrong to say that simply because an organism has more chromosomes than another it is more sophisticated. For example, potatoes have two more chromosomes than humans (48), chickens have the same number as dogs (78) and some species of fern (e.g. adder's tongue) have over a 1,000. The reasons that this occurs is because during the type of cell division that produces sperm and egg cells (see below) it is possible to include the original genetic material and the copy (in the cell nucleus) rather than just the copy. Consequently, the chromosomes are doubled but the information remains the same (since it is copy). In the case of adder's tongue, it is likely that because this species has existed for such a long period of time in evolutionary terms (thought to date to the Tertiary Period between 1.8 and 65 million years ago) it has had plenty of time to undergo this process on more than one occasion.

CELL DIVISION

Human cells replicate (make a copy of themselves and their DNA) in two ways: mitosis and meiosis. Cells must divide in order for an organism to grow, reproduce and repair itself. The first type of cell division, mitosis, is also referred to as semi-conservative replication. This simply means that when it makes a copy of its DNA, one half of the old strand is always kept in the new strand. It sounds complicated but it isn't. During mitosis, the DNA double helix unzips itself and divides into two strands (imagine a ladder dividing exactly down the middle into two halves). Facing one another are the rungs of the ladder or the nucleotide bases (A, T, C, G) in various combinations

along each side (Figure 2.3). Since we know that A can only bond with T, and C can only bond with G, it is possible to add new bases to each side of the unzipped strands of DNA. This results in two identical copies of the original DNA ladder – very clever. During mitosis, therefore, the cell duplicates all of its contents, including its chromosomes, and splits to form two identical daughter cells. Some cells divide more rapidly than others. Hair follicle cells, for example, have one of the highest rates of mitosis and an average hair grows about 0.3 mm a day or 1 cm per month. Other cells that divide rapidly are those that line our digestive tract and mucous membranes (e.g. gums). The second type of cell division, meiosis, only applies to the production of male and female sex cells or gametes (sperm and egg cells). This is sometimes referred to as reductive division since the number of chromosomes is halved from 46 to 23. When the male and female gametes unite (during conception) they produce a fertilised cell (zygote) containing the full complement of 46 chromosomes. This is why sexual reproduction produces offspring that resemble their parents but are not identical to them (the child has half of each parent's genetic material). More of this in Chapter 14.

MITOCHONDRIA AND CELLULAR RESPIRATION

So far, we have seen that (on the whole) human cells require three essential components. Firstly, a cell membrane to ensure structural integrity and to facilitate the transport of substances in and out of the cell. Secondly, the liquid component of the cell, cytoplasm, that provides a medium for transport and the many chemical reactions that take place within the cell. Finally, the cell nucleus that contains DNA tightly wound into 46 chromosomes. DNA directs cellular activity and provides a blueprint for protein synthesis. At the same time, however, the cell also contains a number of other structures (located in the cytoplasm) called organelles that carry out highly specialised functions. These include: mitochondria, ribosomes, endoplasmic reticulum, the golgi apparatus and lysosomes (Figure 2.4). Mitochondria are often described as sausage-shaped and produce chemical energy for the cell in the form of adenosine triphosphate (ATP). We observed earlier in the chapter, how important ATP is for the active transport of potassium and sodium ions in and out of the cell. Mitochondria work as the power plant of the cell to generate ATP through the catabolic process of cellular respiration. This process has three main stages: glycolysis (glyco + lysis = sugar + splitting), the citric acid cycle (also known as Krebs cycle) and electron transport. The first of these stages, glycolysis, refers to the process by which enzymes catabolise or split glucose, a six-carbon sugar ($C_6H_{12}O_6$), into two three-carbon molecules of pyruvic acid (Figure 2.5). Glycolysis can occur with or without oxygen but if no oxygen is present,

only a small amount of ATP is produced (fermentation). The second stage of cellular respiration, the citric acid cycle, commences after pyruvic acid (produced during glycolysis) is converted into another compound called acetyl coenzyme A (abbreviated to acetyl CoA). Acetyl CoA then combines with oxaloacetic acid to form a six-carbon molecule of citric acid. The citric acid undergoes a number of different reactions that produce ATP as well as two further compounds with the heroic names nicotinamide adenine dinucleotide (NAD) and flavin adenine dinucleotide (FAD). The citric acid cycle only occurs when oxygen is present but it doesn't use oxygen directly. It also results in the liberation of carbon dioxide (CO_2) and hydrogen atoms (H) which are accepted by NAD (as NADH) and FAD (as $FADH_2$).

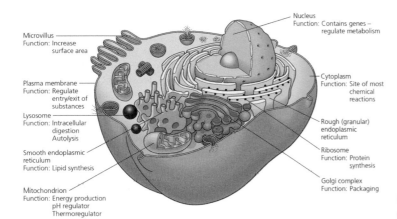

Figure 2.4 Structure and function of a typical cell.

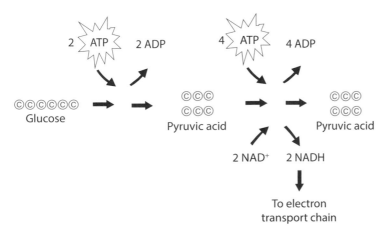

Figure 2.5 Glycolysis.

CELLULAR ENERGY

The final stage of cellular respiration is electron transport which also requires oxygen to be present. During this phase, carrier molecules on the inner lining of the mitochondrial membrane bond with electrons from the hydrogen atoms carried by NADH and $FADH_2$. These carrier molecules transport the electrons through a series of oxidation-reduction reactions in the mitochondria. Oxidation refers to the loss of electrons, and reduction (in chemistry) refers to the acquisition of electrons. For example, when NADH and $FADH_2$ are oxidised, they lose electrons which flow into the electron transport chain. These electrons ultimately encounter and bond with oxygen, thereby 'reducing' it to water (H_2O). Oxygen plays an important role in the electron transport system by attracting electrons along the chain of carriers. However, the key point is that this series of reactions liberates the energy contained within the electrons and generates ATP (chemical energy). During aerobic respiration (in the presence of oxygen) one molecule of glucose yields 38 molecules of ATP. The net (overall) gain is slightly less (36) since some ATP molecules are expended during this process. Mercifully, the production of ATP in the mitochondria is often simplified as the following equation:

$$\text{Glucose} + O_2 \rightarrow \text{ATP (energy)} + CO_2 + H_2O$$
$$or$$
$$C_6H_{12}O_6 + 6O_2 \rightarrow \text{ATP} + 6CO_2 + 6H_2O$$

This is certainly how I tend to think about cellular respiration from a practical point of view. However, it is still useful to look at the three stages of this process (glycolysis, citric acid cycle and electron transport) since it helps to explain where carbon dioxide (CO_2) and water (H_2O) have suddenly materialised from. We also noted that ATP can be produced in the absence of oxygen (anaerobic respiration) but that it is much less efficient than aerobic respiration since it only yields two ATP for each molecule of glucose. This is important since it helps to explain why hypoxia (poor oxygen supply to the cells), and oxygen debt during intense exercise, can interfere with normal cellular activity (see Chapter 9). Anaerobic respiration also produces a number of waste products including lactate which, if not cleared from the blood, can result in acidosis (abnormal increase in the acidity of blood plasma and other body fluid).

RIBOSOMES AND RNA

The next category of intracellular organelles are ribosomes (Figure 2.4). These tiny granular structures consist of two unequal parts (one large and one small subunit) that fit together in order to manufacture proteins from amino acid building blocks using a ribonucleic acid (RNA) template from the nucleus. The name ribosome (ribo + some) is derived from ribonucleic acid and the Greek word for body *soma*. Ribosomes are produced in a specialised part of the nucleus called the nucleolus and made from protein and RNA. We have already spent quite a lot of time poking around in the nucleus looking at DNA but what is RNA? In many ways it is very similar to DNA but it differs from its close relative in a number of important respects. Firstly, RNA is built from the sugar ribose instead of deoxyribose hence ribonucleic acid instead of deoxyribonucleic acid (DNA). Secondly, DNA has a double helix and RNA consists of a single strand of nucleotides (bases). Thirdly, the nucleotide thymine (T) in DNA is replaced on the RNA strand by uracil (U) which also binds with adenine. Finally, RNA is able to transfer genetic material, needed for protein synthesis, from the nucleus to the ribosomes (also constructed from RNA) in the cytoplasm. This feature is extremely important for the maintenance of normal cellular activity.

MANUFACTURING PROTEINS

There is a direct relationship between the linear sequence of nucleotides that make up a gene, and the linear sequence of amino acids in a protein molecule. That is to say, it is possible to copy the information stored on DNA in order to produce new proteins. This is known as the one gene – one protein (or one gene - one polypeptide/chain of amino acids) hypothesis. The process begins when the genetic information necessary for protein synthesis (a particular series of nucleotides/bases) is copied or transcribed from a strand of DNA onto a strand of RNA. This is known as transcription (Figure 2.6). The new RNA strand is referred to as messenger RNA (mRNA) since it carries the coded information out of nucleus and into the cytoplasm of the cell. When mRNA arrives at the ribosome it reassembles itself so that the large and small parts (subunits) are arranged around the mRNA strand. They then proceed to 'translate' the information coded on the mRNA into a specific protein. In order to do this, the ribosome relies on the interaction between mRNA and another type of RNA called transfer RNA (tRNA). As its name suggests, tRNA transfers

or transports individual amino acids to the mRNA (within the ribosome) where they are incorporated into the growing amino acid chain.

TRANSLATION

Translation occurs in three phases: initiation, elongation and termination. During initiation, the small ribosomal subunit sticks to the mRNA and unites with the large ribosomal subunit. The mRNA is now ready to receive the first amino acid and a tRNA molecule aligns with the start codon (three-letter sequence of nucleotides). The next stage, elongation, sees the mRNA slide through the ribosome one codon at a time (imagine a conveyer belt). As each new codon enters the

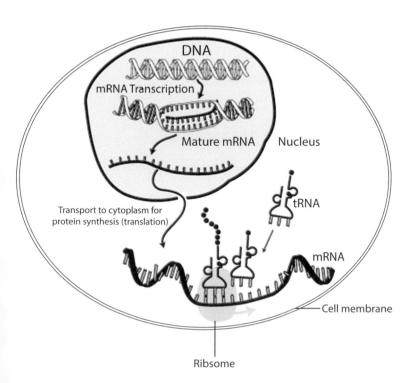

Figure 2.6 Transcription, translation, mRNA and tRNA.

ribosome, a complementary tRNA provides a new amino acid. When the amino acids are aligned next to one another, the ribosome constructs a peptide bond between them. The resulting protein chains can be hundreds of amino acids in length and synthesising these molecules requires a great deal of chemical energy (ATP). Finally, when the last part of the mRNA enters the ribosome (the stop codon), translation ends and the ribosomal subunits, mRNA and protein, separate. The protein is then folded into the correct shape and is ready to be transported to wherever it is required. If a coding error occurs during the elongation phase of this process it can produce an entirely different protein. For example, because each section of the polypeptide chain is constructed using codons, consisting of three nucleotides (e.g. adenine/thymine/adenine), if a single nucleotide is 'deleted' it will change the entire sequential arrangement after that point. This type of nucleotide 'spelling mistake' helps to explain why we exhibit different physiological characteristics and variations. Blood type A and blood type B, for example, both possess the same number of nucleotides (1,062) but blood type B has a slightly different sequence of amino acids (7). This simple difference in 'spelling' has important implications for transfusion compatibility as we will see in Chapter 5.

ENDOPLASMIC RETICULUM AND GOLGI BODY

The next intracellular organelle is the wonderfully named endoplasmic reticulum (ER). ER is a series of interconnecting membranous canals that are continuous with the nuclear membrane and encompass a large amount of space within the cell (Figure 2.4). ER is classified as either rough or smooth. Rough ER is studded with ribosomes on the cytoplasmic side of the membrane and contributes to the production of proteins (as described in the preceding section). In pancreatic cells, for example, the rough ER produces insulin (a peptide hormone). Smooth ER, on the other

hand, has no ribosomes and manufactures lipids and steroid hormones (see Chapter 13). It is also associated with the detoxification of some drugs and compounds particularly in the cells of the liver. In muscle cells, the ER is known as the sarcoplasmic reticulum and releases calcium ions during muscular contraction (and absorbs and stores them during relaxation). The golgi body (also referred to as the golgi complex or golgi apparatus) is also found in the cytoplasm and is often compared to a pile of flattened sacs. These sacs are actually a series of flattened membranous canals known as cisternae and they manufacture, store and transport cellular products (particularly those from the ER). One end of the golgi body (the *cis* face, usually closest to the ER) acts as the receiving area whilst the other end (the *trans* face) acts as the 'shipping' area. I can't help thinking of a giant warehouse where 'goods' are transported in and shipped out again. Proteins and other substances are conveyed to and from the golgi body in tiny, fluid-filled, membranous sacs called transport vesicles. Some of these are used within the cell and some extruded into the extracellular compartment (exocytosis). Depending on the type of cell, there may be many golgi bodies or there may be very few.

LYSOSOMES

The final intracellular organelle discussed in this chapter is manufactured in the golgi body and is called a lysosome (lyse + soma = splitting + body). As its name suggests, it is not the friendliest of the intracellular community. Lysosomes are small vesicles that contain hydrolytic enzymes used to digest cellular molecules. The enzymes themselves are produced in the ER and transported to the receiving (*cis*) face of the golgi body. Lysosomes then 'bud off' the shipping (*trans*) face and patrol the cytoplasm for macromolecules (large molecules) or bacteria which may have been ingested by the cell via endocytosis. Earlier we observed how lysosomes combine with food vacuoles or phagosomes in order to digest the particles contained within it. Lysosomes also fuse with old organelles (e.g. mitochondria) in order to degrade and recycle their components for use in the manufacture of new structures. If the lysosome's membrane ruptures for any reason, enzymes are released that can damage or destroy the cell which is why they have acquired the nickname 'suicide bags'. Consequently, lysosomes seem to play an important role in the process of programmed cell death or apoptosis.

AGEING

We have observed that most somatic or body cells (with a few notable exceptions) reproduce via mitosis. During mitosis the cell nucleus divides, resulting in the formation of two daughter cells, each with exactly the same chromosome/DNA content as the original parent cell. So why don't they continue to divide over and over again, producing perfect copy after perfect copy? Or, to put it another way, why do we age and die? This is actually a very sensible question and a huge amount of money is invested into researching why we get older and what can be done about it. There are various theories as to why we age, including physiological, cellular and genetic explanations. One physiological theory suggests that ageing is simply the result of cumulative wear and tear and is strongly linked to chance environmental factors. Another physiological explanation proposes that as metabolic waste products accumulate in the cell (and elsewhere) they become inappropriately attached to one another (cross-linked) and increasingly difficult to break down and remove. For example, the amino acids that make up collagen eventually cross-link leading to loss of flexibility in the skin, joints and blood vessels. Cell doubling theory, on the other hand, is based on the idea that cells are only capable of replicating a certain number times. Eventually, therefore, cell numbers decline to the point where normal cell functioning is difficult to maintain. Free radical theory proposes that, over time, the body becomes less able to withstand the effects of free radicals on its DNA and phospholipids, leading to genetic and cellular damage. Free radicals are unstable molecules (including oxygen ions)

that 'attack' the nearest stable molecule in order to steal an electron from its outer shell (remember bonding from Chapter 1). In normal circumstances, molecules called antioxidants neutralise free radicals before they can do significant damage to the cell. As we age, however, fewer antioxidants are produced/available and free radical mediated damage becomes more common.

PROGRAMMED CELL DEATH

The final theory listed here (there are many others) is programmed cell death (apoptosis) initiated and executed by lysosomes and lysosomal enzymes. This theory is genetic in nature and proposes that our cells are programmed (after conception) to age and die. That is not to say that environmental factors are irrelevant. If you smoke twenty cigarettes a day you are undoubtedly increasing your chances of developing cardiovascular disease, chronic obstructive pulmonary disease (COPD) and lung cancer – all of which may shorten your projected lifespan. However, even though the genetic mechanism that is responsible for ageing remains unclear at the present time, it seems likely that genetic makeup is an important factor in determining longevity. The genetic argument for ageing is supported by the existence of rare genetic conditions such as Progeria and Werner's syndrome (adult Progeria). Progeria derives its name from the Greek for 'prematurely old' and causes physiological changes that resemble accelerated ageing. The development of symptoms is comparable to ageing at 6–8 times faster than normal and is characterised by limited growth, alopecia (hair loss) and progressive degeneration of the cardiovascular system. Symptoms typically commence during the first years of life (although diagnosis may occur later) and those with the disease rarely live beyond their mid-teens. Werner's syndrome is also characterised by premature ageing but growth and development are often normal until puberty. Diagnosis is typically made in the early 20s and life expectancy is about 50 years.

PREDICTING DEATH

A team of scientists at Stockholm's Karo-linska Institute analysed data from almost half a million UK adults aged 40 to 70 years, of whom 8,352 died in the following five years. They then worked out which factors were most strongly linked to risk of death and developed a test to predict the percentage risk of dying in the next five years for those in this age range. Their report is published in *The Lancet*[1] and the test can be taken online at www.ubble.co.uk if you are interested (and aged 40–70). On a less serious note, if you would like to predict your day of death for 'fun' you can take the test at the appropriately named website: The Death Clock. It uses a number of modifiable variables to provide a personalised day of death. You can then share your day of death with your friends via social media or download your own 'death clock' to your computer or blog (relentlessly counting down to the appointed hour). Apparently, my day of death is Tuesday, 24 October 2045 (at least I know not to buy tickets for Fireworks Night that year). I would stress that this will not accurately predict your day of death (although statistically it must get it right every so often) but it does provide some useful motivation to get assignments, jobs, etc. finished as you watch the seconds of your life tick away.

TISSUE TYPES

So far we have looked at the body on an atomic, molecular and a cellular level. In terms of size and complexity, the next functional unit of the body is tissue. Tissue is simply a collection or aggregation of cells acting cooperatively to perform one or more specific function in the body. There are four distinct categories of tissue: epithelial, connective, muscular and nervous. The first type, epithelial, has three important functions: protection, secretion and absorption. The best way to imagine epithelial tissue is as a continuous sheet of cells that cover the outside and the inside surfaces of the body. For example, the skin, the lining of the cardiovascular system,

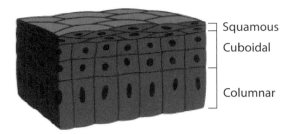

Figure 2.7 Epithelial cells.

the digestive tract, the urinary tract, the respiratory tract and the reproductive tract are all composed of epithelial cells. Epithelial tissue that covers the outer surfaces of the body (including the mucous membranes of the gastrointestinal and urinary tracts that communicate with the outside of the body) is referred to as epithelium. Whilst epithelial tissue that is only found on inner surfaces of the body, such as within the blood and lymphatic vessels, is known as endothelium. In either case, the cells are arranged in a number of ways. The simplest way to classify them is by shape (Figure 2.7). They can be columnar (like columns – upright), cuboidal (like cubes) or squamous (from the Latin for 'fish-scale' – flat). Just pause to remember that they are cells like any other and exhibit exactly the same characteristics discussed above (they have a plasma membrane, nucleus and cytoplasm, etc.).

EPITHELIAL CELLS

Columnar (column-like) cells are typically found in the lining of the stomach and digestive tract where they absorb and secrete a number of substances/molecules. They are also found in the nose, ear and tongue (taste buds) where they help to transmit sensory information towards the brain. 'Goblet cells' are specialist columnar epithelium that secrete mucin, a substance that dissolves in water to produce mucus (picture a goblet of mucus). Others are covered in fine hair-like structures called cilia (ciliated epithelium). These are capable of rapid, rhythmic wafting in order to propel mucus out of the respiratory tract or, in the case of those found in the female reproductive tract, they waft the egg cell (ovum) along the fallopian tube towards the uterus (see Chapter 14). Cuboidal (cube-like) epithelial cells are often found in glandular (secretory) tissue and in the lining of the tubules of the kidney (nephrons). They also make up the germinal cells which produce the ova in the female ovary and the sperm in the male testes. Finally, squamous (flat) epithelial cells make up the outer layer of the skin and line a number of cavities and internal structures including the mouth, blood vessels, cervix and lungs. You may have heard of squamous cell carcinoma which refers to a type of cancer or neoplasm that derives from these cells. Examples include skin cancer, some forms of lung cancer and the most common type of cervical cancer. Epithelial cells can also be classified in terms of their structure or arrangement. They can be simple (in a single layer), stratified (one on top of the other – in strata) or pseudo-stratified (in a single layer but appear to be stratified). For example, simple squamous epithelium can be found on the inside of blood vessels or lining the air sacs (alveoli) of the lungs. This simple arrangement allows rapid diffusion of gases such as oxygen and carbon dioxide between cell membranes. Stratified squamous epithelia, on the other hand, are found in the cornea of the eye or lining the oral (mouth) cavity. Stratified epithelium is well suited to areas of the body that are subject to abrasion since the layers can be shed and quickly replaced before the basement membrane is exposed.

CONNECTIVE TISSUE

The next type of tissue is connective tissue and, as it name suggests, it connects and supports a number of internal structures. Examples of connective tissue include cartilage, tendons, ligaments, fat (adipose), bone and blood. Yes, blood, it seems odd but I'll explain later. There are three broad categories of connective tissue: loose, dense and specialised. Loose connective tissue is typically found beneath epithelial membranes and glandular epithelium. It binds these tissues to other tissues and

contributes to the formation of organs. The cells and fibres that make up loose connective tissue tend to have large spaces between them and contain a high proportion of fluid. It is the most common type of connective tissue and includes fat or adipose tissue (which, at the risk of contradicting myself, has a low percentage of water). Fat is located in a number of key places including beneath the skin (subcutaneous fat), around internal organs (visceral fat) and in the yellow bone marrow. It is made up of adipocytes (fat cells) which store energy (as triglycerides), preserve heat and act as a shock absorber for the structures they surround.

DENSE AND SPECIALISED CONNECTIVE TISSUE

Dense connective tissue has a much greater concentration of fibres and tends to provide structural and mechanical support. One of the most important connective tissue fibres is collagen and although it is found in loose connective tissue, there is a much greater abundance in dense connective tissue. For example, in ligaments and tendons, collagen fibres are thick, long and tightly packed together in order to provide the tensile strength necessary to connect and move bones. In cartilage and bone, however, collagen fibres are coated in calcium and phosphate salts in order to provide solidity and strength (see Chapter 4). Dense connective tissue also makes up the lower layers of the skin (dermis) where it is arranged in sheets. Finally, bone, cartilage and blood are all examples of specialised connective tissue (see Chapters 4 and 5). Blood is classified as connective tissue since it contains proteins mixed with water (plasma) and can form a gel. In Chapter 1, we saw that blood consists of a cellular component (red blood cells, white blood cells, etc.) and a non-cellular matrix (plasma). The liquid plasma allows blood to transport a wide variety of substances around the body dissolved in solution or attached to cells. In this sense, therefore, it is supremely connective. The only difference with other connective tissue is that it does not contain the fibre elements.

MUSCLE TISSUE

There are three types of muscle tissue: skeletal (voluntary), smooth (involuntary) and cardiac (heart muscle or myocardium). Skeletal or 'voluntary' muscle is the most abundant muscle type in the body and accounts for about 40% of total body weight. In almost all cases (there is always an exception to the rule) it is attached to the skeleton and is under voluntary control. For example, as you are reading this book or tablet, the skeletal muscles of your arms and shoulders are keeping it steady whilst the external skeletal muscles that control your eyes allow you to read the sentences on this page/screen. It is estimated that if you read for an hour (which I hope you do) your eyes will make nearly 10,000 coordinated movements. Anyway, skeletal muscle is composed of long cylindrical fibres that are banded at regular intervals with fine red and white lines called striations (stripes). These striations are actually very fine contractile fibres called myofibrils which not only give the muscle its striped appearance but also enable it to move or contract (shorten in size). Myofibrils are bathed in sarcoplasm (a type of cytoplasm) and bound together by a plasma membrane called sarcolemma. These bundles of muscle cells are organised into larger bundles called fascicles (enclosed by a sheath of connective tissue called perimysium). Skeletal muscle can perform a short, single contraction (twitch) or a long, sustained contraction (tetanus). You have probably heard of the condition tetanus that is caused by a nerve toxin (neuro-toxin) produced by the bacteria *clostridium tetani* (found in soil and manure). If infection occurs, it results in prolonged contraction of skeletal muscle (tetanus) including those of the jaw which is why it is often referred to as 'lock-jaw'.

VOLUNTARY MUSCLE

I mentioned at the beginning of the previous paragraph that there was an exception to the rule regarding the 'voluntary' status of skeletal muscle. The intercostal muscles (located between the ribs) and the diaphragm are collectively known as the muscles of respiration since they allow us to breath. However, although both are composed of skeletal muscle, they are not strictly 'voluntary' in the true sense. This is fortunate, since, if skeletal muscle were purely voluntary, every time we went to sleep we would asphyxiate. Consequently, although breathing is typically an unconscious activity, controlled by the autonomic (automatic) nervous system (Chapter 12), we have the ability to consciously determine the rate and depth of respiration if required. This capacity to override automatic control is very useful since it allows us to hold our breath underwater, sing (sustain a note) or play a wind instrument (force air in an 'unnatural' fashion through a narrow aperture or reed). Voluntary control of our respiratory muscles also allows us to read out loud badly punctuated sentences such as the one that I am now writing which just go on and on and on without any indication where to pause or take a short breath and just make the readers more and more uncomfortable as their lungs slowly and progressively empty of air and I had better stop now before the world starts to spin and fade from vision. If you managed to read all of that in one breath, well done for showing your autonomic nervous system who is boss.

SMOOTH MUSCLE

Smooth or involuntary muscle lacks the striped or striated pattern of skeletal muscle and consists of long spindle (fusiform) shaped cells that appear smooth when examined under a microscope. It is also under the control of the autonomic nervous system and, unlike skeletal muscle, cannot be influenced voluntarily. Smooth muscle has the ability to stretch and maintain tension for a long period of time. This makes it perfect for use in organs such as the stomach and urinary bladder. Smooth muscle can also be found in the walls of the blood vessels, the female reproductive tract, the oesophagus and the iris of the eye (see Chapter 12). It may surprise you that the iris contains smooth muscle fibres but if you look into a mirror, shut your eyes for a few seconds and then open them again, you will see your pupils involuntarily constrict (get smaller) in response to the sudden increase of light. Although the pupils change size, it is the contraction of the circular smooth muscle of the iris that provides the appearance of smaller pupils. Some drugs interfere with this process and the action of other smooth muscle groups. For example, opiates, such as diamorphine (heroin), cause involuntary constriction of the pupils known as miosis (not to be confused with the type of cell division meiosis). Cocaine and amphetamines, on the other hand, cause involuntary dilation of the pupil known as mydriasis. However, research has also shown that if someone is strongly attracted to you, they may also experience involuntarily dilation of the pupils. So next time you see someone looking at you with large, dilated pupils they may be (a) taking cocaine, (b) desperately in love/attracted to you, or (c) just noticed something utterly terrifying over your shoulder. If you go on a date with someone with abnormally constricted pupils, on the other hand, they may really dislike you or have taken some kind of opiate to get through the evening (either way, probably best not to exchange numbers). There are of course many other reasons (and medications) that may explain abnormal pupillary shape and size (e.g. cataract surgery and inflammation of the iris).

CARDIAC MUSCLE

The final type of muscle tissue is cardiac muscle or myocardium (myo + cardium = muscle + heart). This is a specialised type of striated (striped) muscle that is under involuntary control. The heart itself is essentially a muscular pump and, for obvious reasons, it is crucial that it doesn't stop working. Unlike skeletal muscle, that is only intended to contract for a limited period of time, cardiac muscle must continue to work in an uninterrupted fashion for about 80 years or so. It can't suddenly decide that it needs a little break and stop working for two or three minutes (occasionally it does of course – see Chapter 7). In order to ensure endurance and consistency, therefore, cardiac muscle demonstrates characteristics of both skeletal and smooth muscle. For example, it can stretch in a limited way like smooth muscle and contract (twitch only) with the force of skeletal muscle. One of the reasons it is able to endure for so long is because myocardial cells (myocardiocytes) contain a higher than normal proportion of mitochondria. These sausage-shaped organelles produce cellular energy in the form of ATP that enables the heart to continue working and step-up activity if required (e.g. in the event that an ill-tempered bear takes a dislike to you and you need to run for your life). Another unique feature of cardiac muscle is that myocardiocytes are able to generate and transmit electrical impulses (intrinsic conductivity). However, this will be discussed in more detail in Chapter 7.

NERVOUS TISSUE

The final type of tissue is nervous tissue (not in the 'worried' sense). Nervous tissue comprises nerve cells (neurons) that generate, transmit and receive electrical impulses (action potentials), and supporting cells (glial cells) that nourish and protect the nerve cells. The two functions are often expressed as excitable and non-excitable. Nerve cells are highly specialised in their function and vary greatly in length. However, they still exhibit many of the same characteristics as other cells (e.g. nucleus, mitochondria, cytoplasm, etc.) and require oxygen and glucose to produce cellular energy (ATP). In this sense, they are susceptible to the same challenges as other, less-specialised cells and a few more besides. One interesting feature of 'excitable' neurons is that, for the most part, they are unable to undergo mitosis following maturation. Supporting cells, on the other hand, are capable of dividing mitotically and are essential for the maintenance of their more excitable neighbours. There are a number of different types of glial cells including astrocytes (cellular repair and clearance of neurotransmitters), microglia (clearance of cellular debris), oligodendrocytes and schwann cells (both produce an insulating material called myelin). However, we will look in much more detail at how neurons and glial cells work in Chapter 12.

ORGANS AND ORGAN SYSTEMS

The next level of structural sophistication after tissue is the organ. Just as a tissue can be defined as a group of cells acting collectively to perform one or more specific function in an organ, an organ can be defined as a collection of tissues acting together to perform one or more specific function in an organism. The tissue of the organ if often said to consist of parenchyma (functional tissue) and stroma (secondary framework). In Greek, the word *stroma* means anything spread out for sitting or lying upon and essentially refers to the supporting framework of an organ. For example, the parenchyma of the heart is the myocardium or heart muscle whilst the stroma refers to nervous and connective tissues (including the blood). There are a large number of organs within the body organised into different organ systems. These systems work collaboratively to ensure a stable internal environment. We will look in detail at the organs and organ systems in the following chapters but some of the more notable and familiar include: the cardiovascular system (heart and blood vessels), the digestive system, the respiratory system, the immune (lymphatic) system and the reproductive system. I cannot overemphasise, however, that these organs and organ systems function in a highly cooperative fashion. If there is a problem with one organ or system, it is usually reflected in the functioning of another. In some cases, the body is able to make compensatory changes in order to offset the immediate consequences of abnormal functioning. However, whilst this may work in the short term, it often results in maladaptive changes that can increase the problem in the long term. One of the common misconceptions regarding the terms acute and chronic is that the former is always worse than the latter. Acute disease simply refers to a condition where the signs and symptoms appear rapidly. It is correct that, in the worst case scenario, it might kill you! However, typically, the symptoms alert you to the fact there is a problem, persist for a short period of time and disappear following treatment (or of their own accord). Chronic disease, on the other hand, develops slowly and lasts for a long period of time (possibly the extent of your life). The problem with chronic illness is that you may not realise you have the disease (and therefore do not seek treatment) until you become symptomatic. By this time, however, the disease may be so far advanced that treatment is less effective. For example, chronic renal failure (long-term deterioration of kidney function) typically does not become apparent (symptomatic) until about 75% of the kidney is no longer functioning. This, as we shall see in Chapter 10, has significant implications for a number of other systems. However, before we do so, it is important to understand the concept of homeostasis or how the body maintains a stable internal environment in health (Chapter 3).

CHAPTER 2: TEST YOURSELF

Q. How many different types of cell are there in the human body?
A. About 200.

Q. What are the three principle constituents of a cell (in most cases)?
A. Nucleus, cell membrane and cytoplasm.

Q. What is the human cell membrane made from and what does it do?
A. The human cell membrane consists of two layers of phospholipids sometimes referred to as a fatty bi-layer. This provides a barrier that ensures water and ions remain in the correct concentrations within the cell (cytoplasm) and outside the cell (interstitial fluid).

Q. What is the function of the protein molecules (gates) embedded into the cell membrane?
A. They transport ions (and other substances) in and out of the cell.

Q. What is the most abundant ion in the intracellular fluid and what is the most abundant ion in the extracellular fluid?

A. Potassium (K⁺) is the most abundant ion in the intracellular fluid, and sodium (Na⁺) in the extracellular fluid.

Q. What is meant by the term active transport?

A. Active transport requires the expenditure of chemical energy (adenosine triphosphate/ ATP) to transport a substance from an area of low concentration to an area of high concentration.

Q. There are two types of bulk transport: endocytosis and exocytosis. What is the difference between the two?

A. Endocytosis refers to the process where the cell membrane surrounds or engulfs something from outside the cell and transports it inside. Exocytosis refers to the process by which waste and other products are exported out of the cell by secretory vesicles.

Q. The nucleus of the cell contains genetic material known as deoxyribonucleic acid (DNA). In simple terms, what is the function of DNA and how is it stored?

A. DNA is essentially 'information' necessary to control the activity of the cell and produce proteins. It is comprised of paired nucleotides/bases – adenine (A), thymine (T), cytosine (C) and guanine (G) – that are arranged in sequences of three called codons (e.g. CTG) in a unique double-helix configuration.

Q. How many chromosomes does a typical human cell contain?

A. Forty-six chromosomes (23 pairs).

Q. There are two types of cell division: mitosis and meiosis. What is the difference between the two?

A. During mitosis the cell duplicates all of its contents, including its chromosomes, and splits to form two identical daughter cells (each with 46 chromosomes). Meiosis is sometimes referred to as reductive division since the number of chromosomes is halved, from 46 to 23, and contributes to the production of male and female sex cells (sperm and egg cells).

Q. What is the function of the intracellular organelle mitochondria?

A. Mitochondria use oxygen and glucose to produce chemical energy for the cell in the form of adenosine triphosphate (ATP).

Q. Complete the following equation: Glucose + O_2 → ATP + ? + ?

A. Glucose + O_2 → ATP + CO_2 + H_2O

Q. What do ribosomes manufacture (using messenger RNA and transfer RNA)?

A. Proteins.

Q. What is the difference between smooth and rough endoplasmic reticulum (ER)?

A. Rough ER is studded with ribosomes that contribute to the production of proteins and peptide hormones. Smooth ER has no ribosomes and manufactures lipids and steroid hormones.

Q. What is the function of the golgi body?

A. The golgi body manufactures, store and transports cellular products (e.g. from the ER).

(Continued)

(Continued)

Q. What is the principle role of lysosomes?
A. Lysosomes (lyse + soma = splitting + body) are small vesicles that contain hydrolytic enzymes used to digest cellular molecules.

Q. What are the four tissue types?
A. Epithelial, muscular, connective and nervous.

Q. What are the three types of epithelial cell (named after their shape)?
A. Cuboidal (like a cube), columnar (like a column) and squamous (flat like a 'fish-scale).

Q. What type of tissue is blood?
A. Connective.

Q. What type of muscle is the diaphragm and why is it unusual?
A. The diaphragm is voluntary (skeletal) muscle but is under autonomic control most of the time.

NOTE

1 Ganna, A. and Ingelsson, E. (2015) 5 year mortality predictors in 498,103 UK Biobank participants: a prospective population-based study. *The Lancet*, 386(9993): 533–540.

Contents

CHAPTER 3

HOMEOSTASIS

T he term homeostasis is derived from the Greek words for 'same' (homo) and 'standing still' (stasis). It refers to the way in which the body maintains a stable internal environment despite constant changes and variation to the internal and external environment. In Chapter 1, we discussed how the body is constantly catabolising (breaking down) large molecules in order to make them available for cellular respiration and the liberation of energy (ATP). At the same time, it is using the products of catabolism, and other simple substances, to manufacture complex molecules necessary for normal functioning (anabolism). This cyclical process requires a constant supply of oxygen and glucose and generates large amounts of waste products that must be rendered harmless and excreted from the body. Homeostasis is a general term, therefore, that describes how the body is constantly adjusting in order to ensure that it continues to function in the most efficient and effective manner. In simple terms, the cells in our body work best when their surroundings are kept constant. Internal factors, such as the pH of our blood plasma, can have a profound effect on their ability to perform many important tasks and, in Chapter 1, we saw that plasma pH is maintained in a very narrow range (7.35–7.45) using a number of physiological mechanisms. If any of these mechanisms fail or are interfered with (e.g. kidney failure or persistent vomiting) it can result in acidosis or alkalosis (both of which may result in severe ill health). However, it is not just internal factors that upset the balance; external variables such as temperature and environment also require careful physiological adjustment.

FUEL – ENERGY – WASTE

A useful analogy for homeostasis is driving a car. In order to function properly, a car needs fuel, water in its radiator and a fan to prevent overheating. The amount of fuel it uses depends on the driving conditions. For example, if you are driving in heavy traffic (stop-start-stop-start) the car consumes a lot of fuel, gets very hot and pumps out a lot of exhaust fumes (waste product). If you see a gap in the traffic and make a break for freedom, you will also consume a lot of fuel and generate a great deal of heat as you accelerate. As soon as you find yourself on an empty road, however (and assuming you can avoid the temptation to speed), your fuel consumption will decrease as you drive more economically. The same applies to the human body. The more activity you undertake the greater your fuel (oxygen and glucose) consumption will be, the more heat you will generate (as cellular activity increases) and the more waste products you will manufacture (carbon dioxide and lactic acids). In order to compensate for these changes, the various organ systems must cooperate to increase the available oxygen and glucose to the cells, lose heat and excrete potentially harmful waste products.

In short, they must maintain homeostasis or risk an altered health state. To use the analogy of the car again – if it runs out of petrol, the engine will cough, splutter and quickly grind to a halt. Similarly, if the body cannot provide sufficient oxygen and glucose to the cells they will switch from efficient aerobic respiration to inefficient anaerobic respiration before also grinding to a (possibly painful) halt. This is why our respiratory and heart rate both increase during exercise in order to ensure a constant supply of oxygen to the blood and cells. Glucose is also liberated from its stored form (e.g. in the muscle and liver) in order to avoid a deficit. The body simultaneously maintains homeostasis at a chemical, cellular and systemic level.

NEGATIVE FEEDBACK

Homeostasis is maintained by a variety of control systems which detect and respond to changes in internal and external environment. A control system has three basic components: a sensor (or detector), a control centre (or integrator) and a number of effector mechanisms.

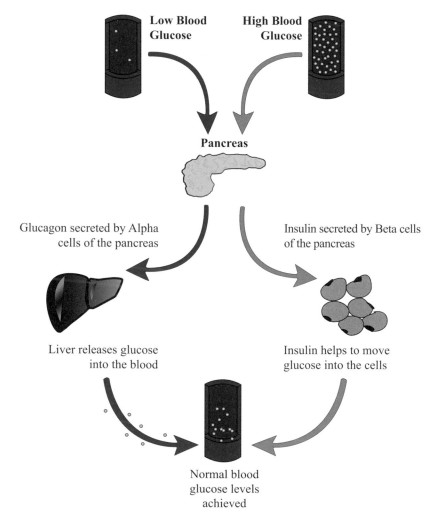

Low Blood Glucose

High Blood Glucose

Pancreas

Glucagon secreted by Alpha cells of the pancreas

Insulin secreted by Beta cells of the pancreas

Liver releases glucose into the blood

Insulin helps to move glucose into the cells

Normal blood glucose levels achieved

Figure 3.1 Negative feedback: blood glucose levels.

The sensor identifies when a variable (something that changes or varies) is no longer within normal limits. The control centre determines whether an adjustment is required or whether it can be ignored. If an adjustment is required, the control centre informs an effector mechanism (the thing that actually does something) to make the necessary correction. There are two ways in which the body can make an adjustment: by negative feedback or by positive feedback. In the case of the former, the body responds in such a way to reverse the direction of change (hence the fact it is negative feedback). A good example of negative feedback is the regulation of blood glucose. Following a meal, high levels of blood glucose are detected by cells in the pancreas (see Chapter 13). The pancreas secretes the hormone insulin which stimulates cells to take up glucose for cellular respiration and storage (Figure 3.1). This reverses the direction of change since glucose is transported out of the blood (into the cell) and levels return to within the normal range. Alternatively, if blood glucose levels become low because you are unable to eat, the pancreas secretes another hormone

called glucagon which releases stored glucose from the liver (and fat cells if necessary). The amount of glucose in the blood rises and the direction of change is once again reversed. The two hormones work collaboratively to ensure that balance (homeostasis) is maintained. Most of the homeostatic adjustments made by our body are the result of negative feedback and include heart rate, blood pressure, fluid balance, respiratory rate and blood glucose levels (all discussed in later chapters). However, probably the best example of negative feedback is temperature regulation (thermoregulation) which will be discussed later in this chapter.

POSITIVE FEEDBACK

Positive feedback is much less common and occurs when the body responds to a change (in a given variable) by increasing that change even further in the same direction. This sounds illogical until you look at the type of physiological processes that are being

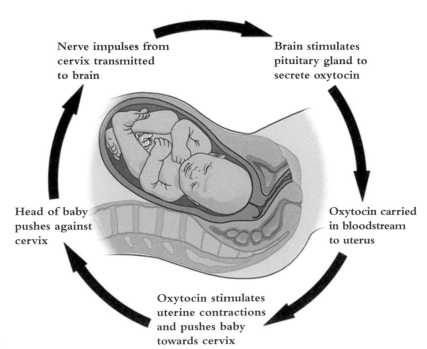

Nerve impulses from cervix transmitted to brain

Brain stimulates pituitary gland to secrete oxytocin

Head of baby pushes against cervix

Oxytocin carried in bloodstream to uterus

Oxytocin stimulates uterine contractions and pushes baby towards cervix

Figure 3.2 Positive feedback: labour.

regulated by this mechanism. Labour (giving birth) is probably the best example of positive feedback since it is self-evident why negative feedback is not an appropriate mechanism to return the female body to its non-pregnant state. Having gone to all the biological trouble of conceiving a child and then carrying it for nine months, it is not practical or desirable to 'reverse' this process in any sense. In order for the body to return to a 'normal' non-pregnant state, therefore, the child has got to come out some way or other. Of course, as any parent knows, there is no returning to 'normal' once a child is born. You say goodbye to sleep for at least two years of your life, and then goodbye to all of your time and money for the rest. I have frequently compared my own children to parasites in the past which either elicits nods of agreement or outright horror (usually from non-parents). According to the *Oxford English Dictionary* a parasite is defined as 'an organism which lives in or on another organism (its host) and benefits by deriving nutrients at the other's expense'. Sounds like a child to me. Anyway, how to get the baby safely out of the mother so that it can continue to grow, prosper and spend its parent's money? Positive feedback of course. When sustained pressure is applied to the internal surface of the cervix (neck of the womb) by the baby's head, it drives a nerve impulse towards the brain where it is interpreted by the hypothalamus (the control centre). The hypothalamus, in turn, sends a signal to the posterior pituitary gland (located close by) to secrete a hormone called oxytocin into the blood (Figure 3.2). Oxytocin acts on the muscle of the womb (uterus) and causes it to contract. The contractions apply increased pressure to the cervix and vaginal wall which stimulate the secretion of more and more oxytocin (a process known as the Ferguson reflex). The direction of change is gradually amplified, therefore, in keeping with the principle of positive feedback, until the baby is finally delivered and there is no longer any pressure applied to the cervix, etc. Oxytocin can also be used to induce or strengthen weak contractions if labour in not progressing. Once the baby has been delivered, the mother can take a well-deserved rest

until the next example of positive feedback is required – breastfeeding.

OXYTOCIN AND BREASTFEEDING

The newly arrived baby will quickly become hungry and announce this fact to its parents through the medium of crying. When the baby suckles on the mother's nipple it drives a nerve impulse towards her brain that stimulates the secretion of oxytocin from the pituitary gland. This time, however, oxytocin acts principally upon the mammary tissue of the breast, contracting the smooth muscle layer that surrounds it and squeezing the milk into the ductal system. It does not actually produce the milk (that is done by another pituitary hormone called prolactin – see Chapter 13) but it is responsible for what is known as the 'letdown' reflex. Once the milk is released from the nipple, the baby continues to suckle, which of course stimulates more oxytocin to be secreted. The process eventually stops when the baby is satisfied and stops feeding (removing the stimulus for oxytocin production). The mother then puts her baby over her shoulder and winds him/her – at which point they vomit all over her back and require another feed (natures little joke). We'll come across a few more examples of positive feedback later in the book (e.g. blood clotting and the transformation of pepsinogen into pepsin) but the overwhelming majority of mechanisms used to maintain homeostasis in humans are negative.

INTEGUMENTARY SYSTEM

The term 'integument' describes an outer covering or layer. The integumentary system, therefore, simply refers to the tissue layer that surrounds and protects the human body and consists of the skin, hair, nails and a number of exocrine glands. It also plays an important role in sensory perception (e.g. touch and pain) and temperature regulation (thermoregulation). Although the skin is only a few millimetres thick it is the largest organ of the body

(a)

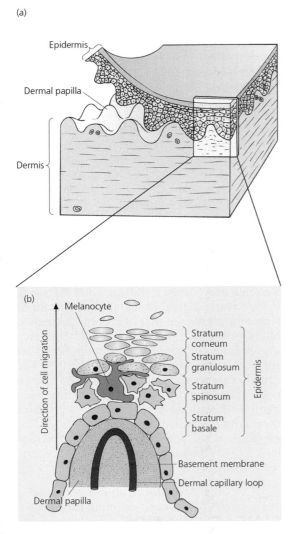

Figure 3.3 (a) Epidermis and dermis. (b) Cell layers.

important component of hair and nails and derives its name from the Greek for 'horn'. When the keratinised cells reach the surface they form a water-resistant barrier called the stratum corneum (this time Latin for 'horned layer') before being shed and replaced by new cells underneath (Figure 3.3). This process is known as desquamation and comes from the Latin *desquamare* meaning to scrape the scales from a fish (not a very romantic vision). It is estimated that we lose a staggering 30,000–40,000 skin cells every minute or so (millions per day). There is no need to worry, however, since (a) cells are incredibly small and (b) they are being constantly replaced and renewed. Cell renewal is most efficient during childhood and declines with age – this has obvious implications for skin integrity and wound healing.

MELANOCYTES

In addition to keratinocytes, a number of other specialised cells can also be found in the epidermis including melanocytes, merkel and langerhans cells (Figure 3.3). Melanocytes produce the brown/black pigment melanin that helps to protect the skin from ultraviolet (UV) radiation present in sunlight. The presence or absence of melanin is also the primary determinant of skin and hair colour associated with ethnicity. In those with pale skin (little melanin) the sun stimulates more melanin to be produced (melanogenesis) resulting in sun-tanning and/or the production of freckles (small clusters of concentrated melanin). It would seem logical that sunlight also made hair darker but, as you know, the opposite is often true. This is because the shaft of the hair that is visible on the head is technically dead (see below) and sunlight can break down the melanin within it which produces a lighter appearance in some people. High levels of UV light also increase the likelihood of developing the skin condition melasma (or chloasma) which causes irregular areas of pigmentation to develop, often on the face. Melasma is more common in women and is thought to result when melanocytes secrete additional melanin in response to raised levels of oestrogen or progesterone. Consequently, it

and accounts for about 16% of your total body weight. It has three layers: epidermis, dermis and subcutaneous fat (adipose). The outermost layer, the epidermis (lit. above the dermis), is composed of stratified squamous ('fish-scale') epithelium. These cells originate just below the surface in a germinal layer and are pushed upwards as mitotic cell division occurs. As they progress towards the surface they are coated in a tough, protein-based substance called keratin which is produced by cells called keratinocytes. Keratin is also an often results during pregnancy or when taking oral contraceptives. The dark line that runs vertically along the midline of the abdomen during some pregnancies (linea nigra), and the darkening of the areolar around the nipples, is due to a similar process. The skin condition vitiligo, on the other hand, results in depigmentation when melanocytes stop producing melanin in a particular area. Albinism refers to widespread or complete loss of pigmentation in the skin, hair and eyes due to the absence of an enzyme involved in the production of melanin (*albus* means 'white' in Latin). It is an inherited (genetic) condition and often results in visual problems and increased susceptibility to sunburn and skin cancer.

MERKEL AND LANGERHANS CELLS

Another type of cell found in the epidermis are merkel cells. These respond to gentle, localised pressure and are particularly abundant on the palmar surface of the fingers. Because they are continually active when a stimulus is present, they are well adapted to determine fine detail such as Braille text. Langerhans cells have a completely different function and work collaboratively with white blood cells to recognise and destroy pathogens (disease-causing microorganisms) that attempt to enter the body via the skin. Finally, it is important to note that the epidermis does not contain any blood or blood vessels. The cells of the epidermis receive all of their nutrients via diffusion of plasma from the dermis below. The surface of the epidermis is uneven and ridged which creates the pattern of our fingerprints. These ridges are formed by cells within the dermis called papillae which also aid the nutrition of the epidermal cells. They are also thought to prevent the dermis and epidermis from separating when sheering forces are applied to the skin (e.g. falling off your bike and sliding along the ground).

DERMIS

The dermis is the inner layer of the skin and is often referred to as the 'true skin' since it is thicker than the epidermis and contains most of the structures and appendages that we associate with this organ. It is dense connective tissue made up of collagen and elastin fibres intertwined with blood vessels, lymph vessels and nerve endings. The collagen and elastin fibres provide structural support and help to ensure that the skin returns to its normal shape after stretching. We saw in Chapter 2 that the amino acids that make up collagen eventually cross-link, leading to loss of flexibility in the skin. This process is also exacerbated by the fact that collagen and elastin production decreases with age, resulting in wrinkles and further reduction in skin elasticity. It is easy to measure the natural elastic recoil of skin and if you pinch the back of your hand the skin should flatten almost immediately. If it is slow to return to its original position (maybe a couple of seconds) it indicates a reduction in these natural elastic fibres. It is important to remember, however, that other organs (such as blood vessels, alveoli, tendons, ligaments, etc.) also contain collagen and elastin fibres and are subject to the same degenerative changes. You can also get an idea of the rigidity and 'chewiness' of collagen by eating fruit pastilles, hard gums or any other type of 'jelly' sweet since they contain boiled collagen (gelatin). This explains why vegetarians, understandably, look horrified when offered a wine gum: 'care for some sugared connective tissue?'

SWEAT GLANDS

One of the most abundant structures in the dermis are the sweat (or sudoriferous) glands (Figure 3.4). Most sweat glands are exocrine (or eccrine) glands and release a clear secretion onto the surface of the skin through a pore. This secretion is primarily water since it is derived from the blood plasma (one of the three fluid compartments). It also contains a small proportion of dissolved substances and ions including sodium and chloride (which accounts for its salty taste). The main function of sweat glands is to regulate temperature and when sweat is evaporated from the surface of the skin it results in heat loss. However, we will discuss this in greater detail later in the

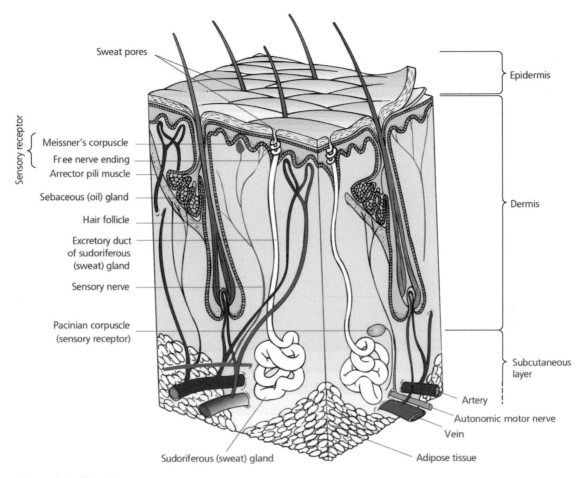

Figure 3.4 The skin.

chapter. Sweat also contains an enzyme that helps to destroy undesirable bacteria that may attempt to colonise the skin (see Chapter 6).

APOCRINE GLANDS

The other type of sweat glands are called apocrine glands and are found mainly in the armpit and groin (the hairy areas). They are not active until puberty when they begin to secrete a fat-infused sweat onto the hair follicles rather than directly onto the surface of the skin. This 'thicker' sweat provides a degree of nourishment for 'friendly' bacteria living on the skin and, as they break it down, produces

the acrid smell we associate with body odour. Apocrine sweat is produced most abundantly during times of anxiety and sexual activity and is thought (by some) to contain a pheromone-like substance that may heighten sexual desirability. However, pheromones are not consciously perceived (if they are perceived at all in humans) and smelling strongly of apocrine sweat will probably not make you more attractive per se (unless your partner likes that sort of thing). In some areas of the body, apocrine glands produce specialised secretions such as the milk produced by the mammary glands of the breast and the wax (cerumen) produced in the ear canals. Cerumen helps to clean and protect the ear canal from water, foreign bodies, bacteria, etc. Some animals use their apocrine glands in even more creative ways and horses produce large amounts of lathery sweat from their apocrine glands to ensure rapid cooling after exercise. Skunks use theirs to . . . well . . . squirt stinky liquid at animals/people they feel threatened by. If you have a few minutes to spare, I thoroughly recommend searching the web for 'recipes' to remove skunk smell. Writing this book has been a real eye-opener for me (apparently tomato juice doesn't work very well but a mixture of baking soda, peroxide and soap seems popular amongst those in the know).

HAIR

It is estimated that the average adult has about 5 million hair follicles of which approximately 100,000 are on their head (Figure 3.4). This sounds an implausibly high number but there are two different types of hair, the most abundant of which are very difficult to perceive. The thick hair that we find on our heads, under our armpits and around the genital area is known as terminal hair. The short, colourless hair found (almost) everywhere else is known as vellus hair. In fact, the only places that hair is not found on the human body are the palms of the hand, the soles of the feet, the lips, the back of the ears, the very end of the penis (glans), the clitoris and the labia minora (inner lips of the female genitalia). In normal circumstances, vellus hair is very difficult to see and it is often further obscured by terminal hair (e.g. on the arms). Before birth, babies are completely covered in a special fur-like hair called lanugo which is thought to aid temperature regulation in the womb. By the time they are born, however, it has usually transformed into vellus hair. Interestingly, those who suffer from severe anorexia or anorexia nervosa may also develop lanugo (usually on the face, arms and back) as a result of profound malnutrition. Since they have lost a significant proportion of insulating body fat (adipose tissue) it may represent a heat conservation mechanism. In health, hair helps to trap warm air next to the skin but it is also a physical barrier to protect the skin from foreign material and UV light.

HAIR STRUCTURE

Hair itself is composed of three different parts: the follicle, the root and the shaft (Figure 3.4). The term follicle simply refers to a small body cavity or sac (in this case, the one in which the hair develops). At the base of the hair follicle is a cluster of cells called the bulb. The bulb is nourished by blood vessels in the dermal papillae that enable cell division to take place. As the newly formed hair cells push upwards and away from their source of nourishment, they quickly die and are keratinised (waterproofed) and coloured by either melanin (black, brown or blond hair) or carotene (red or auburn hair). The part of the hair below the skin is known as the root whilst the portion above the skin is the shaft. It is fortunate that hair cells die as they progress towards the surface, otherwise having a haircut would be a potentially excruciating experience. However, the bulb of the hair is surrounded by nerve endings and if you pluck a hair from your head, eyebrow or elsewhere it is momentarily (and often acutely) painful. There is a rare condition called trichotillomania (cause unknown) which includes the urge to pull out your own hair. It is also known that hair absorbs a number of substances that can be identified in the shaft including poisons such as arsenic. Finally, before we move on, it is worth noting that we also have tiny 'hair-like' structures called cilia projecting from epithelial cells in the respiratory tract and elsewhere. They are not hairs in the true sense but they can provide a physical barrier and trap foreign particles in the same way as body hair.

TINY MUSCLES

Attached to the side of the hair follicle is a small bundle of smooth or involuntary muscle called an erector pili muscle (Figure 3.4). When stimulated by cold (or fear) these tiny muscles contract to allow the hair to stand upright (an involuntary or autonomic response). This process also raises the skin around the hair to form goose-bumps and helps to trap an insulating layer of air next to the skin to slow the rate of cooling. In animals, it also acts as a warning mechanism when they are startled or alarmed. Cats, for example, demonstrate a very obvious erector pili response and, when surprised or frightened, the fur on their back stands on end to make them appear bigger. The same thing happens to porcupines but with even more impressive results as you can imagine. Humans also experience an involuntary goose-bump reaction in response to fear, surprise and other strong emotions (e.g. listening to a particularly 'sad' or emotive piece of music). All of these sensations encourage the sympathetic nervous system to secrete adrenaline and noradrenaline which stimulates the alpha 1 cells situated on the erector pili smooth muscle. Although this doesn't make us appear bigger or more intimidating to a potential aggressor it does alert or orientate us to our situation. From a survival point of view, therefore, it is very useful mechanism even when a potentially hazardous situation proves to be perfectly safe. 'Better safe (and slightly embarrassed) than sorry.' We will discuss this in greater detail when we look at 'flight-or-fight' in Chapters 7, 12 and 13. It does seem odd, however, that listening to music should stimulate this essentially protective mechanism. Part of the reason for this is thought to be that music stimulates the primitive areas of the brain involved with memory, emotion, reward and motivation (see Chapter 12). This results in the secretion of a number of chemical messengers including adrenaline, noradrenaline, dopamine and endorphins that not only result in goose-bumps but also the pleasurable 'tingling' sensations we experience when listening to a particular melody or musical phrase. Although it often seems that our response to music (physiological and emotional) is a deeply personal experience, it is actually a shared or collective reaction thought to have developed over thousands of years as a means of reinforcing social organisation and unity. Safety in numbers, after all, is an essentially protective mechanism.

SEBACEOUS GLANDS

Another structure that is attached to the side of some hair follicles are sebaceous glands (Figure 3.4). These are most abundant on the face, neck, scalp and back. They secrete a waxy substance called sebum onto the hair follicle or, in some cases, directly onto the surface of the skin. Sebum derives its name from the Latin word for tallow (rendered animal fat) and provides a water-resistant coating that helps to keep hair and skin supple. This waterproofing property is particularly evident before birth where sebum, old skin cells and lanugo combine to provide the developing baby with a waxy covering called vernix. Cold water swimmers often cover themselves in a thick layer of grease to insulate themselves against the cold and to keep their skin from macerating (the wrinkly appearance that appears after skin has been immersed in water for too long). The sebaceous glands become particularly active during puberty and an excess of sebum can make the skin and hair oily and greasy. If the hair follicles become blocked with sebum it can lead to the development of acne. If bacteria are present, inflammation and rupture of the follicle may also occur leading to the pitted appearance of the skin. Blackheads (also known as open comedones) occur because the blocked follicle is wider than normal and a plug of sebum can be seen protruding from the epidermis. The black colour is not dirt as commonly thought but oxidised melanin. Whiteheads (closed comedones) are exactly the same but since the follicle is not open to the air, the plug is not oxidised and remains white. The term sebaceous cyst, somewhat confusingly, refers to epidermal or pillar cysts which tend to be blocked with a cheesy, keratin-based substance rather than sebum as the name suggests. Infected sebaceous cysts often require incision and drainage and can produce an impressive quantity of thick, white discharge (not dissimilar to squeezing a tube of toothpaste but not as minty).

NERVE ENDINGS

The dermis also contains a number of different nerve endings which are sensitive to touch, temperature, pressure and pain. The abundance of these receptors varies greatly from location to location, with the face and hands most densely innervated (supplied with nerves). For example, it is estimated that in the fingertips alone there are approximately 2,500 receptors per cm². The information gathered from these nerve endings is relayed (via the spinal cord) to the brain where the sensations are interpreted (see Chapter 12). We have already seen that merkel cells in the epidermis respond to localised sensations of pressure including the perception of closely situated elevated points such as Braille script. The dermis also contains a number of nerve endings that are sensitive to pressure and touch known as mechanoreceptors since they respond to mechanical stimulation and pressure. Meissner's corpuscles, for example, are situated immediately below the epidermis and (like merkel cells) are well represented on the palmar surfaces of the fingers. They are sensitive to light touch and play an important role in controlling handgrip. For example, when you are holding a wine glass you must apply enough pressure to stop it slipping through your fingers but not too much or it will shatter in your hand (giving people the impression that you are slightly unhinged). These nerves are only active when a stimulus is first applied to the surface of the skin and when it is removed again. This explains why we are conscious of our clothes when we first put them on but not after they have been in place for a short period of time. Ruffini's corpuscles, on the other hand, are continually active when a stimulus is present and are sensitive to vibration, stretching of the skin and heat. Finally, Pacinian corpuscles are located deep within the dermis and subcutaneous fat and are sensitive to rapid vibration and pressure (Figure 3.4). Like Meissner's corpuscles, they are only active when a stimulus is first applied to the skin but are not as discriminatory.

PAIN RECEPTORS

The next type of nerve ending found in the dermis (and epidermis) are pain receptors or nociceptors. The term nociception is derived from the Latin word *nocere* meaning 'harm' or 'injurious'. As the name suggests, they are activated in response to potentially harmful or tissue-damaging stimulation although it is the sensory cortex of the brain that actually interprets the information as 'painful' (see Chapter 12). The reason sunburn (a first-degree burn) is more painful than a full thickness burn is, paradoxically, because it is so superficial. Overexposure to UV light and radiation damages the epidermis of the skin and stimulates excessive production of a protein that irritates the nociceptors below. Full thickness burns, on the other hand, destroy the epidermis, dermis and possibly the subcutaneous fat and underlying structures. Consequently, since the nerves themselves have been destroyed, the wound is often painless. One of the major complications of partial and full thickness burns (second and third degree burns) is fluid loss. If the waterproof barrier of the skin is breached, plasma and plasma proteins are lost. This can result in such severe fluid loss that the heart is unable to pump enough blood to the tissue resulting in circulatory collapse (hypovolemic shock). Fluid replacement therapy for burns victims is calculated, therefore, according to the percentage of body surface area affected.

THERMORECEPTORS

The final type of nerve ending found in the dermis are thermoreceptors which, as their name suggests, respond to changes in temperature. There are two types of thermoreceptor: hot and cold. Although both are found throughout the body, there are about four times as many cold receptors as there are hot. The parts of the body with the greatest concentrations are the face and ears which explains why they often feel cold before the rest of the body on a chilly winter's day (unless or course you are wearing that item of 1970s chic – the knitted balaclava). Cold receptors (also known as Krause's end bulbs) start to perceive cold when the surface of the skin reaches about 35°C (normal skin or shell temperature is about 36°C). Maximal rate of firing occurs at temperatures between about 20-30°C. As temperature declines further, firing becomes less frequent which explains why we experience numbness, particularly to our extremities (hand, feet and face). Hot receptors (Ruffini's corpuscles), on the other hand, begin to respond when the temperature of the skin reaches about 30°C. Once it rises above about 45°C, pain receptors (nociceptors) will be activated to prevent tissue damage from occurring. Thermoreceptors can provide seemingly contradictory information, however, and you may have wondered why you sometimes feel cold when first standing under a hot shower. This is because cold receptors can also be activated by skin temperatures of about 45°C resulting in a brief sensation of cold followed by a prolonged sensation of heat (and possibly pain).

THERMOREGULATION

The internal temperature of the human body is maintained at around 37°C. Strictly speaking, however, body temperature can be divided into two values: core temperature and shell temperature. Core temperature is the temperature of the internal organs and the blood (about 36.5–37.5°C). Shell temperature, on the other hand, is the temperature of the skin's surface and may vary considerably according to the temperature of the surrounding environment. The homeostatic regulation of core temperature allows humans to live in a variety of climatic environments including extreme cold and intense heat. It also ensures that normal cell function and metabolic process are maintained. For example, an increase in body temperature also increases the rate of cellular respiration (the rate at which the cells use oxygen and glucose to produce chemical energy/ATP) and the speed at which many other chemical reactions takes place. This is one of the reasons why people often lose weight when feverish (the other being that they are not eating and the body must liberate glucose through destructive metabolism/catabolism of fat, etc.). A decrease in body temperature, on the other hand, will slow the rate of cellular respiration and many other chemical reactions. Some surgical procedures artificially induce whole-body hypothermia (low temperature) to slow the pace of oxygen consumption in order to protect cellular and tissue health. There are also a number of well-documented cases where young children

have been successfully resuscitated after prolonged submersion in freezing water. It is thought that the reason they have survived in these unusual circumstances is because of rapid heat loss (and the induction of hypothermia) following submersion (see below). As we will see in Chapter 7, however, the likelihood of surviving cardiac arrest in normal circumstances is low.

CIRCADIAN RHYTHM

A number of natural variations (beyond conscious control) also affect our core or internal temperature. For example, during a typical 24-hour period, our body temperature fluctuates considerably in accordance with what is known as the diurnal or circadian rhythm (Figure 3.5). Temperature tends to be at its lowest between about 3 and 5 in the morning and at its highest in the early evening. One of the reasons for this pattern of temperature activity is cellular respiration (I told you cells were important). Once we wake up and become increasingly active, we require more chemical energy to drive the various systems of our body. Added to this, most people eat breakfast of some description which kick-starts the cells of our digestive tract. In short, increased cellular activity produces heat which is added to the core, leading to an increase in temperature. As cellular activity winds down in the evening, less heat is produced which is why we often feel cold at night (particularly in the early hours of the morning). Other things

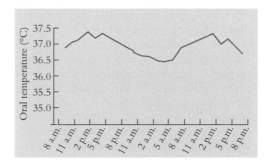

Figure 3.5 Oral temperature over 36 hours.

are happening too of course and we will discuss some of these in this and later chapters. The other natural variation that may affect core temperature in women is the menstrual cycle. Following ovulation, it is common for core temperature to rise between 0.5 and 1°C in response to increased secretion of the hormone progesterone. This spike in temperature can be a useful indicator of fertility for women who are trying to maximise (or minimise) their chances of conception (see Chapter 14).

HEAT EXCHANGE

Regardless of whether our temperature is too hot or too cold, the body will always attempt (in health) to reverse the direction of change in accordance with the principle of negative feedback. Earlier in the chapter we saw that negative feedback requires three components: a receptor, an integrator and an effector mechanism/s. In the case of thermoregulation, the sensors that detect whether a change has taken place are chiefly the hot and cold receptors of the skin and thermoreceptors located in the hypothalamus of the brain. The integrator (or control centre) that receives information from the sensors, and organises an appropriate response, is also the hypothalamus. Finally, the effector mechanisms that carry out and reverse the direction of change are many and varied as we shall see. A good way to visualise the role of the hypothalamus is to think of it as a household thermostat controlling radiators and air-conditioning in order to maintain a comfortable internal temperature. If the thermostat is set to 20°C and room temperature falls to 17°C it will activate the radiators until the ambient temperature returns to 20°C. If, on the other hand, temperature rises to 25°C the air-conditioning will be activated until temperature, once again, returns to its original set point. In the case of the human body, the hypothalamus sets internal (core) temperature at about 37°C. However, before we look at the different effector mechanisms that ensure it remains at (or around) this set point we first need to discuss the ways in which heat can be transferred or exchanged.

RADIATION

The first heat exchange mechanism is radiation which simply refers to the transmission of heat (or energy) from a central point outwards. For example, the sun radiates heat (and energy) from a high concentration (a large thermonuclear reaction in the centre of our solar system) to a lower concentration everywhere else. The body also radiates heat from a high concentration at its core (37°C) to a lower concentration elsewhere (normal room temperature of about 20°C). This is of course why we need to wear clothes (the more layers the better) in order to slow the rate of radiation to a manageable level. The body loses about 65% of its heat through radiation at temperatures below 20°C. In the unlikely

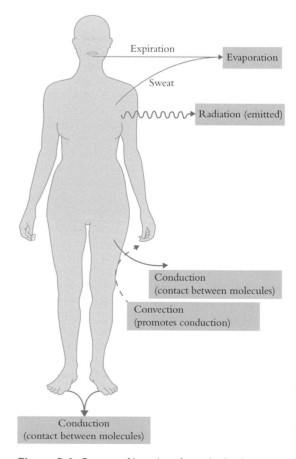

Figure 3.6 Routes of heat loss from the body.

event, therefore, that you had the sudden urge to strip off, run outside and stand motionless in the cold night air you would radiate heat away from your body much more quickly than if you were fully clothed (Figure 3.6). Once you had reached the conclusion that this was a bad idea and returned inside (looking nervously around to see if the neighbours had noticed) you may stand next to a fire or radiator (the clue is in the name) to warm yourself up again. Heat will radiate towards you from a high concentration to a low concentration, adding heat to your core (and the room).

CONDUCTION

The next type of heat exchange mechanism is conduction or the direct transfer of heat between two objects or substances. For example, a hot iron bar will conduct heat into your hand much more quickly than air since it is denser. Obviously, in this case, it is a bad thing since it will result in tissue damage but the same applies to the warming effect of a hot water bottle or the cooling effect of sleeping on a cold surface such as concrete (Figure 3.6). Another good example is water which conducts heat towards or away from the body about 25 times faster than air (radiation). If you slip into a nice hot bath the water envelops you and conducts heat into your skin and core. If on the other hand, you have the bad fortune to fall into the North Atlantic you are in big trouble. The cold water will rapidly conduct heat away from your core body temperature resulting in hypothermia, muscle paralysis and cellular death. A normal person without survival clothing/apparatus can survive in water of 5°C for about 10–20 minutes before drowning. The likelihood, therefore, of Jack Dawson from the film *Titanic*, making such a long and articulate final speech to his soon to be ex-lover, whilst submerged in the icy waters of the North Atlantic, is unlikely to say the least. As soon as he plunged into the sea, his body would undergo what is known as the cold-shock response. A sudden cold stimulus of this nature can cause cessation of breathing (or at the very least a reflex gasp) followed by involuntary hyperventilation for

several minutes. Assuming that Jack did not swallow and/or inhale water when he plunged into the freezing sea from the sinking *Titanic*, he may have been able to have a brief conversation (all the while shivering violently) for a few more minutes before muscle paralysis, disorientation and hallucinations rendered him completely insensible (I can only apologise if I have spoiled the end of this film for you). The principle of conduction also helps to explain why it is important to remove clothing from those who have been submerged in cold water for any period of time. If wet clothing remains in situ following rescue, heat will continue to be conducted away from the core at a much faster rate than if by radiation alone (contributing to ongoing hypothermia). Dry clothing (or a blanket) should be applied immediately to offset further heat loss by radiation, convection and evaporation. In normal circumstances, however, the body does not lose a great deal of heat through conduction.

CONVECTION

The third type of heat exchange mechanism is convection. Convection describes the process where heat is transferred in a gas or liquid by the circulation of currents from a region of high temperature to a region of low temperature (Figure 3.6). For example, when a gas is heated, its molecules move more rapidly and begin to expand (think of water vapour coming out of a kettle). The heated gas is now less dense than unheated gas (whose molecules remain close together) and will rise towards the colder area. At the same time, the unheated (dense) gas will fall towards the heated (expanded) gas resulting in heat exchange and the creation of a convection current. In terms of heat loss, convection can also be forced. For example, when a cool breeze passes over exposed skin it 'carries' heat away with it and encourages the rate of water (sweat) evaporation. The same effect can be achieved by fanning your skin, providing the air is cooler than the temperature of the skin and you are not too vigorous with your fanning motion (producing additional heat as a result of cellular respirational/ATP production). The rate of heat loss from a surface via convection depends on the wind speed and explains why wind-chill temperatures are always lower than air temperatures. Convection can also be used to slow down the rate of heat loss from the body (via radiation) and to add it the core. For example, a temperature management device known as a Bair-hugger is often used to reheat hypothermic patients and keep surgical patients warm during an operation. It delivers warm air into a synthetic inflatable blanket that contains hundreds of tiny perforations which distribute the warmed air evenly across the skin (when inflated it looks a bit like a lilo).

EVAPORATION

The final heat-loss mechanism is evaporation. As liquid evaporates, the change of state (into vapour) requires the use of heat which, in the case of the human body, is lost to the atmosphere (Figure 3.6). The rate at which evaporation occurs depends upon a number of factors including ambient temperature, humidity and air currents (convection). If you have been swimming in the sea on a hot day you will feel cold as you leave the water and try to locate your towel on the beach. This is because water is evaporating from your skin taking heat with it (probably exacerbated by convection currents). Once you towel the water off, however, evaporation slows down and you begin to enjoy the radiated heat from the sun once again. For this reason, sweating is an extremely important heat-loss mechanism and during intense exercise the body can lose up to 85% of its heat in this way (see below). Evaporation does not have to occur from the surface of the skin and dogs cool themselves using their tongue! Although they possess sweat glands on the pads of their feet, water mostly evaporates from their mouth as a steady stream of air passes over their tongue during panting. We also lose water vapour from our mouth during expiration but sticking out your tongue and panting is not a particularly dignified method of heat exchange and may cause people to stop and stare.

WARMING UP

Radiation, conduction, convection and evaporation are all very well but what actually happens when we get cold? Firstly, thermoreceptors in the dermis of our skin send nerve impulses (action potentials) to the hypothalamus of the brain to tell it that temperature has dropped. The hypothalamus recognises that a response is required to reverse the direction of change and employs a number of thermoregulatory effector mechanisms to ensure core temperature remains at 37°C. One of the first autonomic heat-creating (thermogenic) responses to be employed by the body is constriction (narrowing) of the blood vessels that provide the dermis with blood. This process is known as vasoconstriction (vessel narrowing)

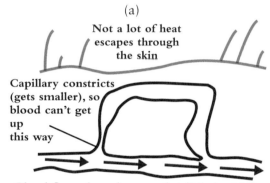

(a)

Not a lot of heat escapes through the skin

Capillary constricts (gets smaller), so blood can't get up this way

Blood flows deep down so that little heat is lost

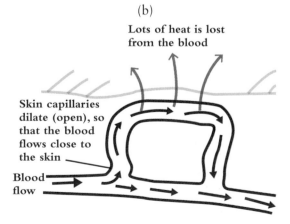

(b)

Lots of heat is lost from the blood

Skin capillaries dilate (open), so that the blood flows close to the skin

Blood flow

Figure 3.7 (a) Cutaneous vasoconstriction. (b) Cutaneous vasodilation.

and ensures that nice warm blood continues to flow within the subcutaneous fat but not to the dermis above (Figure 3.7). Consequently, the heat carried by the blood is added back to the core rather than lost to the atmosphere via radiation. Cold receptors in the dermis will continue to report that temperature is low (since heat is unable to penetrate the insulating fat) until the core returns to its set point of 37°C and vasodilation (vessel widening) occurs. This process also explains why skin appears pale (or blue) when cold since blood is less abundant in the dermis.

SHIVERING AND PILOERECTION

The next mechanism employed by the hypothalamus to reverse the direction of change is shivering. Shivering is simply the rapid, alternate contraction and relaxation of skeletal muscle in order to generate heat via cellular activity (i.e. the harder your muscle cells work the more heat they produce). This is an involuntary response that stops when sufficient heat has been added to the core. It should not surprise us that skeletal (voluntary) muscle can, in certain circumstances, be controlled by our autonomic (automatic) nervous system since, in Chapter 2, we saw that the diaphragm and intercostal muscles are subject to voluntary and involuntary control (when breathing). Although shivering is a very important thermogenic (heat producing) response, it can only be sustained for a limited period of time. As hypothermia (temperature below 35°C) progresses, shivering becomes increasingly violent resulting in further production of heat but also further expenditure of energy. In the same way that skeletal muscle can only perform a limited number of contractions in the gym before seizing up, therefore, shivering cannot be sustained indefinitely and eventually movement becomes slow and laboured. Another thermoregulatory response to cold is the contraction of erector pili muscles (described above) which pull the hair follicle upright and trap a layer of warm air next to the skin. Although this helps to slow down radiation of heat from the body, it is not particularly effective in humans on its own. The final mechanism employed to reverse the direction of change in severe cold is the secretion of additional thyroid hormones by the thyroid gland (see Chapter 13). Since these hormones increase cellular activity throughout the body they also increase the production of heat. In adults, however, increased secretion of thyroid hormones is only activated in response to prolonged exposure to cold and cannot be sustained for very long. In addition to the autonomic responses described, the brain will also encourage appropriate behavioural responses such as seeking shelter, putting on additional clothing and increasing physical activity (to encourage cellular generation of heat). It is only when these combined mechanisms fail (usually because of prolonged exposure to cold) that hypothermia becomes life-threatening.

HYPOTHERMIA

Hypothermia occurs when core temperature falls below 35°C. This is only cause for concern if the compensatory mechanisms described above (e.g. shivering) fail and are unable to reverse the direction of change. Hypothermia is often subdivided, therefore, into mild, moderate and severe categories. Mild hypothermia typically occurs when core temperature is between about 32.2 and 35°C and is characterised by shivering, vasoconstriction, raised blood pressure and increased respiratory rate as cellular activity increases to provide additional heat. Moderate hypothermia occurs when temperature is between about 30.0 and 32.2°C and is accompanied by more violent shivering which will eventually decline as glucose stores are exhausted, resulting in muscle rigidity. The person will appear increasingly pale (blue-tinged) as further vasoconstriction occurs to prevent radiation of heat away from the body (Figure 3.7). Movement will also become progressively uncoordinated and mild confusion may be apparent. Severe hypothermia is said to occur when temperature is below 30°C. At this point, cellular metabolic processes begin to decline and movement becomes increasingly difficult. Blood pressure and respiratory rate also decrease and cardiac arrhythmias (irregular heart rhythms) may occur. Below 27°C over 80% of people are comatose. Before this occurs, however, those with hypothermia may also experience mental confusion, hallucinations and may demonstrate a number of abnormal behaviours including terminal burrowing (a kind of hide-and-die response) and something known as paradoxical undressing. For reasons not fully understood, it is not uncommon in those with severe hypothermia to remove all of their clothes before terminal burrowing and death. It is thought that it may be the result of cold-induced thermoregulatory malfunction of the hypothalamus or because cutaneous (skin) vasoconstriction can only be sustained for so long and, when muscle tone relaxes, blood floods back into the dermis, providing the sensation of heat. At any rate, it clearly hastens the rate of overall heat loss and cardiac arrest (heart + stop) will result shortly after. However, because hypothermia slows cellular activity it is difficult to assess whether brain death has occurred at low temperature even when the heart has stopped. This is why many hypothermia management flow-diagrams display the following warning in large capital letters: NOT DEAD UNTIL WARM AND DEAD. Earlier in the chapter we discussed the fact that young children have been successfully resuscitated after prolonged submersion in freezing water and a 7-year-old Swedish child (found in the ocean on Christmas day 2010) was successfully resuscitated with a temperature of 13°C! Although this case is exceptional (it is highly unlikely that any adult could survive in such circumstances) it does demonstrate the point.

TREATING HYPOTHERMIA

There are different management regimes for the hypothermic patient depending on whether they are being treated in situ (outside) or in a clinical environment (inside). However, preventing further heat loss and incremental rewarming are important in both cases. Contrary to popular belief, a shot of brandy (or other alcoholic drink) is not recommended in severe hypothermia. This is because alcohol stimulates cutaneous vasodilation (widening of the blood vessels in the skin) and although it provides the sensation of warmth in the skin it actually results in increased radiation of heat away from the body. In health, this mechanism is facetiously referred to as wearing a 'beer coat' and can be observed most Friday and Saturday nights as men and women cheerfully wander from pub to pub wearing surprisingly few clothes. They feel warm because of alcohol-induced cutaneous vasodilation but are in fact cooling at a rapid rate. Anyway, alcohol greatly contributes to the risk of developing hypothermia since, in small quantities, it prevents accurate assessment of the true risk of cold and, in large quantities, interferes with normal thermoregulatory mechanisms. For the health care professional, it also makes it very difficult to assess whether a person is unco-ordinated and disorientated because they are hypothermic or because they are intoxicated (or both). Finally, and I apologise in advance for this nerdy cultural reference, perhaps the best example of how to care for a hypothermic patient when trapped on a fictional ice planet with a dead space-creature is provided by the film *The Empire Strikes Back*. Luke Skywalker is found hypothermic and in a semi-conscious state by his friend Han Solo. Moments later, the large rodent-like animal (Tauntaun) that Han was riding to search for Luke keels over and dies (presumably from cardiac arrest secondary to hypothermia). Not discouraged by this seemingly unfortunate event, the ever quick-thinking Han (always my favourite as a child) takes Luke's light sabre and slices open the dead creature's belly to reveal its steaming intestines. As Han begins to stuff his friend inside the creature's abdominal cavity he utters the immortal line: 'this may smell bad kid, but it will keep you alive until I can get the shelter up'. In actual fact, there is a great deal of physiological sense to this unpleasant cause of action. The dead animal may be hypothermic itself but its core temperature is still warmer than the atmospheric temperature outside. Consequently, heat will be conducted into the 'enveloped' Luke Skywalker. It will also protect him from the forced convection of the icy wind and slow the rate of radiation of heat from his own body. From a utilitarian perspective, the sacrifice of the Tauntaun ensured that Luke was able to survive and go on to defeat the evil Empire (if you hate Star Wars you may wish that Han hadn't bothered or that the Tauntaun had lived a little longer). On a slightly more high-brow note, there are reports of Napoleon's troops doing much the same thing with dead horses during the winter retreat from Moscow in 1812–13. Survival is a very powerful instinct.

COOLING DOWN

We have looked at what happens when we get cold, but what happens when we get hot? In short, much the same thing but in reverse. Firstly, the hypothalamus encourages appropriate behavioural responses such as seeking shade, taking off unnecessary clothing, decreasing physical activity (to minimise cellular generation of heat), fanning, etc. Involuntary autonomic responses include cutaneous vasodilation (widening of the blood vessels in the skin) resulting in additional heat loss from radiation (Figure 3.7). The increased blood flow to the skin also explains why some parts of your body, such as the face, often appear red and flushed when hot. The other important heat-loss mechanism is of course sweating. As observed earlier in the chapter, heat is lost as sweat changes state from a liquid to a vapour and evaporates from the skin's surface. Humans possess about 2.5 million sweat-producing (exocrine) glands and during strenuous exercise they produce between 0.8 and 1.5 litres of sweat per hour. However, an athlete competing in a triathlon (or other extreme events) may produce in excess of 4 litres of sweat per hour. This level of sweating is not sustainable, however, and may result in dangerous fluid and sodium (Na^+) loss. Fluid and electrolyte replacement is essential, therefore, to avoid dehydration and maintain blood pressure. The rate at which sweat evaporates from the skin depends upon a number of factors including temperature and humidity (moisture of the air). If temperature is high and humidity is low, sweat will evaporate quickly from the surface of the skin (providing it is exposed). If temperature and humidity are both high,

however, it is difficult for sweat to evaporate and cooling is reduced. Sweat is still produced but simply runs off the body leading to dehydration, electrolyte imbalance and circulatory collapse if uncorrected. Another good way to overheat during exercise is to undertake a 'fun-run' dressed in a full-sized novelty animal or fruit costume. This not only reduces the amount of heat radiated away from the body (by providing an additional physical barrier and preventing skin cooling via convection) it also increases the humidity within the suit by trapping moisture from evaporated sweat. The term 'boil in the bag' seems rather apt.

FEVER

Finally, it is worth taking a few minutes to briefly examine what makes our core temperature rise during illness and why we feel cold during fever (a seemingly contradictory response). In simple terms, core temperature begins to rise following the release of chemicals called pyrogens (pyro + gen*esis* = fire + creation) from damaged tissue as a result of bacterial or viral infection. This triggers the secretion of another chemical called prostaglandin (see Chapter 13) that resets the body's thermoregulatory control centre, the hypothalamus, to a higher point (i.e. above 37°C). Let's imagine that the body's thermostat has been raised to 39°C, any temperature below this new fixed point is considered to be low and the body immediately implements heat-generating mechanisms such as vasoconstriction and shivering. The person experiencing the fever will also feel cold (despite being hot) because vasoconstriction reduces blood flow to the dermis and the thermoreceptors located there. Shivering and vasoconstriction ensure that heat is added to the core, and temperature continues to rise until the new thermostatic set point is met (in this case 39°C). However, the big question is why does the hypothalamus put us through this thoroughly unpleasant process? In simple terms, raising temperature above the normal range (pyrexia) generates a hostile environment for invading microorganisms which helps to inhibit their replication and spread. At the same time, however, pyrexia can interfere with our own cellular health and temperatures above 40°C often result in confusion, irritability and delirium. If temperature continues to rise and is uncorrected, it can result in brain damage and febrile convulsion (seizure associated with pyrexia) in young children. Normally, the body's immune system will destroy the microorganisms long before this occurs and temperature will return to normal in the absence of prostaglandin/pyrogen production. It may be necessary or prudent, however, to provide antipyretic (heat reducing) medication such as paracetamol (which inhibits the production of prostaglandin) in order to quickly return temperature to normal. In both cases, the hypothalamic set point is returned to normal (37°C) and the body implements heat-loss mechanisms in order to reduce temperature. When this first occurs, there is heavy sweating and widespread vasodilation (the face often appears red and flushed) and we often comment that 'the fever has broken'. Although it is possible to rationalise this seemingly contradictory process on paper it is much more difficult to convince a feverish person that what they actually require is cooling down when they are shivering violently and clutching desperately at their blankets (with a temperature of 39°C or above).

CHAPTER 3: TEST YOURSELF

Q. Briefly explain what is meant by the term homeostasis.
A. Homeostasis refers to the way in which the body maintains a stable internal environment despite changes to the internal and external environment.

Q. What is meant by the term negative feedback in relation to homeostasis?
A. Negative feedback refers to the way the body responds to reverse the direction of change in order to main homeostasis.

Q. The body requires three basic components to achieve negative feedback. What are they?
A. The three components necessary to maintain homeostasis are a sensor (or detector), a control centre (or integrator) and an effector mechanism/s.

Q. Most of the homeostatic adjustments made by our body are the result of negative feedback. Provide at least two examples.
A. Examples of negative feedback include thermoregulation, heart rate, blood pressure, fluid balance, respiratory rate, plasma pH and blood glucose levels.

Q. What is meant by the term positive feedback?
A. Positive feedback occurs when the body responds to a change by increasing that change even further in the same direction.

Q. Provide an example of a positive feedback mechanism.
A. Labour (childbirth), breastfeeding, coagulation (blood clotting) and the transformation of pepsinogen into pepsin.

Q. What are the three layer of the skin (from most superficial to deepest)?
A. Epidermis, dermis and subcutaneous fat (hypodermis).

Q. Melanocytes, keratinocytes and merkel cells are all found in the epidermis. What do they do?
A. Melanocytes produce the brown/black pigment melanin that helps to protect the skin from ultraviolet (UV) radiation present in sunlight. Keratinocytes produce keratin which helps to waterproof the epidermis and is an important component of hair and nails. Merkel cells respond to gentle, localised pressure and are particularly abundant on the surface of the fingers.

Q. Where would you find erector pili muscles and what is their function?

A. Erector pili muscles are found in the dermis attached to the side of a hair follicle. When we are cold, they contract to allow the hair to stand upright and trap an insulating layer of air next to the skin.

Q. Where would you find sebaceous glands and what is their function?

A. Sebaceous glands are found in the dermis attached to the side of a hair follicle. They secrete a waxy substance called sebum onto the hair follicle (or directly onto the skin) which provides a water-resistant coating.

Q. Explain the difference between shell and core temperature?

A. Shell temperature is the temperature of the skin's surface and may vary considerably according to the temperature of the surrounding environment. Core temperature is the temperature of the internal organs and the blood (about 36.5–37.5°C).

Q. Name the four ways in which the body gains/loses heat?

A. Radiation, conduction, convection and evaporation.

Q. Which part of the brain controls thermoregulation?

A. The hypothalamus.

Q. What is meant by the term vasoconstriction and how does this help to retain heat when we are cold?

A. Vasoconstriction refers to narrowing (constriction) of the blood vessels that provide the dermis with blood. This process ensures that heat carried by the blood is added back to the core rather than lost to the atmosphere via radiation.

Q. What is meant by the term vasodilation and how does this help to lose heat when we are hot?

A. Vasodilation refers to widening (dilation) of the blood vessels in the dermis resulting in increased blood flow to the skin and additional heat loss via radiation.

Q. How does sweating cause heat loss?

A. After sweat has been secreted onto the surface of the skin it evaporates. The change of state, from a liquid to vapour, requires the use of heat which is lost to the atmosphere.

Q. What is the definition of pyrexia?

A. Pyrexia refers to a temperature above the normal range that is not the result of exercise or increased environmental temperature.

Contents

CHAPTER 4

SKELETAL SYSTEM

MUSCLE

The muscular-skeletal system consists of muscles, bones, cartilage, tendons, ligaments and other connective tissue that helps to stabilise and support the skeleton. In Chapter 2, we identified that there are three types of muscle (skeletal, smooth and cardiac) and briefly observed how they differ from one another in structure and function. In this chapter we will only discuss skeletal muscle since, as its name suggests, it is directly or indirectly attached to the bones of the skeletal system by bands of fibrous connective tissue called tendons. This enables coordinated movement of the skeletal system and allows us to undertake activities such as walking and exercising, as well as fine movement of the fingers, facial muscles and eyes. Skeletal muscle also allows us to maintain body posture through sustained contraction (shortening) of spinal and neck muscles. This is demonstrated in dramatic fashion when you fall asleep in class and your head falls forward (waking you up) as you lose muscle tension. Contraction of skeletal muscle also generates heat as muscle cells (myocytes) convert oxygen and glucose into cellular energy (see Chapter 2). This explains why your temperature rises during exercise and also why respiratory and heart rate increase to provide' more nutrient-rich blood more nutrient-rich blood to the muscles (see Chapters 7, 8 and 9). Finally, the abdominal organs (and other structures) are protected from injury by several layers of skeletal muscle. One of the signs clinicians look for when examining the abdomen is tensing of the abdominal muscles to 'guard' against pain caused by pressure on the inflamed organ/s below.

ORGANISATION OF SKELETAL MUSCLES

Skeletal muscle is the most abundant type of muscle in the body and accounts for about 40% of total body weight. There are about 700 skeletal muscles in total and, for convenience, they are often divided into two complementary divisions or groups: axial muscles and appendicular muscles. Axial muscles are responsible for supporting and moving the head/face, spine, rib cage and pelvis (of the axial skeleton – see below) and protecting the abdominal cavity. Appendicular muscles, on the other hand, support and move the arms and legs. Both axial and appendicular muscles vary greatly in size, shape and function. They are named according to a number of criteria including size, shape, location, structure and action (Figure 4.1). For example, the term maximus (largest) is used to describe the largest (and most superficial) of the three gluteal muscles (gluteus maximus) that helps to define the size and shape of your bum. Other muscles are named because they have a distinctive shape and the deltoid muscle, located at the top of your arm/shoulder, is roughly triangular

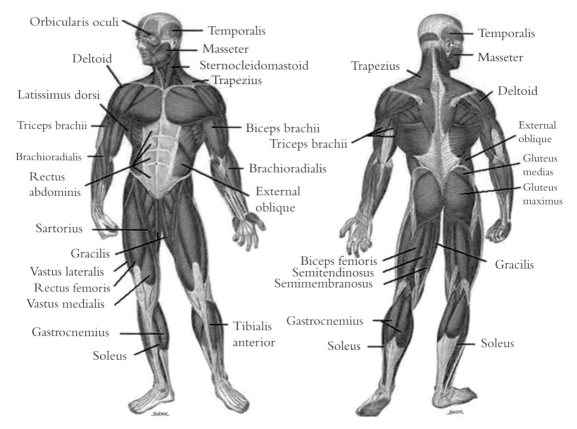

Figure 4.1 Major muscles.

(the Greek letter delta = Δ). Some muscles are named according to their location and the intercostal muscles are found between the ribs (the Latin word costa means rib). Other muscles are named according to the direction of their fibres and the name rectus femoris, for example, describes the muscle that runs vertically along the length of the femur or thigh bone (the Latin word rectus means straight). Similarly, the name rectus abdominis describes the long, flat muscles that extend vertically on either side of the abdomen. Finally, many muscles are named according to their action or function. For example, there are extensor muscles that increase the angle between two bones connected by a joint (see below). There are also flexor muscles that reduce the angle of two bones connected by a joint. Abductor muscles allow the skeleton to move away from the midline of the body whilst adductor muscles allow it to move towards the midline.

Muscles are enclosed, separated from one another and/or connected to other muscles/organs by a thin layer of connective tissue called fascia (plural = fasciae). Fasciae provide a supportive and flexible covering (imagine a sheet of cling film) for nerves and blood vessels as they pass through and between muscles. They also help to reduce friction during movement and provide a degree of elastic recoil.

SKELETAL SYSTEM

The skeletal system accounts for about 20% of total body weight and consists of 206 bones of varying shapes and sizes (some of which are represented in Figure 4.2). The largest of these is the femur or thigh bone and the smallest are the ossicles of the middle ear. Like skeletal muscle, the skeletal system is typically divided

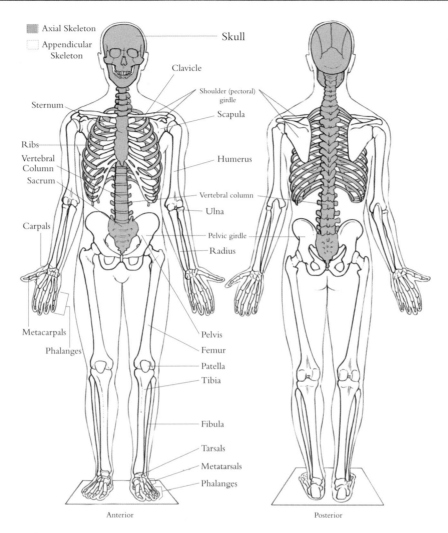

Axial Skeleton
Appendicular Skeleton

Skull
Clavicle
Shoulder (pectoral) girdle
Sternum
Scapula
Ribs
Humerus
Vertebral Column
Sacrum
Vertebral column
Ulna
Carpals
Pelvic girdle
Radius
Metacarpals
Pelvis
Phalanges
Femur
Patella
Tibia
Fibula
Tarsals
Metatarsals
Phalanges

Anterior   Posterior

Figure 4.2 Axial and appendicular skeleton.

into two complementary parts: the axial skeleton (the part that contains and protects the organs) and the appendicular skeleton (the part that moves). The axial skeleton consists of 80 bones and includes those of the skull (cranium), the spine (vertebrae) and the rib cage. At birth, the bones of the cranium are soft and flexible in order to allow the baby's head to mould to the shape of the birth canal during delivery. The longer its head remains in the birth canal, the more 'peanut-shaped' it will be following birth. It is also common for fluid to accumulate in the baby's scalp at this time (caput succedaneum) which protects and

further distorts the appearance of the head. However, both tend to resolve after a few days and the baby's head quickly returns to normal. The bones of the cranium do not completely fuse together until the child is between 12 and 18 months old and it is possible to feel a 'soft-spot' at the front of the skull called the large or anterior fontanelle during this time. There is also a soft spot at the back of the skull (posterior fontanelle) but this has usually closed by the time the baby is about two months old or possibly earlier. It is perfectly safe to gently touch the anterior fontanelle and it should feel flat and firm. If it appears sunken, it can indicate that the child is dehydrated. A bulging or protuberant fontanelle, on the other hand, may be a sign of raised intracranial pressure and should be investigated further. However, it is normal for the fontanelle to bulge slightly during crying (which frankly happens a lot) and pulsations may reflect the pulse of the cerebral arteries.

SKULL AND SINUSES

By adulthood, all 22 bones of the skull have fused together and the fibrous joints between the bony plates (cranial sutures) can be seen on X-ray as thin lines. In total, the skull consists of 8 cranial bones (4 each side) and 14 facial bones (Figure 4.3). The names of the

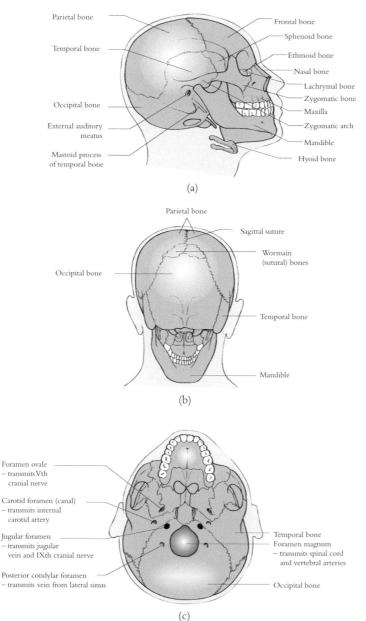

(a)

(b)

(c)

Figure 4.3 Principles bones of the adult skull. (a) Lateral view. (b) Posterior view. (c) Inferior view.

cranial bones (frontal, parietal, occipital and temporal bones) correspond to the lobes of the brain (cerebrum) that are located beneath them (see Chapter 12). There is a large hole at the base of the skull (occipital bone) called the foramen magnum (Latin: great hole) that allows the brainstem to attach to the spinal cord below. There are also a number of smaller foramens (holes) in the skull and facial bones that allow access for blood vessels and nerves (including the optic nerves to the eye and the mental nerves of the jaw). Finally, the skull contains a number of air-filled cavities around the nose called sinuses. These reduce weight at the front of the skull, provide a buffer against facial trauma and increase the resonance of the voice amongst other things. They are also connected to the nasal cavity by small openings or pores called ostia which are easily blocked when the lining of the sinus becomes inflamed (sinusitis). When this occurs, fluid can accumulate in the sinus which causes the unpleasant sensation of nasal congestion and can affect the timbre and resonance of the voice.

SPINE AND RIBS

The axial bones of the spine (vertebrae) are subdivided into 7 cervical (neck), 12 thoracic (chest), 5 lumbar (lower back), 5 sacral (fused bones of the posterior pelvis) and 4 coccygeal (tail) (Figure 4.4). Those of you who are good at mental arithmetic will already have worked out that there are 33 spinal bones in total. Collectively, they support the skull, surround and protect the spinal cord (see Chapter 12) and allow us to stand and sit in an upright position. The coccygeal or 'tail' bones are not as redundant as they are often portrayed and remain an important attachment for a number of muscles, tendons and ligaments. They also provide a degree of support when a person is sitting and leans backwards (a common posture during a boring lecture, tutorial or staff meeting). There are three classic ways to fracture the coccyx: sit down quickly after somebody has pulled the chair out from behind you (not funny), slip down the stairs on your bottom (bump, bump, bump . . . ouch) or

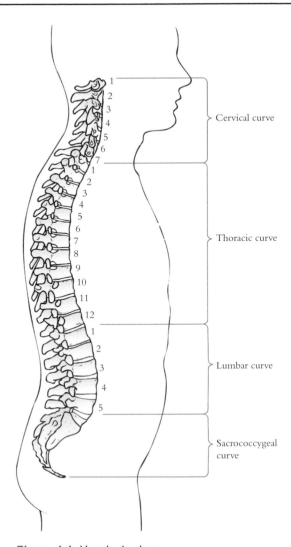

Figure 4.4 Vertebral column.

relive your childhood days by sliding down a playground slide and fly off the end onto your coccygeal bones (I have done this). The axial bones of the rib cage protect the thoracic and upper (superior) abdominal organs. There are 12 pairs of ribs all of which are attached (posteriorly) to the 12 thoracic vertebrae. Pairs 1–7 are often referred to as 'true ribs' and are attached at the front (anteriorly) to the sternum (breast bone) by costal cartilage (Figure 4.2). Pairs 8–10 ('false ribs') are not attached directly to the sternum but to the costal cartilage of rib 7. Cartilage is a highly flexible material (see below) that allows expansion of the lungs and thoracic cavity during breathing. Finally, pairs 11–12 are known as 'floating ribs' since they have no anterior attachment to the sternum at all.

OSSICLES AND HYOID BONE

The remaining bones of the axial skeleton are the tiny ossicles of the ears and the singular hyoid bone of the neck. There are three ossicles in each ear: the malleus, the incus and the stapes (better known as the hammer, anvil and stirrup). They are situated in the middle ear and collectively transmit sound from the ear drum (tympanic membrane) to the fluid-filled inner ear and auditory nerve (see Chapter 12). The final bone of the axial skeleton is the hyoid bone and is the only bone in the body that is not directly attached to another. Instead, it is anchored in place at the base of the tongue by a series of muscles and ligaments. The hyoid bone is U or horseshoe-shaped and is also known as the lingual (tongue) bone since it supports the weight of the tongue and allows us to articulate words during speech. Fractures of the hyoid bone are rare and are usually caused by strangulation or traumatic injury to the neck.

APPENDICULAR SKELETON

The remaining 126 bones of the skeleton belong to the appendicular skeleton and allow movement of the axial skeleton and the manipulation of objects (Figure 4.2). They include the shoulder blades (scapulae), the bones of the upper and lower arm (humerus, radius and ulna), the pelvic girdle (ilium, ischium and pubic bone) and the bones of the upper and lower leg (femur, patella, tibia and fibula). The remaining appendicular bones can be found in the hands, feet, wrists and ankles. The way in which the bones of the hand/wrist and foot are organised is quite similar in many ways. The wrist is made up of eight carpal bones which enable flexible positioning and movement of the hand (Figure 4.5). There are a number of useful mnemonics to help memorise this eccentric group of irregularly shaped,

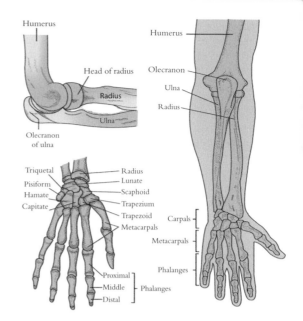

Figure 4.5 Bones of the right forearm and hand.

interconnected bones. I was taught the rather boring: Sally (scaphoid) left (lunate) the (triquetral) party (pisiform) to (trapezium) take (trapezoid) Cathy (capitate) home (hamate). However, I quickly learned (from more disreputable colleagues) the far more memorable: 'Some Lovers Try Positions That They Cannot Handle' and 'Sally Lowers Tim's Pants, Then Things Can Happen'. There are many other mnemonics that are even more explicit but now is not the time or the place (needless to say, Sally has more on her mind than simply showing Cathy home). Anyway . . . the eight carpal bones articulate with the five metacarpal bones of the hand. The bones of the finger and thumb are known as phalanges (phalanx singular) and there are two in the thumb and three in each finger. The fingers and thumb are capable of a wide range of movement including flexion and extension, abduction and adduction (outward and inward movement from a central point) and circumduction (circular movement). Long tendons attach to the phalanges and are pulled – like puppet strings – by the muscles in the palm of the hand and forearm. If you turn your hand palm-upwards and wiggle your fingers, you should be able to see the tendons moving in the wrist as the muscles of the forearm contract and relax. It can be slightly disconcerting to observe how 'machine-like' we are at times.

FOOT BONES

The bones of the proximal (near) foot are known as tarsal bones (Figure 4.6). The largest of these are the talus and the calcaneus (heel bone). Both are connected to the distal (far) end of the tibia and fibula (and to one another) by a series of ligaments. If you are unfortunate enough to twist your ankle, it is usually the talo-fibular and calcaneo-fibular ligaments that are torn or damaged. As a rule of thumb: ligaments attach bones to other bones, and tendons attach bones to muscles allowing movement. For example, the Achilles tendon is attached to the calcaneus (heel bone) at its distal end and two large calf muscles (gastrocnemius and soleus) at its proximal end. Flexing these muscles pulls the Achilles

tendon attached to the heel (plantar flexion) and enables us to stand on our toes, walk, run and jump. The five remaining talus bones (navicular, cuboid and x 3 cuneiform bones) are smaller than the talus and calcaneus and articulate with the five metatarsals. These long bones of the foot are similar to the metatarsals of the hand and are frequently considered newsworthy when a famous footballer breaks one immediately prior to a major tournament. Finally, the bones of the toes are also known as phalanges and, like the hand, there are two in the big toe (also known as the hallux) and three in toes 2–5.

BONE TISSUE

In addition to support, protection and movement, bones also perform a number of other important homeostatic functions. These include buffering the blood against excessive pH changes by absorbing and releasing alkaline salts, blood

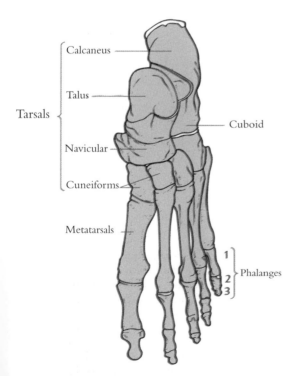
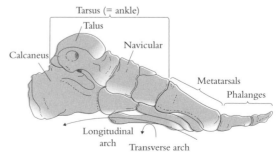

Figure 4.6 Bones of the foot. (a) Superior view. (b) Medial view.

cell formation (haemopoiesis) and fat storage in the bone marrow (see below). Bones also store a number of important minerals including calcium and phosphate. In Chapter 2, we observed how collagen fibres were coated with calcium and phosphate salts to provide bone with solidity and strength. However, this is by no means a static process and bone is constantly being constructed, broken down and reconstructed depending on the metabolic requirements of the body. In Chapter 1, we also saw that plasma calcium was a positively charged ion (cation) and that phosphate was a negatively charged ion (anion). Small amounts of both are necessary to ensure that blood clotting, nerve cells (neurons) and muscles all function normally. It is useful, therefore, to think of bone as a bank where precious minerals can be deposited until circulating levels are depleted and a withdrawal is required. 99% of the body's calcium, and 85% of its phosphate, is stored in the skeleton as crystals of calcium phosphate and it is estimated that 20% of the skeleton is replaced each year by the coordinated activity of three types of cell: osteoblasts, osteocytes and osteoclasts. These cells are constantly at work depositing and withdrawing minerals from our bones in an ongoing process known as bone remodelling. Osteoblasts (the Greek word *blastos* means 'to sprout') are responsible for the formation of new bone and secrete a protein-rich matrix called osteoid. Osteoid is predominantly made from collagen (95%) and provides the scaffolding onto which calcium, phosphate and other minerals crystallise to form a substance known as hydroxylapatite. If osteoid does not mineralise (as the result of vitamin D deficiency for example) it leads to osteomalacia in adults and rickets in children. In both cases, bones become less rigid and skeletal pain, deformity and muscle weakness occur. As osteoblasts form new bone tissue, they often become embedded within the osteoid matrix and are transformed (differentiated) into osteocytes (bone cells).

OSSIFICATION

The process of laying down new bone tissue is known as ossification and takes place in one of two ways: intramembranous ossification and endochondral ossification. Intramembranous ossification refers to ossification in and around a membrane and is responsible for the formation of the flat bones of the skull and mandible (jaw). Endochondral ossification, on the other hand, involves the transformation of cartilage into bone (endochondral = within cartilage) and is responsible for the formation of the long bones of the arm and leg. Both processes are essential for normal bone growth and repair in adults and children. They are also responsible for the ossification and development of the foetal skeleton. For example, by the second month of pregnancy, the embryonic skeleton of the skull and jaw consist of a series of thin membranes (about the thickness of a sheet of tissue paper) consisting largely of collagen and blood vessels. Osteoblasts start to attach themselves to the membrane and begin to secrete osteoid from the centre of the membrane outwards. As observed earlier in the chapter, the edges of the skull bones don't completely ossify until much later to allow for moulding of the head during birth and expansion as the child grows. The embryonic skeleton below the skull is essentially composed of cartilage and during the second and third month of pregnancy it is progressively transformed into bone by endochondral ossification. This commences with the death of cartilage cells (chondrocytes) to provide room for osteoblast activity. However, some bones, such as those of the wrist and ankle, don't ossify until after birth. I remember looking at an X-ray of a baby's ankle and foot for the first time and thinking 'Where are all the bones?'

GROWTH PLATES

Most short bones have a single ossification centre near the middle whilst long bones typically have three (one at the centre and one at each end). Ossification begins in the shaft (diaphysis) of the long bone and progresses towards the two extremities (epiphyses). The physis (or growth plate) is situated between the diaphysis and epiphysis and extends the length of the bone as new chondrocytes (cartilage cells) are produced and are progressively ossified.

At puberty, increased secretion of oestrogen and testosterone leads to gradual 'closure' of these plates and bone growth slows down and eventually stops during the teenage years (see below). Up until this point, the physis is quite clear on X-ray (as a gap) and could be mistaken for a fracture if you were not expecting to see it. The final type of cell involved in the bone remodelling process are osteoclasts (the Greek word *klastos* means 'broken in pieces'). These cells remove bone tissue by breaking down the mineralised matrix (a process known as reabsorption). Osteoclasts anchor themselves to the surface of the bone to create a micro-environment beneath the cell known as the sealing zone. They secrete hydrogen ions (H^+) into the sealing zone to dissolve the mineralised matrix. Once this has been achieved, osteoclasts then release hydrolytic enzymes to remove the collagen and remaining organic material. Osteoclasts play an important role in liberating minerals such as calcium and phosphate for use elsewhere in the body and remodelling bone following traumatic injury (see below).

BONE STRUCTURE

Bones are usually classified by their shape. For example, there are long bones such as the femur and humerus, short bones such as the carpal and tarsal bones, flat bones such as the sternum and ribs, irregular bones such as the vertebrae, mandible (jaw) and sesamoid ('shaped like a sesame seed') bones which develop in tendons. The best example of a sesamoid bone is the kneecap (patella) but other (much smaller) examples can be identified in the wrist (pisiform bone), thumb and elsewhere. An adult long bone consists of a diaphysis or shaft at the centre/mid-section and an epiphysis (thickened head) at either end. In childhood, the epiphysis is separated from the main bone by a layer of cartilage to allow growth. It articulates with other bones (as joints) and is protected by a thin layer of smooth hyaline cartilage (see below). The remainder of the bone is surrounded by a double membrane of connective tissue called periosteum. The outer layer of periosteum is known as the fibrous layer since it contains collagen-secreting cells called fibroblasts. The inner layer is known as the cambium or osteogenic (bone creating) layer since it contains progenitor cells that develop into osteoblasts. The periosteum is richly supplied with blood vessels and provides an attachment for muscles and tendons. It is fixed to the outer surface of the bone by bundles of collagenous fibres called Sharpey's fibres (Figure 4.7).

COMPACT AND SPONGY BONE

Directly below the periosteum is compact or cortical bone which is both strong and smooth in appearance. Compact bone is constructed from densely layered column-like structures known as osteons and accounts for 80% of total bone mass. Each osteon consists of concentric layers (lamellae) of compact bone arranged in a cylinder-like fashion (Figure 4.7). At the centre of each osteon is a small duct (the Haversian canal) which contains nerves and blood vessels which supply nutrients to the bone cells (osteocytes). These canals run parallel to the long axis (shaft) of the bone and are connected to one another by perpendicular ducts known as Volkmann's canals. These ensure that blood is provided throughout the compact bone from the periosteum. The osteocytes themselves are embedded in tiny fluid-filled cavities within the concentric lamellae known as lacunae. Beneath the compact bone is spongy or cancellous bone. This layer is less dense and consists of a complex lattice of small beams or struts called trabeculae. The best way to picture trabeculae (without actually snapping a bone in half) is to visualise the pattern inside sponge or honeycomb (simply bite into a Crunchy bar and marvel at the trabecular structure within). The complex micro-architecture of spongy bone ensures that the skeleton remains sufficiently light for us to run, jump, skip, climb and dance the night away should we desire. Consequently, despite the fact that spongy bone has nearly ten times the surface area of compact bone, it only accounts for 20% of total bone mass. In terms of overall body weight, bone represents a mere 14% of the total.

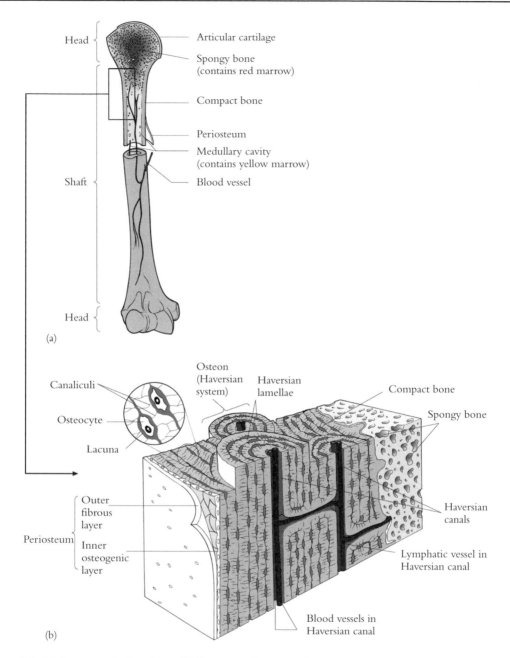

Figure 4.7 (a) Anatomy of a long bone. (b) Structure of compact bone.

BONE MARROW

One of the reasons that long bones are relatively light in comparison to the area they occupy is that the diaphysis is hollow and encloses the medullary or marrow cavity (Figure 4.7). This is lined with a thin vascular membrane known as endosteum and contains yellow bone marrow. In order to prevent bone from becoming unnecessarily thick during growth, osteoclasts reabsorb bone from the endosteal surface as new bone is added to the periosteal side. The epiphyses of long bones also contain a high proportion of spongy bone which provides room for red bone marrow. At birth, all bone marrow is red but as we grow older much of it is transformed into yellow marrow (essentially stored fat). In adults, red marrow is also found in flat bones such as the pelvis (hip bones), sternum (breast bone), scapulae (shoulder blades) and ribs. Red bone marrow produces red blood cells (erythrocytes), platelets (thrombocytes) and white blood cells (leucocytes) and will be discussed in greater detail in Chapter 5. The body can convert yellow marrow back into red marrow to increase blood cell production if necessary. Conversely, those suffering from anorexia or anorexia nervosa may convert red marrow to yellow marrow in order to offset the reduction in body fat elsewhere. However, this is an extreme response to malnutrition and can contribute to calcium and other mineral loss from the spongy bone that results in reduced bone mass (osteoporosis).

BONE DENSITY AND THE ROLE OF HORMONES

Bone growth and remodelling depend on a number of factors including mechanical stress, hormone secretion and adequate dietary intake and absorption of minerals such as calcium and phosphate. Mechanical stress occurs during weight bearing exercise and movement and encourages osteoblast activity and the secretion of osteoid. If you are the parent of a small child/children you have probably wondered why they cannot sit still for more than several seconds at a time and why they feel the need to repeatedly jump on/off the sofa, bed, chair, table, walls, etc. I cannot offer any explanation as to why they leap around with such complete abandon but you can take some comfort from the fact that this activity is both necessary and beneficial for normal bone growth and development (it's still really annoying though). Up until our mid-20s, osteoblasts work hard to build strength into our skeleton. After the age of 30 for women and 45 for men, however, bone density and strength begins to

decline at a fairly steady rate. Since men have a higher peak bone mass than women, the effects take longer to manifest and are typically less severe. Demineralisation primarily occurs in spongy bone and the trabecular matrix becomes increasingly porous – hence the term osteoporosis. Bone mineral density is normally measured using dual energy X-ray absorptiometry (DEXA) or densitometry as it is also known. A calculation called a T-score is produced which compares scanned bone density to that of a young adult (or a Z-score which compares it to an adult of the same age, gender and ethnicity). In essence: the lower the score, the lower bone mineral density and the greater the fragility/risk of fracture. According to World Health Organization guidelines, normal bone density is considered to be within 1 standard deviation (+1 or –1 SD) of the young adult mean. Osteoporosis is diagnosed when the T-score is 2.5 standard deviations (or more) below the mean for the young adult. One of the reasons poor bone mineral density occurs is due to insufficient intake of dietary calcium or the inability to absorb it from the gastrointestinal tract. Absorption of calcium is dependent on the availability of a hormone (chemical messenger) called calcitriol secreted by cells in the kidney (see Chapters 10 and 13). Calcitriol is the active form of vitamin D and is originally derived from calciferol (vitamin D_3) synthesised in the epidermis of the skin following exposure to ultraviolet light. As well as promoting absorption of dietary calcium from the gastrointestinal tract, it also increases the reabsorption of calcium by the kidney (before it is lost in the urine) and stimulates osteoclast activity to mobilise calcium from the bone into the blood plasma.

THYROID AND PARATHYROID HORMONES

The thyroid gland produces the hormones calcitonin, triiodothyronine (T_3) and thyroxine (T_4) which help to increase bone density and promote normal skeletal development. Calcitonin is secreted in response to high levels of plasma calcium and it encourages osteoblasts to deposit calcium in the bone. It also inhibits bone reabsorption by osteoclasts and increases calcium excretion in the urine. T_3 and T_4 are often collectively referred to as 'thyroid hormones' and are essential for normal development of endochondral and intramembranous bone during childhood and the regulation of bone mineral density in adults. Parathyroid hormone, on the other hand, is secreted by the parathyroid glands (situated on the posterior surface of the thyroid gland) in response to low levels of plasma calcium. It stimulates reabsorption of calcium in the kidney and encourages osteoclast activity in the bone leading to demineralisation (in order to make more calcium available to the blood). Parathyroid hormone also converts biologically inert vitamin D_3 into calcitriol in the kidney and is therefore indirectly responsible for absorption of calcium from the gastrointestinal tract. Maintaining constant concentrations of calcium, phosphate and other ions in plasma requires frequent adjustment and regulation. We observed in Chapter 3, that the body is determined to maintain a stable internal environment in spite of constant changes to its metabolic and physiological status (homeostasis). To do this, it frequently utilises two opposing mechanisms. In this case, parathyroid hormone is secreted to increase plasma calcium concentrations when they are too low, and calcitonin is secreted to decrease plasma calcium concentrations when they are too high. This is another example of a negative feedback loop (i.e. the body reverses the direction of change) and we will see many more examples of this phenomenon in both the nervous and endocrine systems.

GROWTH HORMONE, OESTROGEN AND TESTOSTERONE

Another important hormone required for skeletal development and growth is – you won't be surprised to hear – growth hormone (also known as somatotropin). Growth hormone is secreted by the pituitary gland (of the brain) and stimulates cell growth in the cartilage of the epiphyseal plate and elsewhere. The final hormones that play an important role in determining bone density are oestrogen and testosterone. Both help to maintain bone strength by inhibiting osteoclast activity and promoting deposition of bone. Increased secretion of oestrogen, testosterone and growth hormone at puberty combine to rapidly accelerate bone growth (what is known as the pubertal growth spurt). Every time I see my teenage nephews/ niece I embarrass myself (and them) with the words that I dreaded when I was their age: 'haven't you grown'. The look at me in a pitying and slightly disappointed way before finding somebody less old to talk to. It is estimated that enhanced bone growth during the pubertal growth spurt accounts for about 20% of final adult height. However, the rate of bone formation is greater than that of cartilage and eventually the growth plates ossify and close. This occurs more rapidly in response to oestrogen than testosterone which is one of the reasons men are generally taller than women. Following the onset of the menopause, menstruation and ovulation become less frequent and eventually stop as oestrogen production declines. Oestrogen is known to promote osteoclast apoptosis (programmed cell death) and encourage the secretion of osteoid. As levels fall, however, osteoclast activity increases, resulting in progressive demineralisation of spongy bone. This process can be reversed with hormone replacement therapy. However, this is not suitable for all women since it presents a slightly increased risk of developing breast cancer which rises with the duration of the therapy. Consequently, one in three women (compared to one in twelve men) over the age of 50 will develop osteoporosis as a result of hormone deficiency. All of the hormones mentioned above will be discussed in greater detail in Chapters 13 and 14.

CARTILAGE GROWTH

We have seen how important cartilage is in terms of endochondral growth and development but it is also important to recognise and understand the different types of cartilage in terms of functional diversity. Cartilage is composed of a dense network of collagen fibres which provide the tissue with its tensile (capable of being stretched) strength. We observed in Chapter 1, that it also has a very high water content (about 85%) which further contributes to its flexibility and resilience to trauma and compression (living bone, by contrast, contains 10–20% water). Since cartilage contains no nerves or blood vessels it is covered by a fibrous layer of tissue called perichondrium which provides its blood supply and nutrition. In simple terms, cartilage grows in two ways: length-wise (interstitial growth) and width-wise (appositional growth). Interstitial growth involves the rapid division of chondrocytes (cartilage cells) which expand the cartilage from within. Appositional growth, on the other hand, occurs when chondrocytes in the surrounding perichondrium secrete a collagen-based matrix onto the surface of the existing cartilage extending the diameter of the tissue.

CARTILAGE TYPES

There are three different types of cartilage: hyaline, elastic and fibrocartilage. The term hyaline is derived from the Greek for 'glass-like' and describes its translucent blue-white appearance. It is the most abundant cartilage in the body and is found in a wide variety of locations. It protects the epiphyses at moveable joints (articular cartilage), it connects the ribs to the sternum (costal cartilage), it supports the end of the nose (nasal cartilage) and is present in the larynx and trachea (respiratory cartilage). Elastic cartilage is similar to hyaline cartilage but it has a larger number of elastin fibres which provide its yellowish appearance and greater flexibility. Elastic cartilage helps to define and maintain the shape of an area where it is located and provides support for surrounding tissue. For example, it is found in the outer ear (auricle), the auditory (Eustachian) tubes at the back of the nose, and the epiglottis of the voice box (larynx). However, it is possible to transplant cartilage from one area to another and costal cartilage from the ribcage can be used to reconstruct the ear (elastic cartilage).

FIBROCARTILAGE

The final type of cartilage, fibrocartilage, is extremely tough and is found at sites where high pressure is applied such as the meniscus (crescent-shaped pad) of the knee. Its spongy formation makes it an excellent shock absorber and it is also located between the vertebral disks of the spine and the pubic symphysis of the pelvis. The pubic symphysis is also an example of a secondary cartilaginous joint (symphysis) where cartilage connects bone directly to bone. These joints are permanent and allow a small degree of flexible movement. Other examples include the intervertebral joints of the spine and manubrio-sternal joint of the breastbone. Primary cartilaginous joints (synchondrosis), on the other hand, are temporary joints which are only present during bone growth. For example, the epiphyseal plates of long bones form temporary joints until ossification occurs following the pubertal growth spurt. There are two other types of joint present in the human body: fibrous joints and synovial joints. Fibrous joints are typically immovable (or allow only a small degree of movement) and are divided into three categories: sutures, gomphoses and syndesmoses.

SUTURES, GOMPHOSES AND SYNDESMOSES

Sutures are found in the skull and unite the cranial bones with Sharpey's fibres (also used to fix the periosteum to the outer surface of bone). We saw at the beginning of the chapter that the bones of the cranium do not completely fuse together until the child reaches 12–18 months old and that it is still possible to feel the anterior fontanelle during this time. Gomphoses are also known as peg-in-socket joints (*gomphoein* means 'to bolt together' in Greek) and bind teeth to the spongy bone of the mandible (jaw) and maxilla with specialist connective tissue (periodontal ligaments). Gomphoses are the only type of joint, therefore, that do not bind bone to bone. The final type of fibrous joint, syndesmoses, fasten bone together using a band of fibrous tissue or ligament (*desmos* means 'band' in Greek). The amount of movement in this type of joint is variable and depends on the length of the connecting fibres. For example, the ligament connecting the distal ends of the tibia and fibula is short and only permits a small degree of flexibility. The fibrous membrane between the distal radius and ulna, on the other hand, allows a greater range of movement including rotation of the radius around the ulna when you turn the palm of your hand face up or face down.

SYNOVIAL JOINTS

The final type of joint, synovial joints, are the most common in the human body. They are surrounded by a tough but flexible fibrous capsule that facilitates a wide range of movement but prevents dislocation (Figure 4.8). The joint capsule also contains a number of sensory nerve endings (proprioceptors) that provide awareness of movement and position. This is known as proprioception or 'sense of self' and helps us to appreciate the positive of our limbs in relation to other parts of the body. Proprioception also plays an important part in balance. For example, try standing on one foot with your eyes closed. If you quickly put your other foot down to stop yourself falling over it indicates that your sense of proprioception could be improved (practice makes perfect). The inner surface of the joint capsule is lined with the synovial membrane which secretes synovial fluid. Synovial fluid (often compared to egg white) helps to lubricate the joint and acts

as a shock absorber. It also provides nutrition for the joint capsule and contains phagocytes (devouring cells) that help to remove microbes and debris that accumulate as a result of wear and tear. The articular surfaces of the bones (forming the joint) are covered with smooth hyaline cartilage that further reduces friction during movement. Rheumatoid arthritis is an autoimmune disease (i.e. the body attacks itself) that stimulates the synovial cells of the joint to multiply. This causes thickening of the synovial lining and the formation of a sheet of invasive cellular tissue called pannus which progressively erodes the bone and cartilage at the margins of the joint. The joint becomes increasingly swollen, inflamed, unstable and deformed. Rheumatoid arthritis can also result in the formation of subcutaneous (beneath the skin) masses or nodules. The most common site for these rheumatoid nodules is the olecranon bursa located at the elbow. A bursa ('purse' in Latin) is a small sac-like structure filled with synovial fluid that provides a cushion between the skin and the bone at a number of joints (e.g. knee and elbow).

TYPES OF JOINT

Although synovial joints share the same characteristics, there are six different types of joint which are classified by their shape and range of movement. For example, there are ball and socket joints located at the shoulder and hip, hinge joints located at the elbow and knee, pivot joints located at the top of the neck (between the atlas and axis bones), saddle joints located between the base of the thumb and trapezium (carpal) bone of the wrist, gliding joints located between the carpal and tarsal bones and – finally – condyloid bones located between the distal radius and proximal carpal bones. Range of movement is summarised in Table 4.1.

FRACTURES

There are many different bones to break and many different ways to break them. The only bone I have broken (so far) is the rather

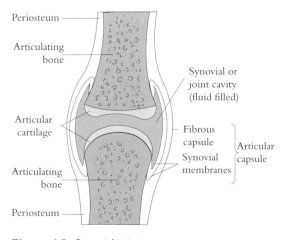

Periosteum

Articulating bone

Synovial or joint cavity (fluid filled)

Articular cartilage

Fibrous capsule

Synovial membranes

Articular capsule

Articulating bone

Periosteum

Figure 4.8 Synovial joint.

TABLE 4.1 Types of synovial joint

Type of synovial joint	Location	Range of movement
Ball and socket	shoulder and hip	flexion, extension, adduction, abduction, internal and external rotation
Condyloid	distal radius and proximal carpal bones	flexion, extension, adduction, abduction and circumduction
Gliding	between the carpal and tarsal bones	gliding movement
Hinge	elbow and knee	flexion and extension
Pivot	between the atlas and axis bones (cervical vertebrae 1 and 2)	rotation
Saddle	between the base of the thumb and trapezium (carpal)	flexion, extension, adduction, abduction and circumduction

unimpressive triquetral bone of the wrist. I jumped over a low wall (in the dark) without realising that the drop on the other side was considerably more than two feet! I distinctly remember thinking at the time 'Where has the ground gone?' before painfully rediscovering it (left hand first). There are many different ways to classify fractures including open and closed (whether the skin is open or closed over/around the broken bone/s), the shape of the fracture (transverse, spiral, wedge, etc.), the mechanism of injury (stress, crush, avulsion, etc.), the position of the fracture (distal, proximal, supracondylar, etc.) or the name of the person who first described it (e.g. a Pott's fracture is named after the 18th-century surgeon Percivall Pott who documented his own painful experience when he broke his ankle). Children's bones are typically much more flexible than adults and they often suffer partial or 'greenstick' fractures. The term greenstick refers to the fact that if you snap a young piece of wood (a green stick) it often snaps on the outer side of the bend but the inner side remains intact. The reason this occurs in children is partly due to the thick fibrous periosteum that surrounds immature bone and partly due to their greater flexibility. Another type of fracture unique to children are those involving the growth plate or physis. There are five common types of growth plate fracture,

first classified by orthopaedic surgeons Robert Salter and Robert Harris in 1963 and known as Salter–Harris fractures. The mnemonic SALTER can be used to remember the presentation of each type:

S   Slipped (type I): fracture of the cartilage of the physis.
A   Above (type II): fractured above the physis or away from the joint.
L   Lower (type III): fracture below the physis in the epiphysis.
TE Through everything (type IV): fracture is through the metaphysis, physis and epiphysis.
R   Ruined or rammed (type V): the physis has been crushed.

It is important that these injuries are correctly diagnosed and treated since they can interfere with normal bone growth and development.

BLEEDING AND HEALING

It is often overlooked that bones are living organs that contain blood vessels, lymphatic vessels and nerves. When a bone is broken we expect to feel pain but often forget that bleeding will also occur. Long-bone fractures that result from high-energy trauma can result in blood loss of 250–3,000mls and an 'open-book' fracture of the pelvis may be higher still. Another possible complication of long-bone or pelvic trauma is the creation of fat emboli (wandering fat fragments). Fat from the bone marrow is able to escape into the bloodstream and eventually becomes lodged in a blood vessel (the Greek word *embolos* means 'plug' or 'wedge'). Fat emboli can also result from severe burns, bone marrow biopsy, liposuction or rib fractures. In order for a fracture to heal with no obvious deformity, the broken ends of the bone must be immobilised and realigned if necessary (a process known as reduction). The first part of the healing process involves the formation of a haematoma as the blood that surrounds the injured bone/s coagulates (clots) and forms a semi-solid mass (see Chapter 5). New blood vessels begin to develop and transport phagocytes (devouring cells) to the area in order to remove debris, tissue fragments and other unnecessary material. Fibroblasts (connective tissue cells) also migrate to the area and secrete collagen which forms a callus around the displaced bones securing them in place. Osteoblasts from the endosteum and periosteum are then able to secrete osteoid into the collagen matrix and bone remodelling begins. The soft callus is gradually transformed into hard callus (similar to spongy bone) and over a period of months the original architecture of the bone is restored. In normal circumstances, the healing bone is usually sufficiently mineralised to remove the immobilising cast within about six weeks of the original injury. Children's bones often heal more quickly than adults because of the high rate of osteoblast activity that occurs during normal growth and the type of fractures they experience.

CHAPTER 4: TEST YOURSELF

Q. What are the three types of muscle?
A. Smooth (involuntary) muscle, skeletal (voluntary) muscle, and cardiac muscle (myocardium).

Q. Explain the difference between axial and appendicular muscles?
A. Axial muscles are responsible for supporting and moving the head/face, spine, rib cage and pelvis (of the axial skeleton). They also protect the organs. Appendicular muscles, support and move the arms and legs (of the appendicular skeleton).

Q. Explain the difference between flexor, extensor, abductor and adductor muscles?
A. Flexor muscles reduce the angle of two bones connected by a joint whilst extensor muscles increase the angle. Abductor muscles allow the skeleton to move away from the midline of the body whilst adductor muscles allow it to move towards the midline.

Q. What is the largest bone of the body?
A. The femur (thigh bone).

Q. Name the four principle bones that make up the cranium?
A. Frontal bone, parietal bone, occipital bone and temporal bone.

Q. What is a sinus and what does it do?
A. A sinus is an air-filled cavity that reduces weight at the front of the skull, buffers against facial trauma and increases the resonance of the voice.

Q. The spine contains cervical (neck), thoracic, lumbar, sacral and coccygeal vertebrae. How many of each are there?
A. Seven cervical vertebrae, 12 thoracic vertebrae, 5 lumbar vertebrae, 5 sacral vertebrae and 4 coccygeal bones (33 in total).

Q. What is the name of the cartilage that connects the ribs to the sternum?
A. Costal cartilage.

Q. Name the eight carpal bones of the wrist (remember the mnemonic: Sally left the party to take Cathy home).
A. Scaphoid, lunate, triquetral, pisiform, trapezium, trapezoid, capitate and hamate.

Q. What is the name for the bones of the finger/thumb?
A. Phalanges (phalanx singular)

Q. Name the bones of the arm and leg (most superior to most inferior).
A. Humerus, radius, ulna, femur, tibia and fibula.

Q. Explain the difference between a tendon and a ligament?
A. Tendons attach bones to muscles to allow movement whilst ligaments attach bones to bones to ensure stability (e.g. of a joint).

Q. What is the principle function of red bone marrow?
A. Blood cell production (haemopoiesis).

Q. In addition to support, protection and movement, what other functions do bones perform?
A. Bones store calcium, phosphate and fat (as yellow bone marrow). They also buffer the blood against excessive pH changes by absorbing and releasing alkaline salts.

Q. What is the difference between compact and cancellous bone?
A. Compact (or cortical) bone forms the outer shell of most bones. It is constructed from column-like structures known as osteons and accounts for 80% of total bone mass. Cancellous (or spongy) bone is less dense and consists of a lattice of small beams called trabeculae. Consequently, although it only accounts for 20% of total bone mass, it has nearly ten times the surface area of compact bone.

Q. What is the difference between osteoblasts, osteocytes and osteoclasts?
A. Osteoblasts are responsible for the formation of new bone and secrete a substance called osteoid (scaffolding onto which minerals can crystallise). During this process, osteoblasts often become embedded within the osteoid matrix and are transformed into osteocytes (bone cells). Osteoclasts remove bone tissue by breaking down the mineralised matrix. They liberate minerals such as calcium for use elsewhere in the body and remodel bone following traumatic injury.

Q. What is meant by the term epiphysis?
A. In childhood, the epiphysis is situated at either end of a long bone. It is separated from the bone by a layer of cartilage to allow growth.

Q. How do the hormones calcitonin and parathyroid hormone influence bone growth and development?
A. Calcitonin is secreted in response to high levels of plasma calcium and encourages osteoblasts to deposit calcium in the bone. Parathyroid hormone is secreted in response to low levels of plasma calcium. It stimulates reabsorption of calcium in the kidney and encourages osteoclast activity leading to demineralisation of bone.

Contents

CHAPTER 5

BLOOD

PLASMA

We already know quite a lot about blood from Chapters 1 and 2. For example, we know that blood is a specialised form of connective tissue since it acts as a vehicle of transport for a variety of substances including oxygen, carbon dioxide, nutrients (such as glucose), waste products, ions and hormones. We also know that blood consists of a cellular component (red blood cells, white blood cells and clotting cells) and a non-cellular matrix or plasma. This can be demonstrated by spinning a sample of blood in a centrifuge. The red blood cells settle at the bottom of the test tube since they are the heaviest. A small band of white blood cells can be identified above the red blood cells and the straw-coloured plasma remains on top since it is lightest. The formed elements of blood (the cells) are also referred to as haematocrit or packed cell volume; 99.9% of haematocrit is composed of red blood cells or erythrocytes as they are also known (the Greek word *eruthros* means 'red'). Haematocrit contributes to the viscosity of blood which, as the proverb says, is thicker than water (about five times). The liquid component of blood (plasma) is about 95% water. The remaining 5% consists of dissolved substances in suspension including ions (e.g. Na^+), nutrients, waste products and plasma proteins. It is estimated that each litre of plasma contains about 75 g of protein. This is almost five time higher than the concentration found in interstitial fluid (between the cells) since the relatively large size of plasma

proteins prevent them from leaving the blood stream (see below).

PLASMA PROTEINS

There are three distinct types of plasma protein: albumin, globulin and fibrinogen. Albumin is made in the liver and accounts for about 60% of the total plasma protein. It is essential for maintaining the osmotic pressure of plasma and if levels fall it can significantly alter the distribution of fluids between different body compartments. For example, one of the side effects of severe liver failure is an accumulation of fluid in the abdominal cavity (ascites – see Chapter 11). There are several reasons why this occurs but one of them is decreased osmotic pressure in the plasma as a result of low albumin levels. This limits the reabsorption of fluid from the abdominal cavity into the circulatory system via the capillaries. In Chapter 1, we defined osmosis as the movement of water from a high concentration (of water) to a low concentration (of water) across a semi-permeable membrane. In this case: the less albumin there is in the plasma, the higher the relative concentration of water, the less oncotic 'pull' the plasma will exert. Albumins also act as transport proteins for fatty acids, fat-soluble hormones (steroids), bilirubin (see below), calcium and many drugs. Globulin has a higher molecular weight than albumin and accounts for about 35% of the total plasma protein. Globulin is subdivided into three types: alpha, beta and gamma globulins. Like albumin, alpha and beta globulins are produced in the liver and act as transport proteins for various substances including fatty acids, hormones and ions. Gamma globulins, on the other hand, are highly specialised proteins also known as immunoglobulins (Igs) or antibodies. They are produced by a type of white blood cell called B cells (see below) in response to foreign proteins and disease-causing organisms (pathogens). The final type of plasma protein is fibrinogen which accounts for about 4% of the total. It is produced by the liver and is important for blood clotting (discussed below).

BLOOD CELL DIFFERENTIATION

All blood cells are produced in the red bone marrow by a process known as haemopoiesis (from the Greek words for 'blood' and 'to make'). The bone marrow contains pluripotent (or multi-potential) stem cells. This sounds very complex but simply refers to the fact that these cells have the ability to produce a variety of different blood cells following a series of cell divisions. For example, a haemocytoblast (haemo + cyto + blast = blood + cell + sprout) produces two types of stem cells called myeloid stem cells and lymphoid stem cells (Figure 5.1). These cells are self-renewing and are capable of undergoing further differentiation to produce mature blood cells. For example, myeloid stem cells differentiate into non-self-renewing precursor cells that eventually produce erythrocytes (red blood cells), thrombocytes (clotting cells or platelets) and a number of leukocytes (white blood cells) that have granules in their cytoplasm (granulocytes). There are three types of granulocyte: neutrophils, basophils and eosinophils (see below). Lymphoid stem cells, on the other hand, produce non-self-renewing

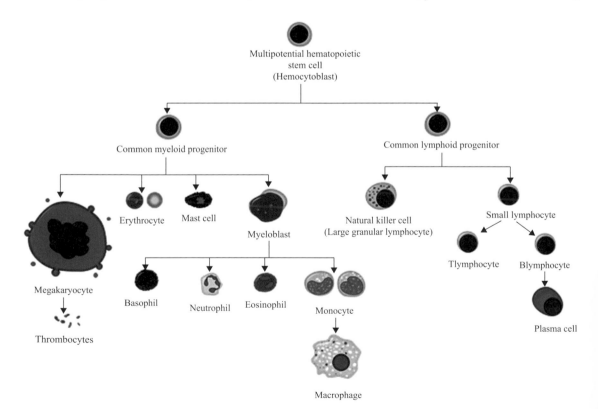

Figure 5.1   Haemopoiesis.

lymphoblasts that differentiate into agranulocytes (lymphocytes without granules in the cytoplasm) such as B cells and T cells, and granulocytes such as natural killer (NK) cells. Some lymphocytes mature in the bone marrow (B cells) whilst others migrate into the circulatory system and make their way to the spleen and thymus gland (T cells). Figure 5.1 provides a simplified diagram of the different pathways or stages of differentiation and the range of mature blood cells produced during haemopoiesis. The number of cells produced at any one time depends on a variety of factors and will be explained below. However, we already know that the most abundant type of blood cell are erythrocytes (red blood cells) which account for 99.9% of packed cell volume. Healthy human blood contains between 4.8 and 5.2 million erythrocytes per microlitre (1 millionth of a litre) compared to 4,000–10,000 white blood cells per microlitre. Erythrocytes are released into the circulatory system from the bone marrow in an immature form called reticulocytes. These quickly mature into erythrocytes (1–2 days) but rarely survive longer than about 120 days. This is because by the time reticulocytes are released from the bone marrow they have lost most of their organelles including their nuclei and ribosomes. As a result, they cannot repair themselves following damage or undergo cell division. The reason for this lack of intracellular content is to increase the area available for haemoglobin (Hb).

HAEMOGLOBIN

Haemoglobin is a complex structure that contains four globular protein chains with a single molecule of the (non-protein) pigment heme attached to each. Heme contains iron (Fe) which forms a weak and reversible bond with oxygen and enables the transport of oxygen (and carbon dioxide) to and from the lungs and cells. Human blood is red in colour due to the iron in haemoglobin. The blood of the horseshoe crab, on the other hand, is blue because it uses copper-based haemocyanin to transport oxygen around its body. In humans, approximately 98.5% of oxygen is bound to haemoglobin as

oxyhaemoglobin (HbO_2) – the remainder is dissolved in the plasma (see Chapter 9).

$$Hb + O_2 \leftrightharpoons HbO_2$$

deoxyhaemoglobin + oxygen $\leftrightharpoons$ oxyhaemoglobin

It is useful at this stage to think of haemoglobin as a taxicab for oxygen and carbon dioxide transport. Four oxygen molecules get into the cab at the lungs and are transported to their destination at a cell (where they are required to make energy). Once oxygen has exited the cab, carbon dioxide molecules jump in for the return fair and are dropped back at the lungs (where they leave the body and begin a new life in the atmosphere). However, this simple analogy doesn't take into account the quantity of 'traffic' required to meet the metabolic demands of the body. For example, each haemoglobin molecule contains four heme units and each erythrocyte contains about 280 million haemoglobin molecules! A quick bit of multiplication (4 × 280,000,000) reveals that each erythrocyte can carry over a billion molecules of oxygen at any one time (1, 120,000,000). That is a lot of gaseous exchange and explains why it is important that erythrocyte numbers remain at a fairly constant level.

CARBON MONOXIDE

It is interesting to note that whilst carbon dioxide binds reversibly with haemoglobin as carbaminohaemoglobin ($HbCO_2$), carbon monoxide (found in car exhaust fumes and cigarette smoke) is much more difficult to shift once attached as carboxyhaemoglobin (HbCO). Carbon monoxide poisoning not only reduces the amount of oxygen available for cellular respiration (since oxygen cannot attach to heme in the normal way), it can also makes the small blood vessels (capillaries) more 'leaky' which may result in cerebral oedema (swelling in the brain). To return to the taxicab analogy, carbon monoxide molecules might be compared to the drunk passengers who refuse/are unable to get out of the cab and let anybody else in. Coincidently, the symptoms experienced by those suffering from carbon monoxide poisoning are quite similar to being drunk/hung-over and include headache, dizziness, vertigo, weakness, nausea and vomiting. Exposure to high levels can result in loss of consciousness, arrhythmias, seizures and/or death.

ERYTHROCYTES

Erythrocytes have a characteristic biconcave appearance often compared to a ring-donut but without a hole (Figure 5.2). This provides a large surface area-to-volume ratio which is beneficial for gaseous exchange. It also provides greater flexibility and enables the cells to squeeze through narrow blood vessels such as capillaries (see Chapter 7). One of the ways they do this is by stacking themselves like dinner plates as they pass through the lumen of the vessel. This avoids damage caused by collision and prevents them from getting stuck which could result in ischaemia (insufficient blood supply to an organ or other part of the body). However, this is precisely what happens when those who suffer from sickle cell disease experience what is known as a 'crisis'. Sickle cell disease is a genetic disorder in which erythrocytes do not develop in the normal way and resemble, as the name suggests, a sickle or crescent (Figure 5.2). This means they have reduced surface area for the transport of oxygen and are more likely get stuck and block small vessels. This causes episodes of severe pain which can last for between five and seven days. Sickle cells also have a shorter lifespan than normal erythrocytes (about 30–40 days) and are not replaced as quickly. This is why the condition is also known as sickle cell anaemia (i.e. the number of cells is deficient). Interestingly, sickle cells offer some protection from the disease malaria (caused by the parasite *plasmodium*) and the gene that causes the disease is thought to have mutated for precisely this reason. We noted earlier in the chapter that, even under normal circumstances, erythrocytes only live for about 120 days before they are engulfed by macrophages (macro + phage = big + eater) in the liver or spleen and recycled. Macrophages 'monitor' the condition of erythrocytes to ensure they are removed from the circulation

before their plasma membrane ruptures and the cell splits open (haemolyses). The heme component of blood is stripped of its iron which is transported to the liver (by the protein transferrin) for the production of new erythrocytes and storage. The remaining heme is broken down (catabolised) and converted into insoluble bilirubin which is transported to the liver (bound to albumin) and excreted as part of the bile (see Chapter 11). The protein component of erythrocytes is disassembled into amino acids which can also be used to produce new erythrocytes in the bone marrow or by other cells elsewhere. It is estimated that about 1% of erythrocytes are removed and replaced each day.

ERYTHROPOIESIS

The process by which new erythrocytes (red blood cells) are produced is called erythropoiesis and is controlled by the hormone erythropoietin (EPO). Erythropoietin is secreted by cells in the kidney (and to a lesser degree the liver) in response to falling or low levels of oxygen in the blood (hypoxaemia). It stimulates the bone marrow to increase the rate of stem cell differentiation and haemoglobin synthesis. This results in the production of greater number of erythrocytes which increase the quantity of oxygen in the blood and slows the secretion of erythropoietin by the kidney. This negative feedback loop ensures that erythrocyte numbers remain relatively constant and that the oxygen-carrying capacity of blood is always sufficient to meet the metabolic requirements of the body. In addition to erythropoietin, folic acid and vitamin B_{12}

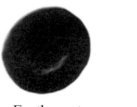

Erythrocyte   Sickle cell

Figure 5.2 Erythrocyte and sickle cell.

are also essential for normal erythrocyte production. If you are a fan of athletics or professional cycling you may know that erythropoietin (EPO) injections have been used by some competitors to increase the oxygen carrying potential of their red blood cells. This is particularly beneficial when competing at high altitude, such as the mountain stages of the Tour de France, since oxygen is less abundant here than at sea level (see Chapter 9). Despite the fact that the use of erythropoietin was banned in 1984, so-called blood doping remains a stubborn problem in professional sport and some athletes have admitted (or been caught) transfusing one or more units of blood immediately prior to an event to increase packed cell volume.

ABO BLOOD TYPES AND TRANSFUSION

A blood transfusion is normally provided to replace intravascular volume following a bleed (e.g. during/after surgery or trauma) or to correct a blood cell or haemoglobin deficit (e.g. anaemia or bone marrow failure).

In these circumstances, the recipient will almost certainly receive blood donated from somebody else. However, not all blood types are compatible and it is essential that transfused blood is appropriately matched to the recipient's blood type or group. There are four blood types (A, B, AB and O) and they are named according to the presence or absence of antigens on the surface of the erythrocyte membrane (Figure 5.3). An antigen is a substance that is recognised as a threat by the immune system and triggers the formation of an antibody or immunoglobulin (Ig) to destroy it. Luckily for us, our immune system ignores the surface antigens on our own erythrocytes (and other cells) and antigens can be considered in much the same way as a badge or security pass. In the case of blood transfusion, if erythrocytes have the correct security pass/antigen, the immune system will ignore them (since they are 'self') and allow access to the circulatory system. If they have the wrong security pass/antigen, the immune system will destroy them in a fairly unpleasant way. However, there is always an exception to the rule and blood type O is able to access the circulatory system without detection since it displays no antigens (very James Bond).

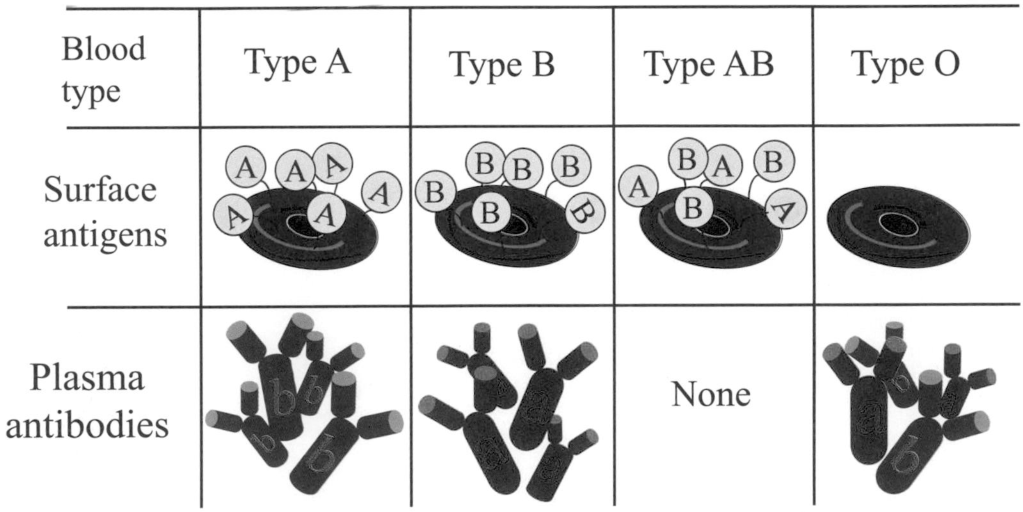

Blood type	Type A	Type B	Type AB	Type O
Surface antigens				
Plasma antibodies			None	

Figure 5.3 ABO blood groups/antigens.

DETECTION AND DESTRUCTION

I have type B blood which means that my erythrocytes have B antigens on the surface of their plasma membranes (Figure 5.3). My immune system, therefore, recognises B antigens as 'self' and does not attack them. This means that I can safely receive transfused blood from another person with type B blood (providing their Rhesus status is compatible with mine as we will see below). In addition to type B blood, it is also safe for me to be transfused with type O blood because, uniquely, it has neither A nor B antigens (badges) on its cell membrane. This allows it to sneak under the immune system radar so to speak (unrecognised) and type O blood is known as the universal donor since it can be safely provided to those with types O, A, B or AB. If, on the other hand, I received transfused blood from a person with type A blood, my immune system would quickly recognise that the new erythrocytes have A antigens on their surface and produce an antibody (anti-A) to destroy these foreign cells. The same is true if I received blood from a person with type AB blood. Although my immune system recognises the B antigens on the erythrocytes surface as 'self' (and wishes them nothing but love and respect) the same cannot be said for the A antigens (which it views with suspicion and dread). The A antigens are considered foreign in exactly the same way as those on type A blood and my immune system will produce anti-A to destroy the cells.

UNIVERSAL DONOR AND UNIVERSAL RECIPIENT

This all seems rather hostile and aggressive but it is important to remember that our body is constantly threatened by pathogenic organisms and material. In order to maintain health and homeostasis, therefore, it is necessary to operate a zero-tolerance policy regarding anything that offers actual or potential threat.

The immune system of a person with type A blood will react equally aggressively to the presence of type B antigens on either type B or type AB erythrocytes. Similarly, type O blood may be the universal donor (since it possesses neither A or B antigens) but this also means it can only accept type O blood itself. Type O recognises both A or B antigens as foreign and produces anti-A, anti-B, or both if transfused with type AB. I like to think that this hostile behaviour is the result of antigen envy and the fact that it is constantly ignored when transfused into those with other blood types. In contrast to type O, type AB blood has both A and B antigens (badges) on the surface of its cell membranes and is known as the universal recipient since people with this type of blood can receive blood from all other types. The immune system of somebody with type AB blood is extremely relaxed regarding blood transfusion and operates something of an open access policy. That is to say, since it identifies A and B antigens as 'self', it is possible to transfuse both type A and type B blood into somebody of this blood group. Type AB can also receive O of course since it is the universal donor (no antigens) and is ignored by all. Table 5.1 (and Figure 5.3) summarise the different surface antigens and plasma antibodies present for all four blood types whilst Figure 5.4

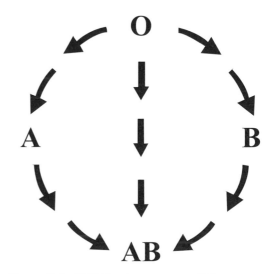

Figure 5.4 ABO blood group compatibility.

TABLE 5.1 Blood groups (antigens and antibodies)

Blood group	Erythrocyte cell membrane antigen	Plasma antibodies
A	A	Anti-B
B	B	Anti-A
AB	A and B	No antibodies
O	None	Anti-A and Anti-B

provides a visual guide to transfusion compatibility (excluding Rhesus status).

ANTIGEN PREVALENCE

Surface antigens are genetically determined and most people in the UK have either type O blood (44%) or type A blood (42%). About 10% of the population have type B and only 4% type AB. However, different populations, in different parts of the world, exhibit different percentage matches for these blood types. For example, the US (taken as a whole) is quite similar to the UK: O: 46%, A: 40%, B: 10%, AB: 4%. In Japan, on the other hand, blood type is distributed roughly as follows: O: 40%, A: 30%, B: 20%, AB: 10%. Japan is particularly interesting since it is widely accepted that blood type has a direct influence on a person's character and behaviour. For example, type A people are thought to be sensible, responsible but a little over-anxious. Type O people are confident and optimistic but stubborn workaholics. AB people are sociable and adaptable but also indecisive and unpredictable. Finally, type B people, such as myself, are apparently creative, pragmatic, selfish, irresponsible and don't always consider other people's feelings or customs (I can picture my wife nodding her head in agreement). In 2011, the Japanese Minister for Reconstruction resigned after being criticised for making insensitive remarks – he blamed it on the fact he has blood type B. This, I feel, will be my excuse for everything from now on.

RHESUS STATUS

In addition to A and B antigens, erythrocytes have at least 50 different other types of surface antigen including (for most people) the Rhesus (Rh) or D antigen (first discovered on the red blood cells of rhesus monkeys). About 85% of the UK population are said to be Rhesus positive since their erythrocytes exhibit the Rhesus antigen. Those who lack the Rhesus antigen and are said to be Rhesus negative (about 15%). The same principles that apply to antigens A and B, also applies to the Rhesus antigen. Those who are Rh negative can donate blood to those who are Rh positive since the immune system of the recipient will not recognise it as a threat (i.e. there is no antigen or 'badge' to detect so it passes under the radar). Conversely, if a person who is Rh negative receives blood from someone who is Rh positive they will produce an antibody (anti-D) to destroy the foreign cells. Consequently, when we describe our blood type, we say that we are either negative or positive. For example, my blood type is B+ which means that that my erythrocytes exhibit both B and Rhesus (or D) antigens on their cell membranes. As a result, I can safely receive blood from the following types: B+, B-, O+ and O-. In the previous section, we talked about type O blood being the universal donor but, strictly speaking, it is O- that is genuinely universal since it can be confidently transfused into any individual without the need to cross match for type. Ideally, it is better to receive type-specific blood but, in an emergency, when time is of the essence, O- is very useful to say the least.

This is why, if you have type O⁻ blood, you will be very popular with your local blood donation service (no pressure).

AGGLUTINATION

So what actually happens if you provide the wrong type of blood to someone? We know that their immune system will produce antibodies but why is this dangerous? In short, it leads to a transfusion reaction that can be mild, severe or potentially life-threatening. When antibodies (immunoglobulins) come into contact with erythrocytes that present opposing antigens (also known as an agglutinins) there is an agglutination reaction (the Latin word *agglutinare* means 'to glue or stick together'). That is to say, the antibodies bind the erythrocytes together into clumps or islands in the plasma. This is followed by the splitting open of the cells (haemolysis) by circulating phagocytes (devouring cells) and the release of their contents into the surrounding plasma. Both agglutination and haemolysis are hazardous events since fragments of the lysed cells can block small vessels in the kidneys (and elsewhere). Leading to possible cell death and tissue damage. The spilled contents of the erythrocytes (including haemoglobin) can also cause pyrexia (increased temperature), chills (for the reasons mentioned in Chapter 3), low blood pressure, raised pulse, nausea and vomiting. During blood transfusion the patient should be closely observed/monitored every 15 minutes for any of these tell-tale signs and symptoms. If transfusion reaction is suspected, the transfusion should be stopped immediately in order to avoid further exposure to the donated blood. It is also worth noting that even if a transfusion reaction does not occur (e.g. type O⁻ blood is transfused into a person with type B⁺ blood) antibodies present in the donor's blood (anti-A and anti-B) may react with the blood of the recipient (B⁺). However, these are so diluted in the recipient's circulation that it does not usually present as a serious problem (naturally this does not occur with type-specific).

RHESUS STATUS AND PREGNANCY

Rhesus status is also very important during pregnancy. As we know, most people (about 85%) are Rhesus positive (i.e. they have the Rhesus antigen on their erythrocyte membrane). If both mother and baby are Rhesus positive or Rhesus negative there is no chance that an agglutination reaction will take place. If the mother is Rhesus positive and the baby is Rhesus negative there is also little risk of harm. Rhesus incompatibility only occurs when the mother's blood type is Rhesus negative and the baby's blood type is Rhesus positive. That is to say, if the mother's immune system recognises the Rhesus antigen on the erythrocyte membrane of the baby's blood it could produce the corresponding antibody (Figure 5.5). This could result in agglutination and haemolysis of the baby's erythrocytes which (depending on the severity of the reaction) may lead to anaemia, hypoxia and brain damage. However, the baby is usually safe since foetal and maternal blood do not mix until delivery (when bleeding occurs at the placenta and uterus). Approximately 20% of Rhesus negative mothers who carry a Rhesus positive child produce anti-Rhesus antibodies within six months of delivery. This is not a problem for the child since it has been safely delivered. However, the antibodies remain in the mother's circulation and pose a potential risk to the NEXT child to be conceived/carried since, unlike erythrocytes, they are small enough to cross into the foetal circulation. Fortunately, haemolytic disease of the foetus and neonate (new-born) is almost entirely preventable. Women who are Rhesus negative are given an intramuscular injection of a substance called anti-D between weeks 28 and 30 of pregnancy (and in some cases also after delivery). Anti-D destroys any Rhesus positive cells that may have entered the mother's bloodstream and prevents her immune system from becoming sensitised to Rhesus antigens. The Rhesus negative mother will require this treatment after each pregnancy including termination and miscarriage.

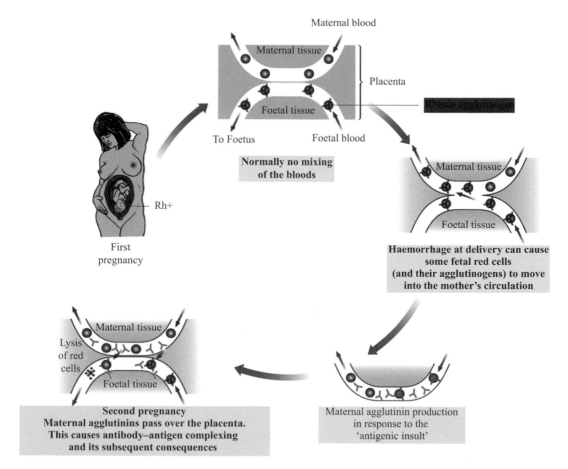

Figure 5.5 Pregnancy and rhesus incompatibility.

THROMBOCYTES AND THE CLOTTING CASCADE

Thrombocytes (clot + cell), or platelets as they are also known, are not actually cells in the strictest sense. They are small membrane-bound fragments of much larger cells called megakaryocytes (mega + karyo + cyte = large + nucleus + cell). Megakaryocytes are derived from myeloid stem cells and undergo a process of extension and rupture which releases cell fragments into the circulation (Figure 5.1). A plasma membrane quickly forms around the cytoplasm of each fragment to produce the irregularly shaped thrombocyte. Thrombocytes are essential to the clotting

process that occurs when blood vessels are either ruptured or their lining (tunica intima) is damaged in some way (see Chapter 7). This process is known as haemostasis (from the Greek words for 'blood' and 'stand still') and also involves a number of chemicals and clotting factors. During haemostasis, three stages occur in rapid succession: vascular constriction, thrombocyte 'plug' formation and coagulation. Immediately following vascular injury, the blood vessel constricts (vasoconstriction) in response to the release of chemicals from the damaged endothelial cells that line the vessel. At the same time, the endothelial cell membranes become 'sticky' which facilitates the attachment of thrombocytes in order to minimise initial blood loss. The thrombocytes begin to collect or aggregate (clump) at the site of the injury and quickly form a plug. They stick to one another and to collagen fibres that have been exposed following damage to the lining of the vessel. This process is assisted by a large plasma protein called von Willebrand factor which stabilises the bond between thrombocytes and collagen. Thrombocytes also release (degranulate) chemical messengers that further stimulate and promote vascular spasm, thrombocyte aggregation (clumping) and cellular repair.

COAGULATION

The final stage of haemostasis is the formation of a stable blood clot or coagulation (i.e. the transformation of blood from a liquid to a solid substance). This involves a complex series of events that results in the transformation of soluble fibrinogen (a plasma protein) into an insoluble mesh of fibrin threads that trap blood cells and plasma. This process is known as the common clotting cascade since each stage facilitates the next and is initiated by two different but interconnected pathways (Figure 5.6). The first pathway is called the intrinsic pathway and is activated when plasma comes into contact with the

damaged vessel wall. The second, or extrinsic pathway, is activated when a substance called tissue factor (factor III)[1] is released by damaged endothelial cells. This may occur at the same time as the intrinsic pathway or independently. Either way, both result in the conversion of clotting factor X (also known as thrombokinase or Stuart-Prower factor) into clotting factor Xa or activated factor X (activated thrombokinase). This converts the plasma protein prothrombin (factor II) into the enzyme thrombin which, in turn, transforms soluble fibrinogen (factor I) into insoluble fibrin. Thrombin also activates a plasma protein called fibrin stabilising factor (factor XIII) which binds the fibrin strands together into a net-like structure which traps blood cells as they try to pass through it. Blood clotting is a good example of a positive feedback loop whereby the body initiates a response which continues in the same direction until balance is restored (Chapter 3). For example, as more thrombocytes aggregate in response to vascular damage, the more chemical messengers they release, the more aggregation that occurs, etc. It is important to note, however, that the body actively prevents the formation of clots in non-damaged blood vessels by releasing anticoagulant (anti-clotting) substances such as heparin, prostacyclin and thrombomodulin. It also dissolves blood clots

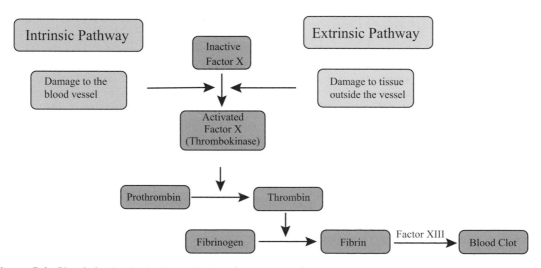

Figure 5.6 Blood clotting: intrinsic, extrinsic and common pathways.

once the vessel has healed itself using a fibrin digesting enzyme called plasmin. This process is known as fibrinolysis (fibrin + splitting) and commences following the secretion of a substances called tissue plasminogen activator (tPA) by the vascular endothelial cells (usually within about two days of the initial injury).

CLOTTING FACTOR DEFICIENCIES

Almost all stages of the coagulation process require the presence of calcium ions (Ca^{++}) and adequate levels of plasma calcium are essential for normal clotting to occur. Clotting factor deficiencies and low levels of other substances, such as vitamin K, can also increase the time it takes for blood to coagulate. For example, most cases (about 80%) of the genetic bleeding disorder haemophilia result because the liver is not able von to produce enough clotting factor VIII (anti-haemophilic factor). Similarly, the most common hereditary clotting disorder, Von Willebrand's disease, is the result of a deficiency of the plasma protein von Willebrand factor which helps to stabilise the bond between thrombocytes and collagen (see above). Finally, vitamin K is essential for the formation of a number of clotting factors including factor II (prothrombin) and factor X. The anticoagulant drug warfarin inhibits the amount of vitamin K available to the liver and prevents the production of these and other factors. This lengthens clotting time and is useful for the management of those likely to develop blood clots (see Chapter 7). One of the great misconceptions about warfarin is that it somehow 'thins' the blood when it actually interferes with the production of clotting factors (e.g. prothrombin). Dietary deficiency of vitamin K can also lead to lengthening of clotting time which is why it is very important to eat delicious green vegetables such as broccoli and spinach.

CHAPTER 5: TEST YOURSELF

Q. What type of tissue is blood?
A. Connective tissue.

Q. List at least four substances transported by the blood?
A. Oxygen, carbon dioxide, nutrients (e.g. glucose), waste products, ions (e.g. Na+) and hormones.

Q. How many litres of blood does an average adult possess?
A. Five litres.

Q. List the cellular components of blood?
A. Erythrocytes (red blood cells), leukocytes (white blood cells) and thrombocytes (platelets).

Q. The non-cellular matrix of blood consists of plasma (about 3 litres) and plasma proteins. List the three principle plasma proteins and briefly explain what they do?
A. Albumin is essential for maintaining the osmotic pressure of plasma and for the transport of fatty acids, hormones, bilirubin, calcium and many drugs. Globulins also act as transport proteins for a variety of substances including fatty acids, hormones and electrolytes. Fibrinogen is a clotting factor that can be transformed into fibrin threads that trap blood cells and plasma.

(Continued)

Contents

TYPES OF IMMUNITY

The human body is constantly exposed to a wide variety of pathogenic and non-pathogenic microorganisms and material. These include bacteria, viruses, fungi, parasites and non-living substances such as toxins, chemicals and drugs. Fortunately for us, our body has a number of external and internal safeguards that prevent most invaders from entering the body or causing lasting harm. They can be conveniently divided into two complementary systems: non-specific immunity and specific immunity. Non-specific immunity is also known as congenital (present from birth) or naturally occurring immunity and is not dependent on previous exposure to harmful substances or microorganisms. That is to say, it does not differentiate between one type of threat and another and all potentially harmful agents are dealt with in the same way. The most obvious type of non-specific immunity is made up of the physical and chemical barriers of our integumentary system. We have already discussed some of the functions that these structures undertake in Chapter 3 but it is worth quickly outlining the very important contribution they make to non-specific immunity.

SKIN AND SECRETIONS

The body's first line of defence is provided by the skin and the mucous membranes that line the digestive, reproductive, respiratory and urinary tracts. The skin is the largest organ of the body and provides both a physical and chemical barrier. The epithelial cells that cover the skin's surface are coated in a tough, protein-based substance called keratin that provides a water-resistant barrier known as the stratum corneum. These cells are constantly shed (desquamated) and replaced by new cells, which helps to prevent bacterial colonisation of the skin. Sebum, secreted onto hair follicles and the surface of the skin, also helps to inhibit fungal and bacterial growth and, when mixed with eccrine sweat, forms a fine acidic film called the acid mantle. It is a common misconception that the pH of the skin is neutral (pH 7) when it is actually quite variable and can range from between pH 4.5 and 6. This is one of the reasons why excessive washing with detergents can encourage opportunistic bacterial and yeast colonisation rather than inhibit it (particularly in sensitive areas). Eccrine sweat also contains an enzyme called lysozyme (splitting + enzyme) that helps to destroy the cell walls of some bacteria. Other secretions, such as tears, saliva and mucus, also contain this bactericidal enzyme. The next time you see a child (possibly your own) crying, with saliva dribbling from their open mouth and a great big snot bubble inflated from one nostril, marvel at the 'sophistication' of natural immunity as you wipe the anti-bacterial 'paste' from their angelic little face.

COMMENSALS

Another important component of our non-specific immune system that you may be wiping away are the 'friendly' microbes (mostly bacteria) which live on the surface of our skin (and elsewhere). These commensal organisms compete with opportunistic and potentially pathogenic bacteria for essential nutrients and also secrete inhibitory chemicals to eliminate them. This relationship is said to be 'symbiotic' since both organisms (us and the bacteria) derive mutual benefit and pose little harm to one another. However, if commensal bacteria migrate to an area they normally do not inhabit (e.g. following a penetrating injury to the skin) it can cause infection. For example, *Staphylococcus epidermidis* is a common type of bacteria present on the surface of the skin and, providing it remains in situ, does not cause infection. However, if it infiltrates the skin following a bite, cut or abrasion it may lead to inflammation and infection of subcutaneous connective tissue (a condition known as cellulitis that usually requires antibiotic therapy). Most bacterial commensals live in our digestive tract and perform a variety of functions. In addition to competing with other potentially harmful bacteria, they also help to ferment complex carbohydrates (such as cellulose) that would otherwise be impossible to digest. They also synthesise a number of vitamins (including folic acid and vitamin K) as well as producing a lot of gas! Antibiotic therapy can damage and disrupt intestinal commensal activity and allow potentially pathogenic bacteria such as *Clostridium difficile* to multiply. If this occurs, it can lead to painful abdominal cramps, fever and severe diarrhoea. Although diarrhoea is extremely unpleasant (and in some instances potentially life-threatening) it serves an important defensive function since it 'speeds' harmful bacteria out of the digestive system and helps to prevent colonisation.

MUCUS

The digestive, reproductive, respiratory and urinary tracts are lined with mucous membranes that, as the name suggests, secrete mucus. We will discuss mucus in Chapters 9 and 11 but essentially it is a sticky substance that helps to trap irritants and pathogenic microorganisms which can then be removed or destroyed. For example, mucus secreted from the nose can go one of two ways. It can sweep trapped material outwards (hopefully into a waiting tissue), or inwards, where the trapped material is swallowed and usually destroyed by hydrochloric acid in the stomach (pH 1.5–3.5). Mucus secreted in the bladder, urinary and reproductive tracts also sweeps trapped microorganisms out of the body. Bacterial colonisation is further inhibited by the pH of urine (about 6) and vaginal secretion (about 4–5). Finally, coughing and sneezing are an effective way of 'ejecting' unwanted material from the body at high speed. Unfortunately, they are also an effective way of spreading large droplets containing potentially contagious material over a wide surface area (often the face of the person standing in front of you). It is estimated that the influenza virus can spread up to 6 feet from a person's head just by talking and breathing – luckily, there is more to our immune system than just physical and chemical barriers.

SELF AND NON-SELF

The key mechanism that enables the immune system to avoid disease and maintain health is its ability to distinguish between the body's own cells (self) and those that represent a potential threat (non-self). In the same way that erythrocytes (red blood cells) possess surface antigens that determine blood type, other cells and substances (e.g. toxins) possess similar markers that enable the immune system to distinguish between its own cells and those that are foreign and potentially harmful. The human body is not a particularly tolerant environment for foreign cells or material and, once detected as non-self, they are attacked and destroyed in a variety of unpleasant ways. Before we look at the internal defence mechanisms of our non-specific immune system it is worth quickly examining the different types of pathogenic microorganism that we encounter on a fairly regular basis. Broadly speaking, they can be classified into four main groups: parasites, fungus/yeast, bacteria and viruses. However, it is important to note that the likelihood that any of these organisms will cause infection or illness is dependent on two interconnected factors. The first is the virulence of the organism and we have already noted that many bacteria offer little threat to us under normal circumstances. The second factor is the resistance of the host (i.e. how strong or efficient the immune system is). For example, the very young and the very old are most susceptible to opportunistic infection since their immune system is either immature or compromised (see below).

PARASITES

In the UK, we are fortunate that parasitic infection is typically limited in severity (unless it has been acquired abroad). There are two main types of internal parasite: protozoa and helminths (worms). The word protozoa is derived from the Greek for 'first' (*proto*) and 'animal' (*zoon*) and refers to the enormous number of single-celled organisms that live freely in soil and water. Not all protozoa are harmful to humans but common pathogenic examples include *trypanosoma* (sleeping sickness), *plasmodium* (malaria), *entamoeba* (amoebic dysentery) and *toxoplasma gondii* (toxoplasmosis). The first two examples are transmitted by insects (the tsetse fly and mosquito) and are not native to the UK. *Entamoeba* is also uncommon in the UK (and other developed nations) and is usually acquired from food or water that has been contaminated by faecal material containing amoebic cysts (it can also be sexually transmitted). Despite the fact that the incidence of amoebic dysentery is more prevalent in the developing world, one of the best-known outbreaks occurred at the Chicago World Fair in 1931. Poor plumbing permitted raw sewage to contaminate drinking water, resulting in about 1,000 cases and 58 deaths.

TOXOPLASMA GONDII

The final example of a pathogenic protozoon, *toxoplasma gondii*, is one of the most common parasitic infections found in humans. It is difficult to estimate how many people have toxoplasmosis since those infected often have no obvious symptoms (they are asymptomatic). Moreover, symptoms such as a raised temperature, sore throat and muscle aches are frequently diagnosed as viral illness since they are so generic. Toxoplasmosis is of greatest concern, therefore, to those with poor or compromised immunity and can cause serious damage to the retina of the eye and in a small number of cases prove fatal (e.g. to those suffering from immunodeficiency disease or, if infection occurs during pregnancy, to the foetus). Transmission typically occurs through hand-to-mouth contamination with cat faeces (e.g. from litter trays or soil) or by eating undercooked meat that contains the *toxoplasma gondii* cysts (acquired when animals accidentally ingest cysts in soil, water or infected tissue). The relationship between cats and *toxoplasma gondii* is an important one since the reproductive phase of this protozoon can only occur in the cells that line the cat's gastrointestinal tract. It has been suggested that the parasite is responsible for subtle but long-term effects on the personality and behaviour of its other hosts (e.g. rodents). For example, *toxoplasma gondii* has been shown to alter the behaviour of infected rats and mice in a way that makes them more likely to be caught – and therefore ingested – by cats (they become more risk averse and are actually attracted to the smell of cat urine). How far it influences human behaviour is contentious but it has been suggested that it may be responsible for a range of behaviours including short attention span, anxiety, neuroticism and schizophrenia with certain population groups demonstrating higher levels of infection than others. This raises the possibility that *toxoplasma gondii* may influence cultural behaviour as well as individual actions.

WORMS

The second type of parasitic organism are helminths or parasitic worms. Like protozoa, they can live both freely and parasitically. Unlike protozoa, they are much more complex organisms and are generally visible to naked eye. Helminths often inhabit the digestive tract and are transmitted by ingestion/faecal contamination. Pathogenic examples include roundworms, hookworms and tapeworms (none of which is prevalent in the UK). The most common parasitic worm encountered in the UK is probably threadworm (also known as pinworm). Threadworms are white and look, as the name suggests, like small pieces of thread. They are particularly common in children under the age of 10 and can be seen around the child's anus or in their faeces. They can be incredibly itchy (particularly at night) and children often scratch their bottom, which transfers the worm's eggs under their finger nails. There is a very good children's book by Babette Cole called Dr Dog that includes perhaps the best advice that can be offered to any child, or adult, on this subject: 'don't scratch your bum and suck your thumb'. Dr Dog provides excellent advice on a number of other common disorders including the management of external parasites such as head lice. Finally, the disease elephantiasis (frequently and incorrectly referred to as elephantitis) is caused by thread-like parasitic worms that block the vessels of the lymphatic system (see below) leading to enlargement and thickening of the tissues of the lower limb and (in men) the scrotum. The worms produce millions of larvae that circulate in the bloodstream and can be transmitted to a new host via mosquitos or black flies.

FUNGUS AND YEAST

Yeast belongs to the fungus family and accounts for about 1% of all fungal species (hence the fact the two are considered together). Yeasts are typically unicellular microorganisms and reproduce via mitosis (Chapter 2). Other types of fungus originate from microscopic spores (from the Greek word for 'seed') and filaments that mature into larger, visible structures. Small amounts of yeast and fungus are present on our skin but growth is usually inhibited by our non-specific immune system (e.g. pH and commensal bacteria). Those with impaired immunity, however, may be at risk of developing opportunistic yeast and fungal infection. For example, candida albicans is a type of fungus normally present on our skin and mucous membranes that grows as yeast. Candida (or thrush) infections are commonly found in parts of the body where two skin areas touch or rub together such as the armpits, groin and toes. The fungus thrives in warm, moist conditions and commonly occurs in the mouth and vagina. Other common (and annoying) fungal infections include ring worm (tinea) and athlete's foot (tinea pedis). Both are caused by a group of fungi called dermatophytes and are highly contagious. Ring worm can be passed from person to person and from animal to person (or vice versa). Its name is misleading since it is not a worm at all and refers to the red, scaly, ring-like pattern that often forms on affected skin. Ring worm can also occur beneath the nails which typically appear yellow, thickened and brittle when infected. For most people, fungal infection represents a minor irritation or inconvenience and is easily treated. For those who are immunosuppressed or immunocompromised, however, it can be much more serious.

BACTERIA

The next type of microorganism, bacteria, is found in every habitat on earth and has even been discovered inside glacial ice in Antarctica and in hot springs at Yellowstone National Park in the US (where water temperature reaches near boiling point). One of the ways some bacteria are able to survive in such harsh conditions for decades or even centuries is that they are able to form dormant spores (different from fungal spores). When these are eaten, inhaled or come into contact with an exposed area on a host they are able to reactivate and multiply. The fact that bacteria are able to survive at such extremes is one of the reasons they are so difficult to eliminate (entirely at least) in hospitals and elsewhere. However, as we have already observed, the human body is colonised (inside and out) by commensal bacteria that, for the most part, don't trouble us a great deal. It is also important to remember that almost everything we touch is covered by millions of these tenacious microorganisms. For example, it has been estimated that in every gram of soil there are typically about 40 million bacterial cells! Bacteria are classified on the basis of a number of different criteria including their shape, ability to form spores, method of energy production (aerobic or anaerobic) and reaction to gram stain. For example, the term 'coccus' refers to any bacterium that has a spherical or round shape (e.g. streptococci are spherical but arranged in chains whereas staphylococci are arranged in clusters). Gram stain simply refers to the process (developed by Danish bacteriologist Hans Christian Gram) where bacterial cells are stained with a purple dye called crystal violet. The preparation is then treated with alcohol or acetone which washes the stain out of 'Gram-negative' cells. The cells' ability to retain the stain differentiates between the types of cell wall that 'Gram positive' and 'Gram-negative' bacteria possess. Bacteria do not have a nucleus but they do possess simple DNA in the form of a chromosomal loop and plasmid rings. Chromosomal DNA contains most of the genetic information and is suspended in the cytoplasm. Plasmid DNA, on the other hand, forms small rings that carry a small amount of information that can help the bacterium survive stressful situations (e.g. exposure to antibiotics – see below).

VIRUSES

A virus (from the Latin word for 'poison') is an incredibly small (sub-microscopic) infectious agent that is unable to grow or reproduce outside of a host cell. Because of this, it is useful to think of viruses as intracellular parasites and they can infect bacterial cells as well as those of plants and animals. Viruses have a very simple structure and only contain one or two strands of DNA or RNA protected by a protein coat called a capsid. The virus injects its genetic material into the host cell and 'hijacks' its intracellular machinery to produce copies. In order to do this, it attaches itself to the surface of the host cell using antigens that protrude from the capsid. When sufficient copies of the virus have been made the host cell ruptures and the new viruses are released into the surrounding tissue (where they can infect new cells). This process always puts me in mind of the film *Alien* where an unidentified space-creature attaches itself to actor John Hurt's face and (unbeknown to him or the audience) injects him with an organism that continues to grow and develop inside his seemingly healthy body. Famously of course the eponymous alien matures and bursts in dramatic fashion from poor John's chest during dinner before going on to wreak havoc with colleague Ellen Ripley's films – obviously viruses are working on a much smaller scale!

STAGES OF INFECTION

The stages of any infectious disease follow a fairly predictable pattern: incubation, prodrome, illness, decline and convalescence (Figure 6.1). The incubation period refers to the time between infection and the first signs and symptoms. This depends upon the virulence of the microorganism and the resistance of the host. The prodromal phase is the short period of mild, generalised symptoms that precede the illness itself. During the illness proper, pathogens (disease-causing organisms) may damage body tissues since the immune system has not responded fully or adequately. Decline refers to the period when the immune system has overcome the pathogen and symptoms begin to ease. Finally, convalescence signals recovery, repair and restoration of function. In the case of both bacterial and viral infections, incubation period can vary enormously. For example, the incubation period for viral gastroenteritis (e.g. norovirus or rotavirus) can be as little as 24 hours. The typical incubation period for influenza (flu virus) is between one and four days. Chickenpox (varicella-zoster virus), on the other hand, has an incubation period of between 14 to 16 days after exposure to a

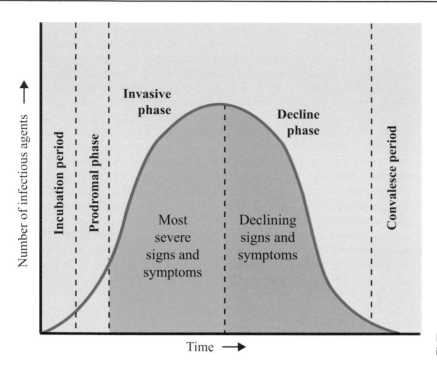

Figure 6.1 Stages of infection.

varicella rash. Varicella is also one of a number of viruses that can remain dormant or 'hidden' in the body after the primary infection has resolved. If reactivation does occur (because the person is immunocompromised or unwell) it causes herpes zoster or shingles. Shingles is an infection of a nerve that causes pain and an itchy rash along the band of skin supplied by the nerve. The same principle applies to the herpes simplex virus which causes small blisters (cold sores) to develop on and around the lips. They typically resolve without treatment within 7–10 days but remain dormant in the nerve until the person is tired, unwell or their immune system is under pressure.

CHEST INFECTION

The main types of chest infection are bronchitis and pneumonia. Most cases of bronchitis are caused by viruses, whereas most cases of pneumonia are caused by bacteria. Consequently, antibiotics (which only kill bacteria) are rarely indicated to treat the former. You

may be thinking: 'but I have received antibiotics for a chest infection and I felt much better'. There are two reasons for this. The first is that you had a bacterial infection in which case antibiotics were the correct treatment. The other, more common, reason simply relates to timing. Most people make an appointment to see their doctor when they are feeling at their worst and not when they have a bit of a sniffle or running nose (the prodromal phase mentioned above). Even when symptoms become more pronounced during the illness proper, most people still think: 'I'll be OK in a day or two.' It is only when the illness is at its worst that they often decide 'enough is enough' and plead with their GP for antibiotics. After several days of taking antibiotics the person will probably begin to feel much better – surely it must be the antibiotics? Maybe but maybe not. The fact that the person is feeling better often simply reflects the fact that their immune system has overcome the pathogen (in this case a virus) and symptoms begin to ease in keeping with the decline phase. The next thing we need to look at, therefore, is how the immune system overcomes pathogenic microorganisms such as viruses once they have breached our physical barriers and entered the body?

INTERNAL DEFENCES (OF THE NON-SPECIFIC IMMUNE SYSTEM)

The body uses a wide variety of non-specific cellular and chemical mechanisms to protect itself from potentially harmful microorganisms and substances. These include leukocytes (white blood cells) with granules in their cytoplasm (granulocytes) mentioned earlier in the chapter. Granulocytes are particularly important for the removal of bacteria and parasites from the body and consist of neutrophils, basophils and eosinophils (Figure 5.1). Neutrophils are the most abundant of the white blood cells and account for 50–70% of circulating leukocytes. They are wandering phagocytes (devouring cells) that digest microorganisms, insoluble particles and other cell debris. Think of a neutrophil as a cellular Pac-Man (the 1980s arcade game character), but rather than eating dots and multi-coloured 'ghosts' they digest bacteria and other pathogens using enzymes within their intracellular granules. Neutrophils are highly mobile and are typically the first on the scene to fight pathogens. They are followed by macrophages (big eaters) about three to four hours later (super Pac-Men). Macrophages are derived from another type of leukocyte called a monocyte (Figure 5.1). These are the largest of all the leukocytes and are released into the circulation from the bone marrow. After a few days they migrate to different tissues (e.g. liver, spleen, lungs, etc.) where they mature into macrophages. There are two principle types of macrophage: fixed macrophages (that remain in certain tissues and organs) and free macrophages (that are able to migrate from tissue to tissue). The lifespan of a macrophage is dependent on its type and ranges from between about 6–16 days for circulating macrophages, to 3 months or more for those in the liver (Kupffer cells). Neutrophils, on the other hand, have a much shorter life span and typically only survive for 5–6 days. People who have abnormally low levels of neutrophils (often because they are immunocompromised following chemotherapy) are said to be neutropenic. Neutropenia is a serious condition that renders the individual highly vulnerable to opportunistic infection and they may need to be reverse-barrier nursed when in hospital. That is to say, they are cared for in protective isolation to minimise exposure to pathogenic microorganisms and substances that could cause infection (remember the correlation between pathogen virulence and host defence regarding the incidence and severity of infectious disease).

BASOPHILS, MAST CELLS AND EOSINOPHILS

The next type of leukocyte that contributes to the body's non-specific immune response are basophils. These cells account for less than 1% of the total leukocyte population and are the least common of the granulocytes. Basophils play an important role during inflammatory reactions and store and release inflammatory chemicals such as histamine. Histamine causes dilation (widening) of small blood vessels and increases the permeability of capillaries (i.e. it allows plasma and some cells to pass through the capillary wall more easily). Histamine also irritates the hell out of nerve endings, leading to itching and/or pain (hence the need for antihistamine medication following inflammation caused by an insect bite). Another type of cell that contains histamine and helps to facilitate the inflammatory response are mast cells. Mast cells tend to accumulate in the lungs, gastrointestinal tract and skin, whereas basophils are usually found in the peripheral circulation where they migrate into extravascular (outside the vessel) tissue. Both cells have surface receptors for immunoglobulin (Ig) E (see below) and play an important role in the mediation of allergic reactions including asthma, eczema, allergic rhinitis (hay fever) and allergic conjunctivitis. The final type of granulocytic leukocyte are eosinophils which account for less than 5% of circulating white blood cells. Like neutrophils, eosinophils phagocytose (devour and digest) pathogenic material and are chiefly responsible for the destruction of parasitic organisms such as helminths (worms). Because worms are too big to be phagocytosed individually, eosinophils collectively attack the outer membrane of the parasite in order to destroy or disable it. Eosinophils also play an important role in fighting viral infection and (with basophils and mast cells) help mediate allergic responses such as asthma (see Chapter 9).

NATURAL KILLER CELLS

The final cells to be discussed as part of the non-specific immune system are the appropriately named natural killer cells. NK cells are large granular lymphocytes (Figure 5.1) that mature in the bone marrow, lymph nodes,

spleen, tonsils and thymus gland (Figure 6.2). They are often described as policing the body since they eliminate a variety of infected and abnormal cells by detecting lack of 'self'. This process is known as immunological surveillance since it allows the body to recognise and destroy previously normal cells that now represent a threat. 'Policing' is perhaps the wrong word therefore, and 'assassination' is probably more accurate. NK cells are not phagocytic – they are much stealthier, as you would expect from an assassin. The way in which they kill cancer and virus-infected cells involves secreting cytotoxic proteins onto the target cell which triggers apoptosis (programmed cell death) before further cell division or viral replication can take place. It also enhances the inflammatory response.

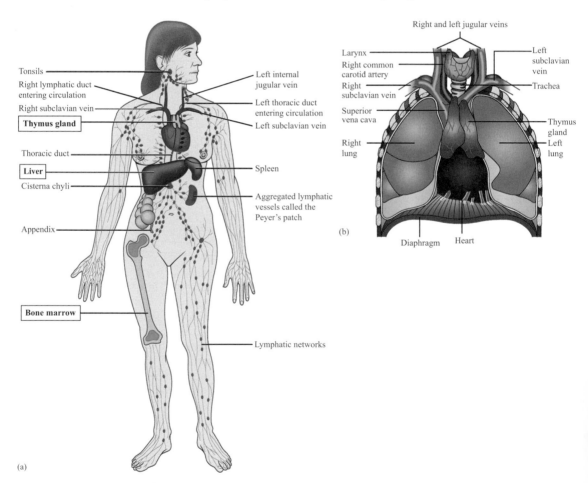

Figure 6.2 (a) Lymphatic system. (b) Thymus gland of a child.

INFLAMMATORY RESPONSE

The inflammatory response is a protective mechanism that is activated when body tissue is injured by trauma, chemicals, radiation, extremes of temperature or infection by microorganisms. It helps to prevent the spread of pathogenic material to other parts of the body and assists in the elimination of harmful agents. Inflammation produces up to five cardinal signs: redness (rubor), heat (calor), swelling (tumour), pain (dolor) and loss of function (e.g. when a joint is involved). These signs and symptoms are triggered by chemical mediators or messengers derived either from the plasma or from leukocytes. Plasma-derived mediators are usually present in a precursory form that need to be activated, whilst cell-derived mediators are normally stored in intracellular granules that need to be secreted or discharged. Plasma is the source of three major mediators: kinins, products of coagulation and proteins of the complement system. Cell-derived mediators include histamine, cytokines, leukotrienes and prostaglandins (see also Chapter 13). They all sound very complicated but – in essence – they simply help to prepare the body to defend itself from potentially harmful material. For example, following injury, many of the chemical mediators mentioned above contribute to the vascular phase of the inflammatory response by encouraging small vessel dilation and increased permeability. This allows more blood to flow to the affected area (hyperaemia) which accounts for the increased redness and heat experienced during inflammation. At the same time, the increased permeability (leakiness) of the vessel wall allows plasma to escape from the circulatory system into the surrounding tissue (hence the swelling, pain and loss of function). Plasma-derived chemical mediators, and those secreted by granulocytic leukocytes or damaged cells (following injury), work in a complementary fashion. For example, basophils and mast cells secrete histamine which contributes to small vessel dilation and increases permeability. They also produce inflammatory mediators called leukotrienes (following the breakdown of phospholipids from their cell membrane). Leukotrienes are complementary in action with histamine but far more potent. They also attract wandering phagocytes and help them to stick onto potential pathogens.

PROSTAGLANDINS, CYTOKINES AND THE COMPLEMENT SYSTEM

Another group of inflammatory mediators derived from the phospholipid membranes of damaged cells are prostaglandins. These intensify the vasoactive effects of histamine and kinins, and stimulate the migration of phagocytes through capillary walls. Unfortunately for us, prostaglandins also intensify and prolong the pain associated with inflammation. Macrophages, mast cells, B cells and T cells (see below) all produce chemical messengers called cytokines (from the Greek words for 'cell' and 'movement'). Cytokines are a broad group of small proteins that signal, attract and activate phagocytes and NK cells. They include alpha-interferons which are produced by virus-infected cells and trigger the production of antiviral proteins within the cytoplasm. These interfere with viral replication and help to stimulate NK cell activity. Proteins of the complement system are found in the plasma and, as their name suggests, they complement the action of leukocytes and antibodies attached to bacterial cell walls. They interact with one another (in a similar way to the clotting cascade) in order to stimulate further histamine secretion, attract neutrophils and other phagocytes to the area and destroy bacteria by interfering with the integrity of their cell walls (they punch a lot of holes in it).

STAGES OF THE INFLAMMATORY RESPONSE

This is all very interesting (in my opinion) but how does all this activity result in a coordinated response by the non-specific immune system? We have seen that the secretion of many of the chemicals described above results (directly or indirectly) in vasodilation and greater permeability of small blood vessels. This leads to increased blood flow to the area (containing neutrophils, etc.) and loss of plasma from the local circulation into the surrounding tissue. This in turn helps to push foreign material into the lymphatic system where it can be eliminated (see below) and delivers plasma-based chemical mediators to the injured area. For example, products of coagulation form a physical barrier (fibrin mesh) that helps to prevent the further spread of pathogenic material and provides a temporary framework for repair. The loss of plasma from the circulation also causes blood viscosity (thickness) to increase which slows down circulation. This is useful since it enables leukocytes (e.g. neutrophils and monocytes) to slow down and accumulate along the endothelial surface of the vessel. This process is known as margination (or pavementing) and always reminds me of paratroopers lining-up by the open door of a plane and waiting to jump

into battle. The next stage of the immune response is called emigration or diapedesis (from the Greek words for 'leap through'). It refers to the relocation of the waiting leukocytes from the plasma into the adjacent tissue as they flatten and squeeze through the widened (more permeable) endothelial junctions of the vessel wall (Figure 6.3). Once the cells have emigrated from the circulatory system to the interstitial space they still need to navigate their way to where the pathogenic material is located. Fortunately, however, we have already observed that a number of cellular chemicals signal to phagocytes in order to attract them to where they are needed (e.g. cytokines and complement proteins). This process is called chemotaxis and refers to the movement or orientation (taxis) of cells in response to chemical stimulation or signalling. The final stage of the cellular response is phagocyte activation and the elimination of the injurious agent. However, this can be a brutal and costly encounter for both sides. Dead and dying pathogens (and phagocytes) litter the battlefield and contribute to the formation of pus. If the immune

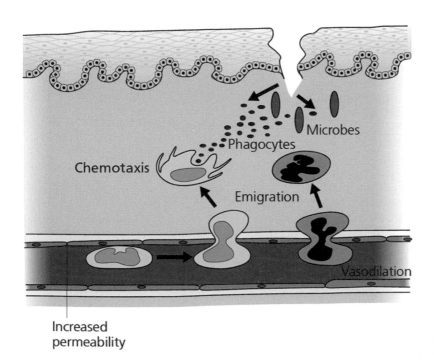

Figure 6.3 Emigration and chemotaxis.

system is unable to clear this cellular debris, it can become enclosed by collagen fibres and forms an abscess (in which case the area may require incision and drainage before healing can take place).

SPECIFIC IMMUNITY AND THE ROLE OF ANTIBODIES

Specific immunity is also known as acquired or adaptive immunity and is only available at birth in an extremely limited fashion (see below). It is acquired following exposure to an antigen and develops in breadth and complexity with each new antigen encounter. Antigens, as we have noted, are present on the surface of a wide variety of microorganisms and foreign materials (e.g. bacteria and toxins). They are recognised as a threat by the body's specific and non-specific immune system and, in the case of the latter, trigger the formation of antibodies. This is known as antibody-mediated immunity (or humoral immunity) and involves the transformation of B cells (lymphocytes) into plasma cells which are capable of producing and secreting large quantities of antigen-specific antibodies into the circulatory system. A small number of B cells also differentiate into memory B cells that survive for many years in the circulatory system and allow the immune system to 'remember' an antigen and respond more rapidly when it is encountered in the future (see below). Both processes allow the body to target and destroy specific microorganisms and pathogenic material with a high level of accuracy and efficiency. There are five main types of antibody or immunoglobulin (Ig) known as IgA, IgD, IgE, IgG and IgM. They are all large 'Y'-shaped proteins that attach to a specific antigen on the basis of their molecular shape. The 'prongs' of the Y are designed to bind to the antigen whereas the upright 'stem' allows it to combine with other immune structures such as complement proteins and mast cells (see below and Chapter 9). When antibodies (Igs) bind to viral antigens they prevent them from attaching to other cells which, in turn, helps to slow viral replication. They are also able to coat or opsonise bacterial cells which allows phagocytes to target them more easily (the Greek word *opsonin* means 'to prepare for eating').

ANTIBODIES

Finally, antibodies help to activate the complement system cascade which results in pore formation (in the cellular membrane), enhanced phagocytosis (via opsonisation) and histamine release from mast cells and basophils. Different antibodies can be found in different locations and perform a number of complementary roles. For example, IgA can be found in a variety of secretions including those of gastrointestinal and respiratory tracts, tears, saliva and colostrum (breast milk secreted in the first week of lactation). It helps to guard against viral and bacterial invasion. IgD acts as a surface receptor on B cells and plays a key role in initiating early B cell activation. IgE protects against parasitic infection and binds to basophils and mast cells to facilitate the release of chemical mediators such as histamine and leukotrienes. In some circumstances, however, this contributes to hypersensitivity and the exacerbation of allergic disease such as asthma, allergic rhinitis, food allergy and dermatitis (see Chapter 9). IgG is the most abundant type of immunoglobulin in the plasma and extracellular fluid, and binds to a wide variety of pathogens including viruses, bacteria and fungi. It is also very small which allows it to access different tissue types with relative ease. For example, it is the only antibody that is able to cross the placental membrane and provides the developing baby with a degree of humoral immunity in utero and for some months following birth (along with IgA which is provided via colostrum). Finally, IgM is the largest antibody and is found primarily in the plasma. It is the first antibody to be produced in response to an antigen and is chiefly responsible for the agglutination (clumping) of erythrocytes when incompatibility is detected (Chapter 5). Although antibodies are grouped into five main types, the number of different antibodies produced by plasma cells is enormous. It is estimated that over the course of our lifetime our body can produce up to 100 million different antibodies in response to pathogens and pathogenic material.

T CELLS

Most lymphocytes in the circulatory system and tissue are T cells (so named because they mature in the thymus gland, Figure 6.2). Their role is to coordinate the activity of other immune cells and to recognise, remember and destroy foreign cells. Consequently, there are a variety of different types of T cell each with different roles and responsibilities. The most important are probably helper T cells which act as the commanding officers or managers of the immune system. Once activated, they secrete a variety of cytokine (cell + movement) chemicals that help to attract and recruit other immune cells to the area. For example, they stimulate B cells to produce and secrete antibodies and activate cytotoxic T cells (see below) to destroy infected target cells. They also attract and potentiate neutrophils (devouring cells) and macrophages (giant devouring cells). As a direct result of helper T cell activity, therefore, the immune response gains momentum as more and more defensive mechanisms are activated and dispatched on the body's behalf.

CYTOTOXIC AND REGULATORY T CELLS

Cytotoxic T cells work in a very different way to helper T cells and are the only T cell that directly attacks other cells. Like natural killer (NK) cells they are not phagocytic and specialise in destroying virus-infected and cancer cells. They achieve this by binding to the foreign cell and injecting a toxic chemical (perforin) into its membrane. This is romantically known as 'the kiss of death' and (less romantically) causes the membrane to rupture and the cell to split open (cytolysis). This mechanism of action is similar to the way in which some complement

proteins perforate bacterial cell walls to achieve cytolysis. After detaching from the target cell, cytotoxic T cells continue to hunt down and destroy other cells that display the same antigen. In contrast to cytotoxic and helper T cells, regulatory (or suppressor) T cells release chemicals that suppress the activity of T and B cells. It is extremely important that the immune system has the ability to step down and restrain the immune response once a threat has been inactivated or destroyed. This helps to prevent uncontrolled or unnecessary immune activity which can lead to autoimmune disease (where the body attacks and destroys its own cells and tissue). Examples of common autoimmune diseases include rheumatoid arthritis, multiple sclerosis and type I diabetes. Although we know what happens during autoimmune disease (e.g. T cells attack insulin producing beta cells of the pancreas in type I diabetes) it remains unclear why it happens in the first place.

MEMORY T CELLS

Finally, memory T cells (like memory B cells) are produced after each new antigen encounter to ensure that the immune system remains in a state of readiness should the same microorganism/antigen be detected in the future. They can remain in circulation for a number of decades and allow the body to launch a rapid immune response before signs and symptoms appear. The importance of T cells to our overall health is perhaps best demonstrated by the effects of human immunodeficiency virus (HIV) and acquired immune deficiency syndrome (AIDS). The HIV virus depletes the number of helper T cells (also known as CD4 cells) which prevents the body from mounting a coordinated immune response and leaves it increasingly susceptible to opportunistic infection and disease. The number of T cells in circulation is used to assess the stage of both diseases and to indicate which treatment option is most appropriate. A healthy helper T cell/CD4 count is considered to be between 500 and 1,500 cells per cubic millimetre (mm^3) of blood. A helper T cell count of less than 200 cells/mm^3 is one of the indications for a diagnosis of AIDS (as opposed to HIV).

PRIMARY AND SECONDARY IMMUNE RESPONSE

When someone is first exposed to an infectious microorganism they rely on their non-specific immune system to mount an initial defence. In many cases, this is successful and depends upon the virulence of the invader and the resistance of the host. For example, new-born infants rely primarily on their non-specific defences since (with the exception of small amounts IgA and IgG provided by their mother) their specific immune defences are still developing. If the infection is severe or tenacious, activated B cells will differentiate into plasma cells and produce antibodies in response to the presenting antigen. This phase is known as the lag phase since it can take weeks to develop and the amount of antibody produced is usually relatively low. The first antibody produced is IgM although small amounts of IgG are usually also secreted. During this time, however, the person will experience the signs and symptoms of the illness as they progress through the stages of infectious disease: incubation, prodrome, illness, decline and convalescence (Figure 6.1). Secondary immune response, on the other hand, occurs following second or subsequent exposure to an antigen and is typically faster and more powerful (Figure 6.4). This is because, following the initial encounter,

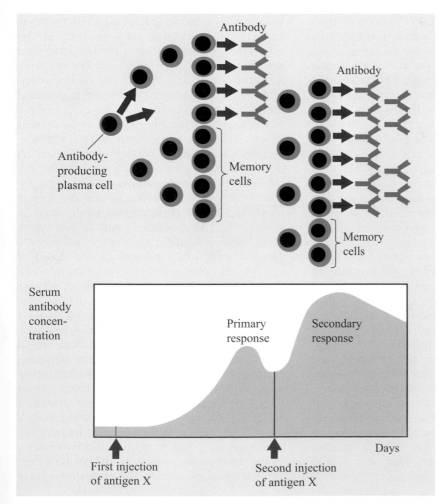

Figure 6.4 Primary and secondary immune/ antibody response.

memory B and T cells recognise the pathogen and launch a pre-prepared defence. The lag phase is shorter and the quantity of antibodies produced is both higher and enduring. The main type of antibody produced during secondary immune response is IgG. It is important to note that this is not an unusual or infrequent occurrence and is happening all the time.

VACCINATION

We experience good health because our body is waging constant war on our behalf to prevent infection and disease. Crucially, the immune system develops and becomes more efficient with each successive exposure to a pathogen. For example, those who contract chickenpox (varicella-zoster virus) will typically not have it because subsequent exposure to the virus triggers the secondary immune response which eliminates the virus before signs and symptoms present. This is also the underlying principle behind vaccination which aims to produce the same immune protection that follows natural infection but without causing disease in the first place. Some vaccines are known as live or attenuated vaccines (e.g. measles mumps and rubella/MMR and Bacillus Calmette-Guérin/BCG). This means that the infectious agent has been altered in such a way to make it harmless or less virulent. The other type of vaccines are known as inactivated or killed vaccines (e.g. tetanus) since the infectious agent has been killed using heat or formaldehyde. They still produce an immune response but require regular boosters to ensure continued protection. Some people worry that vaccination can overwhelm, or somehow compromise, a child's immune system. However, it is important to remember that within hours of birth, a baby's gastrointestinal and respiratory tract are heavily colonised with bacteria. Their immune system is designed to deal with a constant stream of foreign antigens and, rather than overwhelming the immune system, vaccines help stimulate and strengthen it in the same manner as natural exposure to an antigen. That said, a child who is moderately or severely ill on the day of

their vaccination might be asked to return at a later date. We observed earlier in the chapter, that over the course of our lifetime, our immune system will produce up to 100 million different antibodies in response to pathogens and pathogenic material encountered on a day-to-day basis. However, antibody-mediated immunity is only one part of our immune response and it is essential that all three elements continue to work in a coordinated fashion if we are to continue to resist disease and infection.

LYMPHATIC SYSTEM

Although we have already discussed many of the components of the lymphatic system in passing it is important to bring them together in order to recognise and understand the important role that this frequently overlooked system provides. The lymphatic system actually consists of four interrelated components: lymph, lymphatic vessels, lymph nodes and lymphoid organs/tissues (Figure 6.2). Collectively, they provide the physical environment in which the cells and secretions of our immune system develop and operate. If you imagine the different leucocytes and lymphocytes as the soldiers of the immune army, the lymphatic system provides the barracks and the means of transport for these cells. Lymph itself is a clear fluid that contains and carries white blood cells (mainly lymphocytes and macrophages) and, when present in the digestive system, also transports fats (see Chapter 11). Lymph is very similar in character to plasma and is derived from the interstitial fluid that surrounds the cells (the Latin word *lympha* means 'spring water'). Lymph drains from the interstitial space into a network of close-ended tubes called lymphatic capillaries situated next to the 'true capillaries' of the circulatory system. Most lymphatic capillaries (about 70%) are located near the surface of the skin; the remainder are located around the body's deeper structures and internal organs. They converge into larger, thin-walled lymphatic vessels that eventually return the lymph to the venous circulation at the right internal jugular vein (via the lymphatic duct) and left subclavian vein (via the thoracic duct). Lymphatic vessels are similar in structure to veins and have a large number of valves to prevent back flow (see Chapters 7 and 8). The movement of the body, and contraction of the muscles, compress the lymphatic vessels in order to propel lymph through the system in a kind of milking action.

LYMPH NODES

Before lymph returns to the venous circulation, it must also pass through numerous bean-shaped masses of tissue called lymph nodes (Figures 6.2, 6.5). These are situated along the course of the lymphatic vessels and in strategic clusters at key areas such as the neck (cervical nodes), the armpits (axillary nodes) and the groin (inguinal nodes). Each lymph node is surrounded by a fibrous capsule and divided into the cortex (outer layer) which contains B and T cells, and the medulla (inner layer) which contains macrophages and antibody-secreting plasma cells. Any harmful material that has been washed into the lymph is filtered through the white blood cells in the lymph nodes and removed before re-entering the venous blood. Lymph nodes act like barracks or garrisons for the immune cells and enable them to ambush and destroy pathogenic material in a series of killing zones. In total, there are between 600 to 700 lymph nodes dispersed throughout the human body. This system is not infallible, however, and we

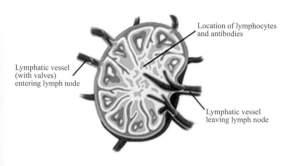

Figure 6.5 Lymph node.

observed earlier in the chapter that the disease elephantiasis is caused by parasitic worms that block the lymphatic vessels leading to thickening of the tissues of the lower limb. Lymphoedema (lymphatic obstruction) can also occur following damage or disruption to the lymphatic system. Finally, lymph nodes frequently become inflamed or enlarged as a result of a wide variety of infections and diseases. These range from simple viral infections such as a sore throat or glandular fever (mononucleosis), to serious cancers such as lymphoma and leukaemia.

LYMPHOID ORGANS AND TISSUES

The final components of the lymphatic system are the lymphoid organs and associated tissues. The most important of these is the bone marrow since, as we have seen, it produces all of the cells of our non-specific/specific immune systems including neutrophils, basophils, eosinophils, natural killer (NK) cells, monocytes, B cells and T cells (Figure 5.1). The thymus gland is also very important since it is where T cells mature and develop a sense of 'self-tolerance' in order to distinguish between self and foreign cells. It is located behind the sternum within the thoracic cavity and partially overlays the heart and aortic arch (Figure 6.2). The thymus is most active during the early years of life since the body is exposed to a constant stream of new microorganisms and foreign substances. It must ensure that T cells mature and are available to participate in the immune response as soon as possible. The thymus continues to enlarge until the child reaches puberty at which point it begins to atrophy (waste away) and eventually only fibrous and fatty tissue remain.

SPLEEN

The largest lymphatic organ is the much misunderstood spleen. Whenever I ask students to pick an organ and tell me what it does, the spleen always seems to be the last one to be identified (followed by a non-committal shrug when asked what it does). It is about the size of a fist and is located on the far left of the abdominal cavity, immediately below the diaphragm and adjacent to the stomach (Figure 6.2). The spleen is a highly vascular organ and is essentially a giant lymph node. It is surrounded by a fibrous capsule and contains red pulp and white pulp. The red pulp is chiefly responsible for the removal and recycling of worn out and damaged erythrocytes (remember they live for about 120 days) and the destruction of blood-borne pathogens. It also stores erythrocytes, macrophages and a large number of thrombocytes (clotting cells) which can be released if bleeding occurs. The red pulp is thought to be the site of erythrocyte production in the foetus but is superseded by the bone marrow after birth. The white pulp, on the other hand, contains T cells, B cells and macrophages which help to destroy blood borne pathogens. If the spleen is severely damaged following abdominal trauma it is sometimes necessary to remove it (splenectomy) since it can cause internal bleeding (haemorrhage) resulting in hypovolaemia (low volume of circulating blood) and hypovolemic shock. If this occurs, the liver and bone marrow are able to take over many of the spleen's functions although the individual is usually prescribed long-term antibiotic therapy in order to compensate for the loss of immune function.

MUCOSA-ASSOCIATED LYMPHOID TISSUE

The final type of lymphoid tissue protects the epithelia of the gastrointestinal, respiratory, urinary and reproductive tracts and is collectively known as mucosa-associated lymphoid tissue (MALT). MALT includes the tonsils, the vermiform (Latin for 'worm-shaped') appendix and clusters of lymphoid nodules called Peyer's patches (Figure 6.2). The tonsils are large lymphoid nodules located at the back of the tongue and mouth (lingual and palatine tonsils) and the back of the nose (nasopharyngeal tonsils or adenoids). Although they are similar to lymph nodes they are not encapsulated in the same way and the mucosa that covers them contains pits or crypts. These tonsillar crypts trap bacteria and other pathogenic material which is then destroyed by lymphocytes as it works its way into the lymphoid tissue. It seems a little reckless to encourage infection in this way and painful inflammation of the tonsils (tonsillitis) is certainly common in childhood. However, it is a calculated risk since frequent exposure to new antigens encourages the production of memory B and T cells that are able to launch a faster and more efficient immune response in the future. It is also no coincidence that lymphatic tissue is found at the entry points to the gastrointestinal and respiratory tract where many foreign substances are either ingested or inhaled. Peyer's patches, on the other hand, are found within the wall of the small intestine (ileum) and work in collaboration with the lymph nodes of the mesentery (see Chapter 11). They are similar in structure to tonsils (i.e. they are unencapsulated) and contain large numbers of B and T cells. Finally, the vermiform appendix is a small 'worm-shaped' pouch or tube located at the junction between the small and large intestines (the caecum). In humans, it is known to contribute to the immune response and may be involved in storing and presenting antigens to the immune system so that it can detect the difference between potentially harmful and harmless substances present in the gastrointestinal tract. It has also been suggested that it may prevent the gastrointestinal tract from becoming inflamed in response to certain foods and medications. Occasionally, however, the appendix itself becomes infected and inflamed (appendicitis) and has to be surgically removed (appendectomy) to prevent or correct rupture which results in the release of intestinal contents into the abdominal cavity (see Chapter 11).

CHAPTER 6: TEST YOURSELF

Q. Explain the difference between non-specific and specific immunity.

A. Non-specific immunity is present from birth (congenital) and is not dependent on previous exposure to harmful substances or microorganisms. Specific immunity is acquired following exposure to an antigen and develops in breadth and complexity with each new antigen encounter.

Q. An important part of our non-specific defence is provided by our integumentary system. What is meant by the term integumentary?

A. Integumentary refers to the tissue layer that surrounds and protects the human body and consists of physical (skin, hair, nails) and chemical (sweat, tears, mucus) barriers.

Q. When sebum and sweat mix on the surface of the skin, it forms an acidic film called the acid mantle. What is the typical pH range?

A. Between 4.5 and 6.

Q. White blood cells (leukocytes) can be broadly divided into two groups: those with granules in their cytoplasm (granulocytes) and those without (agranulocytes). Neutrophils, basophils and eosinophils are all granulocytes. Briefly explain what they do and how they differ from one another.

A. Neutrophils account for 50–70% of circulating leukocytes. They are wandering phagocytes (devouring cells) that digest microorganisms and other cell debris. Basophils account for less than 1% of the total leukocyte population but play an important role during inflammatory reactions since they store/release inflammatory chemicals such as histamine. Eosinophils account for less than 5% of circulating leukocytes and, like neutrophils, phagocytose (devour) pathogenic material. They are also responsible for the destruction of parasitic organisms and help mediate allergic responses.

Q. What is a macrophage?

A. Macrophages are the largest of the leukocytes and are phagocytes (macro + phage = big + eater). They are derived from another type of leukocyte called a monocyte.

Q. In Chapter 5, we saw that lymphocytes are white blood cells produced by lymphoid stem cells. Natural Killer (NK) cells are a type of large granular lymphocyte. Briefly explain how they destroy cancer and virus-infected cells.

A. NK cells destroy cancer and virus-infected cells by secreting cytotoxic proteins onto the target cell which triggers programmed cell death (apoptosis) before further cell division or viral replication can take place.

Q. Explain the role of B cells with reference to specific immunity.

A. When the immune system detects the presence of a foreign antigen/cell, it triggers the transformation of B cells (lymphocytes) into plasma cells which are capable of producing and secreting large quantities of antigen-specific antibodies (immunoglobulins) into the circulatory system. These help to target and destroy foreign cells. A small number of B cells also transform into memory B cells that survive for many years and allow the immune system to 'remember' an antigen and respond more rapidly in the future.

(Continued)

(Continued)

Q. What are the five types of antibody/immunoglobulin and which is the most abundant?

A. IgA, IgD, IgE, IgG (most abundant) and IgM.

Q. Briefly explain the difference between helper, regulatory, cytotoxic and memory T cells.

A. Helper T cells act as the managers of the immune system and, once activated, attract and recruit other immune cells to the area. Regulatory T cells suppress the activity of T and B cells once a threat has been destroyed. Cytotoxic T cells destroy virus-infected and cancer cells by binding to the foreign cell and injecting a toxic chemical (perforin) into its membrane. Memory T cells (like memory B cells) are produced after each new antigen encounter to ensure the immune system remains in a state of readiness should the same microorganism/antigen be detected in the future.

Q. What is meant by secondary immune response?

A. Secondary immune response occurs following second exposure to an antigen and is typically faster and more powerful because memory T and B cells recognise the pathogen and launch a pre-prepared defence.

Q. List the four different types of pathogenic microorganism we encounter on a regular basis.

A. Parasites, fungus/yeast, bacteria and viruses.

Q. What are the two principle factors that contribute to the likelihood of developing a disease from a microorganism?

A. The virulence of the microorganism and the resistance of the host (i.e. how strong or efficient our immune system is).

Q. What is lymphatic fluid (lymph)?

A. Lymph is similar in character to plasma and is derived from interstitial fluid. It circulates around the lymphatic system/vessels and transports white blood cells.

Q. What is the function of lymph nodes and where are they located?

A. Lymph nodes are bean-shaped masses of tissue that house B cells, T cells and macrophages. They are situated along the course of the lymphatic vessels in clusters at key areas including the neck (cervical nodes), armpits (axillary nodes) and groin (inguinal nodes).

Q. Name the three principle organs of the lymphatic system.

A. Bone marrow, pancreas and thymus gland.

Q. Where do B and T cells mature?

A. B cells mature in the bone marrow and T cells in the thymus gland.

Q. What does the acronym MALT stand for and provide one example.

A. Mucosa-associated lymphoid tissue includes the appendix, tonsils and Peyer's patches (clusters of lymphoid nodules located in the small intestine).

Contents

CHAPTER 7

CARDIOVASCULAR SYSTEM

CIRCULATION

The term cardiovascular simply refers to the relationship between the heart (from the Greek word *kardia*) and the blood vessels (from the Latin word *vasculum* for 'small vessel'). Although it is tempting to consider the two independently it is important to remember that they form a closed system or circuit that ensures tissues receive oxygenated blood for cellular metabolism and that deoxygenated blood is returned to the lungs in order for gaseous exchange to occur (see Chapter 9). The heart itself is simply a muscular pump that pushes the blood (specialised connective tissue) through the different vessels in order that the various substances it transports (oxygen, carbon dioxide, nutrients, waste products, ions, hormones, etc.) circulate to where they need to go. The circulation of the blood around the body was first described in detail by the English physician William Harvey in 1628 (building upon the work of earlier scholars). Prior to this, it was thought that the venous circulation was separate from the arterial circulation rather than forming a complete and closed loop. The circulatory system can be broadly divided into two parts: the pulmonary circulation (to and from the lungs) and the systemic circulation (to and from the rest of the body). Each circuit begins and ends at the heart.

ARTERIES AND VEINS

The average adult has approximately five litres of blood distributed throughout the cardiovascular system in a number of different vessels (Figure 7.1). There are three main types of blood vessel: arteries, veins and capillaries. Structurally, arteries and veins are very similar. Both have a fibrous outer layer or membrane called the tunica adventitia or tunica externa (from the Latin for 'outer coat'). Beneath this is a layer of smooth muscle and elastic tissue called the tunica media ('middle coat'). The inner lining (tunica intima) of both vessels consists of a single layer of simple squamous epithelial cells known as endothelium (Figure 7.2). The endothelium is in direct contact with the blood and provides an uninterrupted and non-thrombogenic surface (i.e. it discourages clotting). Although both arteries and veins are constructed from the same three layers of tissue there are a number of distinct anatomical differences between them. Firstly, arteries always travel away from the heart ('A' for 'artery' and 'away') and veins travel towards it. Secondly, arterial walls are thicker than veins since they contain more smooth muscle and elastic tissue in the tunica media. Smooth muscle is necessary for vasoconstriction and vasodilation in both vessels but the quantity reflects the different pressures exerted by the blood against artery and

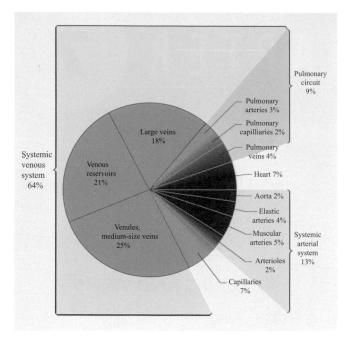

Figure 7.1 Distribution of blood within the circulatory system.

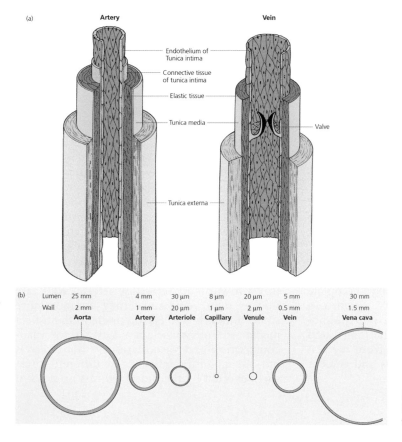

Figure 7.2 (a) Structure of blood vessels. (b) Variations in the thickness of blood vessel walls.

vein walls (see Chapter 8). Finally, since veins return blood to the heart (at low pressure) many, particularly those of the lower limb, contain valves in order to prevent backflow.

CAPILLARIES

The final type of blood vessels are capillaries (from the Latin word *capillaris* for 'hair-like'). These microscopic tubes consist of a single layer of endothelial cells through which plasma and other small molecules can pass. There is no tunica media or adventitia and the diameter of each capillary is only slightly larger than that of a single erythrocyte (remember how they can stack themselves like dinner plates to avoid blockage when travelling through these narrow vessels). Capillaries connect small arteries (arterioles) to small veins (venules) and the capillary network (or bed) between the two is the site of nutrient and waste exchange between the blood and interstitial fluid that surrounds the cells (Figure 7.3). The flow of blood through the capillary bed is known as microcirculation and takes place in two types of capillary. The first type of capillary is known as a metarteriole (or vascular shunt) and directly connects the arteriole to the opposing venule. True capillaries, on the other hand, branch from metarterioles and provide nutrient and waste product exchange between the plasma and interstitial fluid. The entrance to each true capillary is protected by a band of smooth muscle called a precapillary sphincter. This contracts or relaxes in order to control the flow of blood through the capillary bed. For example, when precapillary sphincters contract (close), blood flows directly through the metarteriole and bypasses the tissue. This occurs during vigorous exercise when blood is re-routed from the gastrointestinal tract to skeletal muscle in order to prioritise blood supply to the latter.

HYDROSTATIC PRESSURE

As well as facilitating the movement of nutrients and waste products in and out of the tissue, capillaries also allow fluid (plasma) to move between the blood and interstitial space. This occurs because of the difference in hydrostatic pressure at the arteriole end of the capillary and the osmotic pressure at the venous end. This sounds more complicated than it is. Hydrostatic pressure simply refers to the force exerted by fluid against the wall of the capillary. Osmotic pressure, as we observed in Chapter 1, refers to the concentration of

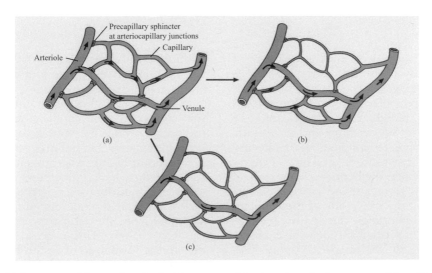

Figure 7.3 (a) Structure of the capillary bed with two possible alterations in the pattern of flow (b) and (c).

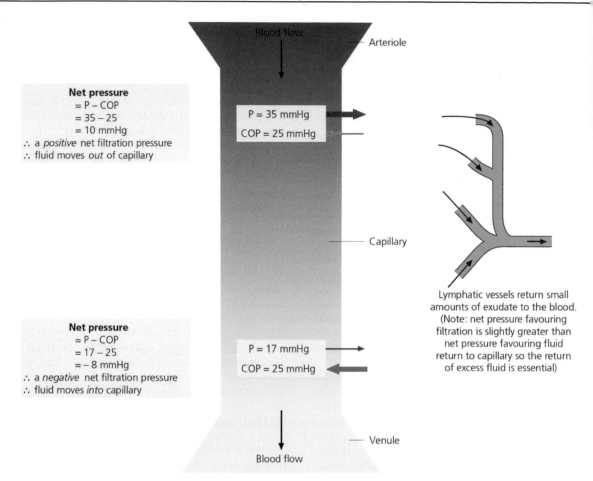

Net pressure
= P – COP
= 35 – 25
= 10 mmHg
∴ a *positive* net filtration pressure
∴ fluid moves *out* of capillary

P = 35 mmHg
COP = 25 mmHg

Blood flow

Arteriole

Capillary

Lymphatic vessels return small amounts of exudate to the blood. (Note: net pressure favouring filtration is slightly greater than net pressure favouring fluid return to capillary so the return of excess fluid is essential)

Net pressure
= P – COP
= 17 – 25
= – 8 mmHg
∴ a *negative* net filtration pressure
∴ fluid moves *into* capillary

P = 17 mmHg
COP = 25 mmHg

Venule

Blood flow

Figure 7.4 Fluid exchange between plasma and interstitial fluid across the capillary wall (P = fluid/hydrostatic pressure, COP = colloid osmotic pressure).

water and is influenced by the quantity of plasma proteins and solutes in the blood (e.g. albumin and sodium). Remember: the 'higher' the osmotic pressure the 'drier' (more concentrated) the blood. When blood enters the arteriole end of the capillary, the hydrostatic pressure is about 35 millimetres of mercury (mmHg) and the osmotic pressure is about 25 mmHg. Because the hydrostatic pressure in the capillary is greater than that of the interstitial fluid (on the other side of the capillary wall) and the osmotic pressure within the capillary, plasma is pushed through the capillary wall into the interstitial space (Figure 7.4). When the blood reaches the middle of the capillary bed, the hydrostatic and osmotic pressure

within the vessels are equal which allows fluid to pass evenly between the capillary and interstitial space. Exchange of gases, nutrients and waste products occurs at this point. Finally, at the venous end of the capillary, the hydrostatic pressure is about 17 mmHg, whilst osmotic pressure remains 25 mmHg (since plasma proteins are too big to pass through the capillary wall). Because hydrostatic pressure in the vessel is less than the osmotic pressure, fluid (as well as carbon dioxide and waste products) is pulled from the interstitial space into the capillary vessels. This process also contributes to the formation of lymph but instead of returning to the capillary/venous circulation, fluid drains from the interstitial space into a network of close-ended tubes called lymphatic capillaries (Chapter 6).

FLUID EXCHANGE

It is also important to note that any changes to osmotic and hydrostatic pressure can upset the exchange of fluid between the blood and interstitial compartment. We have seen (and will see time and again) that the body works best when homeostasis is maintained. For example, if osmotic pressure falls below hydrostatic pressure (e.g. as a result of low plasma protein levels in the blood), fluid is no longer pulled back into the capillaries from the interstitial space and oedema occurs. Similarly, if hydrostatic pressure is too high (e.g. as a result of raised blood pressure) too much fluid is pushed into the interstitial space at the arteriole end of the capillary which may also result in oedema and poor venous return (the quantity of blood returned to the heart). The brain contains a specialised wall of capillaries with very tight epithelial junctions called the blood-brain barrier (see Chapter 12). This prevents pathogens, proteins and a number of

other substances passing from the blood into the brain and causing disease and (potentially fatal) cerebral oedema. Lipid-soluble substances such as glucose, oxygen, carbon dioxide, alcohol and anaesthetic agents are able to cross the blood-brain barrier and other substances can do so very slowly (e.g. most ions). We will discuss selective permeability later in this chapter when we look at the role of the kidney in the long-term control of blood pressure but before we do, it is important to understand how the heart works.

THE HEART

We have already observed that the heart is a muscular pump that propels blood through the circulatory system in order to deliver the various substances it carries to where they are needed. For example, the heart ensures that tissues receive a constant supply of oxygen and glucose for cellular metabolism and that deoxygenated blood (containing carbon dioxide) is returned to the lungs to undergo gaseous exchange. From a functional point of view, therefore, the heart is quite easy to

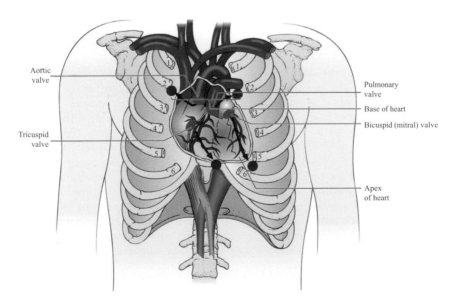

Figure 7.5 Location of the heart, heart valves (green spots) and auscultation sites for heart sounds (red spots) within the mediastinum.

understand. However, the way it maintains an uninterrupted (and appropriate) flow of blood through the circulatory system, and adapts to a constantly changing internal and external environment, is more complicated. In terms of the gross (visible to the naked eye) anatomy of the heart, it is about the size of its 'owners' fist and is situated between the two lungs roughly in the centre of the thoracic cavity (Figure 7.5). This central compartment is known as the mediastinum and also contains a number of large blood vessels, the oesophagus, trachea, thoracic duct, thymus gland and the phrenic and cardiac nerves. The inferior (lower) aspect of the heart is known as the apex because it forms a point that is directed toward the left hip. It rests upon the diaphragm at about the level of the fifth intercostal space (the gap between the fifth and sixth ribs). The superior (upper) aspect of the heart is somewhat confusingly known as the base (since it is flat) and is situated behind the sternum at the level of the third costal (rib) cartilage.

PERICARDIUM

The heart muscle (myocardium) itself is surrounded or enclosed by a double membranous sac called the pericardium (peri + cardium = around + heart). The outer membrane is known as the parietal pericardium and is reinforced by thick connective tissue (the fibrous pericardium) which protects the heart and anchors it to surrounding tissue. The term parietal is used in relation to a number of other anatomical structures within the body and typically refers to an outer layer or boundary (the Latin word *pariēs* means 'wall'). The inner layer of the pericardium is known as the visceral pericardium and adheres to the surface of the heart muscle (the Latin word *viscus* means 'organ'). This layer is sometimes also referred to as the epicardium (epi + cardium = above + heart). Anyway, whilst this is all very instructive, you are probably thinking: 'but what is the point of this double membranous sac?' In simple terms, it suspends the heart muscle (myocardium) in a membranous 'bag' within the mediastinum and allows it to contract in a frictionless environment. The two opposing membranes (one anchoring the heart in place – the other attached to the muscle itself) both secrete lubricating fluid into the thin cavity between them which enables them to glide over one another during myocardial contraction. The normal resting heart rate for an adult is between 60 to 100 beats per minute (bpm) which means that it must contract a minimum of 86, 400 times a day (60 × 60 × 24). Even if it were possible to retain a constant cardiac rhythm of 60 bpm (which, as we shall see, it isn't) this equates to 31.5 million contractions per year. The parietal and visceral pericardium perform an extremely important function, therefore, since they ensure that the heart is able to contract in a continuous fashion without sustaining contact damage as a result of friction or shearing forces. Viral and bacterial infection of the pericardium can result in a condition known as pericarditis where the pericardium becomes inflamed and (painful) friction occurs. In some cases, this may lead to another condition called pericardial or cardiac tamponade where fluid accumulates in the pericardial cavity and puts pressure on the heart. This prevents the heart from functioning properly and can result in a serious (and potentially fatal) reduction in cardiac output (see below).

MYOCARDIUM AND ENDOCARDIUM

The next (and by far the thickest) layer of the heart is the myocardium or cardiac muscle. We discussed cardiac muscle in Chapter 2 when we looked at the four different types of tissue and we already know that it is a specialised type of striated (striped) muscle that demonstrates characteristics of both skeletal and smooth muscle. For example, it can stretch in a limited way like smooth muscle but contracts with the force of skeletal muscle. This helps to ensure that it continues to work in a consistent and uninterrupted fashion over the course of our lives. It must also be able to rapidly increase workload if required (e.g. during fight or flight situations). One of the reasons the heart is able to achieve this is because the myocardial cells (myocardiocytes) have abundant reserves of the protein myoglobin that store oxygen and also contain large numbers of mitochondria. These sausage-shaped organelles (discussed in Chapter 2) are able to produce additional ATP (chemical energy) that enables the heart to step-up activity when necessary. Another unique feature of cardiac muscle is that it contains specialised myocardiocytes and nerve fibres that enable the heart to generate and transmit electrical impulses (see intrinsic conduction below). The final and innermost layer of the heart wall is the endocardium (endo + cardium = within + heart). The endocardium is continuous with the vascular endothelium that lines the blood vessels entering and leaving the heart and serves the same function. It is constructed from a single sheet of squamous epithelial cells (resting on a thin connective tissue layer) and provides a continuous 'non-stick' and non-thrombogenic surface for the blood to flow over within the heart. It lines all four chambers of the heart and covers the valves between them.

FOUR CHAMBERS, FOUR VESSELS, FOUR VALVES

In order to understand how the heart works it is necessary to recognise 12 key structures: 4 chambers, 4 blood vessels and 4 valves. The diagram of the heart below (Figure 7.6) may appear complicated at first glance but when broken down into these three groups (of four) it is fairly straightforward to understand. Firstly, the heart has four chambers: two upper (superior) chambers called atria, and two lower (inferior) chambers called ventricles (from the Latin word for 'belly'). The right and left atria are essentially receiving chambers for venous blood (remember all veins travel towards the heart). Both atria have relatively thin myocardial walls since only a small amount of muscular contraction is necessary to push the blood into the ventricles below (for the most part gravity is usually sufficient). On the anterior

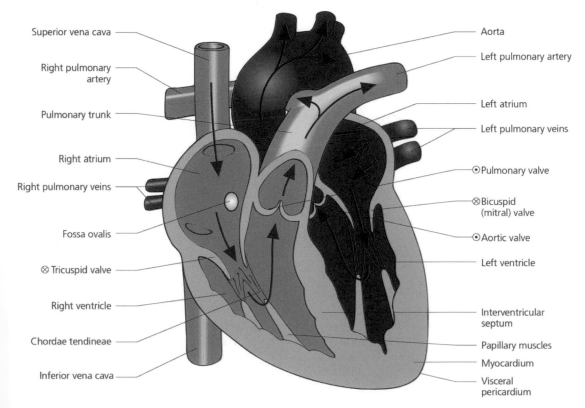

Figure 7.6 Chambers, blood vessels and valves of the heart.

(front) wall of each atria there is also a small wrinkled structure called an auricle (Latin for 'little ear') which helps to increase the volume of blood that each chamber can accommodate. The ventricles, on the other hand, have much thicker muscular walls since they have to pump blood against gravity (upwards) into the arteries (which always travel away from the heart). The heart is divided into right and left sides by a central partition called the ventricular septum. The right side of the heart receives deoxygenated blood from the body (following cellular respiration) which it pumps to the lungs (via the pulmonary circulation) in order that carbon dioxide can be exchanged for oxygen (see Chapter 9). Once this has occurred (in the pulmonary capillaries) the newly oxygenated blood returns to the left side of the heart where it is pumped into the systemic (whole-body) circulation and made available for cellular metabolism.

RIGHT SIDE OF THE HEART

This brings us nicely to the four blood vessels that supply the atria and drain the ventricles, and the four valves that prevent backflow (or regurgitation) of blood into the preceding chamber. The right atrium is supplied with deoxygenated blood by the superior (upper) and inferior (lower) branches of the vena cava (from the Latin words for 'hollow vein'). The superior vena cava drains oxygen depleted blood from the neck and chest whilst the inferior vena cava returns deoxygenated blood from the legs and abdomen. Once inside the right atrium, blood empties into the right ventricle through the first of the four valves: the tricuspid or right atrioventricular valve (since it is situated between the right atrium and ventricle). The term tricuspid simply refers to the fact that the valve has three cusps or flaps (covered in endocardium) which close during ventricular contraction to prevent backflow (Figure 7.6). The tricuspid valve is held in place by a series of strong fibrous cords known as chordae tendineae which are anchored to the walls of the ventricle below (also referred to as 'heart strings'). During right ventricular

contraction the blood is pumped from the lower chamber through another valve called the pulmonary semilunar valve. This is situated at the entrance to the pulmonary artery which, as its name suggests, carries blood away from the heart to the pulmonary system or lungs (the Latin word *pulmo* means 'lung'). The pulmonary semilunar valve consists of three membranous flaps of tissue that prevent backflow of blood from the pulmonary artery into the right ventricle. Although it is structurally similar to the preceding tricuspid valve it is less robust and not supported by chordae tendineae. However, it is still able to prevent backflow because of the pocket-like nature of the cusps on the arterial side of the valve. If blood flows back towards the ventricle, it fills the pockets of the cusp which press against one another to close the valve.

LEFT SIDE OF THE HEART

Once the blood has passed through the pulmonary artery (and gaseous exchange has taken place in the lungs) it is returned to the left side of the heart by the pulmonary vein. As noted above, it is convenient to divide the right and left side of the heart into two pumps: the right side pumping deoxygenated blood to the lungs (pulmonary circulation) and the left side pumping oxygenated blood to the rest of the body (systemic circulation). Unsurprisingly then, we find that the structures found on the right side of the heart are more or less mirrored on the left. Oxygenated blood enters the left atrium via the pulmonary veins (two from each lung, Figure 7.6). It is also worth noting at this point that the pulmonary artery and pulmonary veins are unusual in that the former is the only artery to carry deoxygenated blood and the latter is the only vein/s to carry oxygenated blood. This is the source of much head-scratching and (initial) confusion amongst students who have previously been taught that arteries carry oxygenated blood and veins carry deoxygenated blood. This is certainly true in most cases but not ALL. For example, during pregnancy, the umbilical cord which connects the placenta to the foetus, contains three blood vessels: two arteries and one vein. The umbilical vein carries oxygenated (and nutrient-rich) blood from the placenta to the developing foetus whilst the two arteries carry deoxygenated blood in the opposite direction. We are on much safer ground simply stating that veins always travel towards the heart and arteries away from it. Even in the case of the developing foetus, blood from the umbilical vein is shunted into the inferior vena cava and travels towards the heart, whilst the arteries carry blood away from the heart towards the placenta. However, let's not worry too much about this.

AORTA

To return to the adult heart, once blood has drained from the pulmonary arteries into the left atrium, it passes through the bicuspid or left atrioventricular valve. Functionally, it is exactly the same as the tricuspid valve on the right side of the heart (i.e. it prevents backflow of blood into the left atrium and is held

in place by chordae tendineae). Structurally, however, it only has two cusps (hence bicuspid) rather than three (tricuspid). It is not entirely clear why this occurs but may have something to do with the unique way blood flows through the heart during embryonic and foetal development. In any case, not content with two names, the bicuspid valve/left atrioventricular valve is also known as the mitral valve because of its dubious similarity to a Bishop's hat or Mitre. The final heart valve is the aortic semilunar valve and, as its name indicates, it is situated at the entrance to the aorta (Figure 7.6). Like the pulmonary semilunar valve, it consists of three membranous flaps and prevents backflow of blow from the artery into the (left) ventricle. The aorta itself is the largest artery in the body and is traditionally divided into the ascending aorta (from the left ventricle), the aortic arch (in the mediastinum) and the descending aorta which eventually divides (bifurcates) into two smaller arteries at the level of the fourth lumbar vertebra in the abdomen (Figure 7.7). The aorta not only transports oxygenated blood to the systemic circulation but also to the myocardium

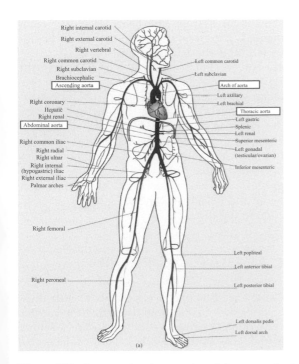
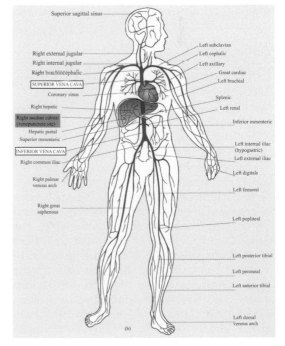

Figure 7.7 Aorta and major arteries of the systemic circulation.

TABLE 7.1 Twelve main structures of the heart

	Blood vessel	Chamber	Valve
1	vena cava (into)	R atrium	tricuspid
2	pulmonary artery (out of)	R ventricle	pulmonary semilunar valve
3	pulmonary vein (into)	L atrium	bicuspid
4	aorta (out of)	L ventricle	aortic semilunar valve

itself. Two coronary arteries originate at the ascending aorta and ensure that the heart muscle receives a continuous and prioritised supply of nutrient-rich blood consistent with the physiological demands placed upon it. The aortic arch supplies blood to the upper body via the brachiocephalic arteries (arms and chest), the carotid arteries (brain) and the subclavian arteries (arms and chest). The thoracic and abdominal aorta supply oxygenated blood to the rest of the body (excluding some parts of the lungs). In summary then, the heart has four chambers (two receiving and two pumping), four main blood vessels (two veins and two arteries) and four valves – all of which prevent backflow into the preceding chamber (see Table 7.1).

THE CARDIAC CYCLE

The function of the heart is to maintain constant circulation of blood to the lungs and body. In order to do this the ventricular myocardium (heart muscle) must contract (become shorter and tighter) to squeeze blood into the pulmonary artery and aorta (typically between 60 and 100 times each minute). This is known as ventricular systole (from the Greek word for 'contract') and is often simplified as 'the heart at work'. The heart then relaxes to allow blood from the vena cavae and pulmonary veins to drain through the atria and fill the empty ventricles before the next contraction occurs. This process is referred to as ventricular diastole (from the Greek word for 'draw apart') and is often simplified as 'the heart at rest'. The two phases of the cardiac cycle (work and rest) are equally important and must remain in balance to achieve efficient circulation and perfusion. The relationship between the two also explains some of the functional differences between the tri/bicuspid valves and the two semilunar valves. For example, during ventricular diastole (the heart at rest) the tricuspid and bicuspid valves are open in order to allow the ventricles to fill with blood in preparation for cardiac contraction. The semilunar valves, on the other hand, are both closed to prevent backflow of the recently ejected blood. Towards the end of this phase, the atria contract in order to force the remaining blood into the ventricles (sometimes referred to as the atrial kick). As ventricular systole (the heart at work) commences, the pressure in the ventricle begins to rise and the tricuspid and bicuspid valves are forced shut to prevent backflow into the atria. They are able to withstand this rapid increase in pressure (without turning inside out) because they are anchored in place by the chordae tendineae which are themselves attached to papillary muscles in the ventricles. In contrast, the unsecured membranous cusps of the semilunar valves are forced open by the pressure exerted by the contracting ventricular walls and blood is propelled into the arteries, completing the cycle.

CARDIAC OUTPUT

Using a stethoscope, it is possible to hear (auscultate) two distinct sounds during the cardiac cycle often described as 'lub' and 'dub'. The first sound (lub) is caused by the closing of the tricuspid and bicuspid valves at the beginning of ventricular systole. The dub sound occurs when the two semilunar valves close at the very end of this phase. Sometimes it is also possible to hear abnormal or unusual sounds when listening to the heart. We refer to these sounds as heart murmurs and they usually occur when normal flow of blood is interrupted. For example, if a valve is not able to close properly it is sometimes possible to hear a 'swishing' sound as blood is pushed back into the preceding chamber. If this occurs, not all of the blood within the chamber is pushed into the artery which results in a decrease in stroke volume. Stroke volume (SV) is defined as the amount of blood in millilitres (ml), pumped from the ventricle in one contraction or heartbeat. For a healthy man of about 70 kilograms (kg), stroke volume is estimated to be about 70 ml (normal range: 55–100 ml). Stroke volume is important since it contributes to cardiac output (CO) or the total amount of blood pumped from each ventricle in one minute. This is calculated by multiplying stroke volume (SV) by how many times the heart contracts per minute or heart rate (HR). This is summarised as:

$$SV \times HR = CO$$

For example, if a healthy man has a heart rate of 75 beats per minute and a stroke volume of 70 ml, his cardiac output will be 5,250 ml per minute (75 × 70 = 5,250). Or, to put it another way, in one minute his heart will pump 5.25 litres of blood around his body (slightly more than his total circulatory volume of about 5 litres).

CARDIAC OUTPUT AND EXERCISE

Using the same arithmetic as above, it is possible to demonstrate why exercise is good for our heart (in the long term at least). Firstly, let's imagine that, like me, you don't enjoy running much and have a perfectly respectable resting pulse (heart rate) of 75 beats per minute. Each day then, your heart beats 108, 000 times (24 hours × 60 minutes × 75 beats). Now let's imagine that you read a really good book (not this one) extolling the virtues of

exercise and begin to run for one hour every day with an average heart rate of 120 beats per minute. Crucially, as you become fitter over time, your resting pulse drops 5 beats per minute to 70. Now, in any given day, your heart contracts:

$$23 \times 60 \times 70 \ (= 96,600) + 1 \times 60 \times 120$$
$$(= 7,200)$$

Making a new total of 103, 800 times per day. By taking up running, therefore, you have 'saved' 4,200 beats per day or 1,533,000 beats per year! That is to say, your heart does not have to work as hard and, theoretically, lasts for longer. Convinced enough to put on your running/cycling/zumba shoes? On the other hand, the heart is described as failing when cardiac output is no longer sufficient to meet the metabolic needs of the body (i.e. the quantity of blood delivered to the tissues each minute is insufficient). This may be because heart rate is too low (or too high) or because stroke volume is poor. However, before we explore this concept further, we need to understand the mechanism that allows the heart to contract (beat) and to speed up and slow down as required.

INTRINSIC CONDUCTION

The contraction and relaxation of the myocardium (heart muscle) is coordinated through the activity of the heart's intrinsic conduction system. This allows the heart to independently initiate and distribute nerve impulses (action potentials) that allow the ventricles (and to a lesser degree the atria) to contract without the involvement of the central nervous system. This unique ability is known as automaticity (or auto-rhythmicity) and requires specialised cells called nodal or pacemaker cells. The main group of nodal cells is found in the wall of the right atrium (close to the entrance of the superior vena cava) and forms the sinoatrial or SA node (Figure 7.8). The SA node generates electrical impulses between 60 and 100 times per minute and sets the pace for the heart. For this reason, it is often referred to as the cardiac 'pacemaker' and the rhythm

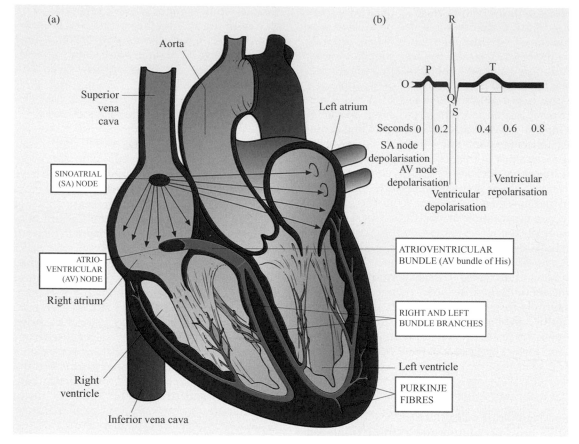

Figure 7.8 (a) Conduction system of the heart. (b) Normal electrocardiogram (ECG) of a single heartbeat.

that it generates (in health) is known as sinus rhythm. Each impulse is transmitted across the atrial surface by cell-to-cell contact within the inter-nodal pathways until it reaches the next bundle or collection of nodal cells. These are situated between the right atrium and right ventricle and form what is known as the atrio-ventricular or AV node. In health, the AV node functions as a distribution centre for the nerve impulses it receives from the SA node and, after a brief delay (approx. 0.1 seconds) to allow the atria to finish contracting, it dispatches the impulse towards the next stage of the conduction system. If the SA node or inter-modal pathways are damaged, however, it can generate impulses at a rate of between 40 and 60 beats per minute. This is not as efficient as the SA node but, given the alternative, it is

better than nothing! We will see later in the chapter how the AV node can also 'coordinate' aberrant and irregular impulses from the nodal cells of the atria (during atrial fibrillation).

PURKINJE FIBRES

Under normal circumstances, the AV node transmits the nerve impulse (action potential) to a bundle of nerve cells located in the ventricular septum called the bundle of His (or atrioventricular bundle). This provides electrical conduction to the ventricles and splits into two pathways: the right and left bundle branches (Figure 7.8). The left bundle branch is larger than the right since the left ventricle is more muscular. Both pathways extend towards the apex (point) of the heart before turning upwards and dividing into a network of filaments known as Purkinje fibres. These are located beneath the endocardium of the ventricular walls and distribute the electrical impulse into the muscle. If you have ever had the misfortune to electrocute yourself you will be aware that electricity stimulates involuntary muscular contraction (a jolt). Unlike this type of unwanted electrical activity, however, the network of Purkinje fibres conduct the electrical discharge in a controlled and coordinated fashion that stimulates myocardial contraction to squeeze the blood out of the chamber into the waiting arteries. Once the nerve impulse has dissipated into the muscle, the cycle begins again. This electrical activity can be observed using a cardiac monitor or electrocardiogram (ECG). A typical ECG has three distinguishable waves or deflections (Figure 7.8). The first P wave arises when the impulse from the SA node sweeps over the atrial walls. It appears small since the nerve impulse is still young and relatively weak. Approximately 0.01 seconds after the P wave occurs the atria contract in order to empty the remaining blood into the ventricles (late ventricular diastole). The PRS complex represents the rapid spread of electricity from the AV node into the Purkinje fibres and the corresponding contraction of the ventricular myocardium. This impressive spike of activity is relative to the quantity of electricity dissipated into the muscle and represents ventricular systole. Finally, the smaller T wave indicates the short resting period (ventricular repolarisation) before the next contraction takes place and coincides with early ventricular diastole.

CONDUCTION PROBLEMS

Changes in the size, duration and timing of P, QRS and T waves reflect problems with the intrinsic conduction system as a result of disease or damage to the heart. For example, an ST segment that is elevated or depressed indicates cardiac ischaemia (insufficient blood supply to the myocardium). One of the most

common reasons for this to occur is partial or complete occlusion of one (or more) of the coronary arteries by a blood clot (coronary thrombosis). If occlusion is complete, it may result in what is known as an ST elevation myocardial infarction or STEMI. This is a prime example of a medical term that appears completely incomprehensible but is actually highly descriptive. ST elevation, as we know, simply refers to the changes observed on the ECG (Figure 7.9). Myocardial, as we also know, refers to the heart muscle. Finally, the term infarction indicates obstruction of the blood supply to an organ (or area of tissue) by a thrombus or other embolus. This is more commonly referred to as a heart attack. Unfortunately, as a result of constant misrepresentation on the big and small screen, the term heart attack is often confused with cardiac arrest. Cardiac arrest refers to the cessation of normal cardiac activity (cardiac output), at which point the unfortunate person is technically dead and requires immediate resuscitation. During a heart attack, on the other hand, the person typically experiences chest pain (often described as crushing) as a result of myocardial ischaemia. In some cases, this can lead to cardiac arrest (either immediately or after the event) but the two are not synonymous. For example, the aim of treatment during a heart attack is to unblock the affected coronary artery, as quickly as possible, in order

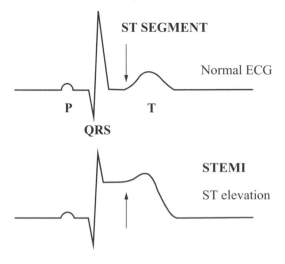

Figure 7.9 Normal ST segment and ST elevation.

to reperfuse the tissue with blood (providing oxygen and glucose) and minimise damage to heart muscle cells (myocardiocytes). If treatment is delayed or unsuccessful, damage to the ventricular myocardium results in inadequate cardiac output and increases the likelihood of cardiac arrest and/or chronic cardiac failure in the future. The aim of treatment during a cardiac arrest, on the other hand, is to 'restart' the heart (whilst providing cardio-pulmonary resuscitation) since there is no cardiac output and therefore no tissue perfusion.

CARDIAC ARREST

Before the heart stops altogether it often exhibits one of two 'tell-tale' pre-arrest arrhythmias (abnormal heart rhythm): ventricular tachycardia and/or ventricular fibrillation. Ventricular tachycardia (VT) occurs when Purkinje or nodal cells generate a series of abnormal electrical impulses (extrasystoles) in the ventricles at a rate of more than 120 beats per minute. These often originate around scar tissue (e.g. following a STEMI) or as a result of ischaemia or electrolyte imbalance. VT can significantly reduce cardiac output and may quickly deteriorate into ventricular fibrillation (VF) and asystole (a complete absence of systolic ventricular activity). During VF, the ventricles quiver or twitch (fibrillate) rather than contract which leads to a fatal deterioration in cardiac output with no audible or palpable (able to be felt) pulse. VT and VF are typically the only arrhythmias that are treated using a controlled 'shock' of electrical energy to the heart via a defibrillator. This is because defibrillation is intended to shock or convert the abnormal electrical activity exhibited by the cardiac muscle back into normal sinus rhythm. If the heart is in asystole, there is, by definition, no electrical activity and therefore nothing to shock (Figure 7.10). It is still possible to successfully resuscitate somebody whose heart has stopped but much more difficult to achieve and prognosis (outcome) is typically poor. Essentially,

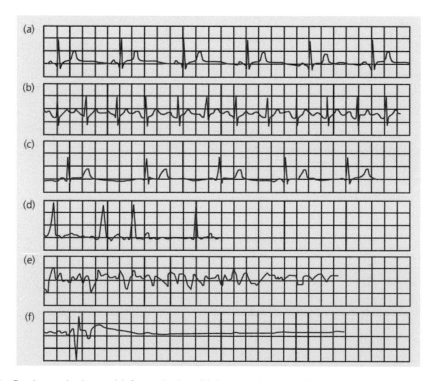

Figure 7.10 Cardiac arrhythmias. (a) Sinus rhythm. (b) Sinus tachycardia. (c) Sinus bradycardia. (d) Atrial fibrillation (AF). (e) Ventricular fibrillation (VF). (f) Asystole.

TABLE 7.2 Eight reversible causes of cardiac arrest (4 Hs/4 Ts)

Four Hs	Four Ts
Hypoxia	Tension pneumothorax
Hypovolaemia	Tamponade (cardiac)
Hypothermia	Toxins
Hyperkalaemia	Thromboembolism

the resuscitation team attempt to convert asystole into a 'shockable' rhythm, such as VT, by treating potentially reversible causes and administering regular doses of intravenous adrenaline (also known as epinephrine). Adrenaline is used primarily to increase blood flow to the heart and brain during cardiopulmonary resuscitation (CPR) but it can also stimulate myocardiocyte activity (automaticity) during asystole. Any electrical activity is better than none! There are a number of potentially reversible causes of cardiac arrest that, for ease of memory, are often presented as the four H's and four T's (see Table 7.2).

SURVIVING CARDIAC ARREST

The best way to survive a cardiac arrest is to have a witnessed arrest (preferably by a healthcare professional) somewhere that has easy access to a defibrillator (hospital, sports centre, school, etc.) since, at the point you collapse, it is likely that your heart will be in VT or VF (Figure 7.10). The worse place to have a cardiac arrest is on the golf course or somewhere equally inaccessible to assistance. Unfortunately, popular literature, film and television drama (medical in particular) consistently overemphasise the probability of successful resuscitation following cardiac arrest/asystole. Two examples of this are provided in the otherwise entertaining films *Casino Royale* and *The Hunger Games: Catching Fire*. In the first film, James Bond actually attempts to resuscitate himself after he is poisoned with digoxin (digitalis). There are so

many inconsistencies in this scene that I won't bore you with nerdy detail but the most obvious error is that Bond seems to defibrillate himself whilst in asystole. Not only is he technically dead when he performs this heroic act, it is also a completely pointless exercise for the reasons discussed above. The *Hunger Games* scene also contains many medical inaccuracies but my main criticism is the speed and vigour with which the character Peeta Mellark recovers following his electrocution and apparent cardiac arrest. He exhibits super-human resilience to his several minutes of technical death and, despite requiring full cardio-pulmonary resuscitation from morally ambiguous Finnick Odair, he staggers to his feet and carries on as if recovering from a nasty stitch (a few hours later he is battling killer monkeys). No wonder Katniss Everdeen secretly harbours deep feelings for him. Anyway, look out for your own examples of miraculous recoveries in film and television (you will know that it is becoming a problem when, like me, you start shouting at the television and making a list of the errors).

ATRIAL FIBRILLATION

The final conduction problem I want to briefly mention is atrial fibrillation (AF). This relatively common condition (it affects around 800, 000 people in the UK each year) occurs because the normal electrical impulses generated by the sinoatrial (SA) node are overwhelmed by disorganised electrical activity that originates in the atria and pulmonary veins. If all of these aberrant impulses were transmitted to the ventricles, the heart would soon tire and cardiac arrest would occur. Fortunately, the atrioventricular (AV) node acts as a natural circuit breaker and coordinates the transmission of an appropriate number of impulses from the nodal cells of the atria to the ventricles. The result is an irregular heartbeat which may occur in episodes lasting from minutes to weeks (paroxysmal AF) or could occur permanently for a number of years. Diagnosis is confirmed by the absence of P waves on ECG (remember that, in health, P waves are created when the impulse from the SA node sweeps over the atrial walls). Atrial fibrillation is not as serious as ventricular fibrillation (VF) since the atria only contract in order to empty about 30% of the blood into the waiting ventricle (the rest drains via gravity). It is frequently asymptomatic but can result in palpitations, breathlessness, fainting, chest pain and, over a period of time, chronic heart failure. It also increases the risk of suffering from a stroke (cerebral thrombosis) since turbulent blood flow in the heart can produce blood clots that are released into the circulatory system and become lodged in the narrow vessels of the brain. This causes ischaemia and tissue damage in the same way as coronary thrombosis or heart attack (which is why it is called 'brain attack' in Canada and the US).

SPEEDING UP

Although the heart can initiate and distribute nerve impulses without the involvement of the central nervous system (automaticity) it is innervated (supplied with nerves) by the autonomic nervous system (ANS). The ANS regulates many key involuntary functions including heart rate, respiratory rate, blood pressure and digestion (see below and Chapter 12). It has two antagonistic divisions: the sympathetic nervous system and the parasympathetic nervous system. The sympathetic division is responsible for our flight-or-fight response (in the most primitive sense, it prepares the body to expend energy to ensure survival). The parasympathetic nervous system, on the other hand, has the opposite effect and is responsible for facilitating 'resting and digesting' activities.

For example, the parasympathetic nervous system decreases heart rate, respiratory rate and blood pressure (e.g. following exercise or during sleep) increases gastrointestinal activity (including salivation) and relaxes sphincter muscles (you get the idea). The fact that the two divisions of the ANS are antagonistic allows them to maintain a stable internal environment (homeostasis) through opposing but complementary activity. In the case of the heart, both sympathetic and parasympathetic activity is controlled by the cardiovascular centre located in the medulla oblongata of the brainstem (see Chapters 8 and 12). For example, imagine that you spot a large, ferocious bear making its way towards you and, in the absence of anywhere to hide, you decide to run rather than fight. In order to provide your skeletal muscle with the additional oxygen and glucose it requires for intensive cellular metabolism, the cardio-acceleratory centre of the brain stimulates the sympathetic nervous system to increase heart rate. Sympathetic nerve endings secrete the neurotransmitter (and hormone) adrenaline which binds to beta-1 receptors on the sinoatrial (SA) node of the heart (the pacemaker). This encourages more sodium and calcium to enter the cells (through ion channels discussed in Chapter 2) and temporarily prevents potassium from exiting the cell. To put it simply: the cells of the sinoatrial node become more 'positive' (since sodium, calcium and potassium are all positive ions: Na^+, Ca^{++}, K^+) and produce nerve impulses at a faster rate than normal. The more nerve impulses that are generated from the sinoatrial node, the more ventricular contractions there are per minute, and the greater volume of blood that is pumped around the circulatory system (HR x SV = CO). This increases your chances of survival by allowing you to run from the bear at a faster rate (providing the bear is not particularly motivated and feeling a little under the weather).

SLOWING DOWN

Assuming that you have escaped from the bear and now stand panting behind a tree, the parasympathetic division of the autonomic nervous system begins to slow your heart rate down again. The cardio-inhibitory centre stimulates the vagus nerve of the parasympathetic nervous system to secrete another chemical messenger called acetylcholine. This decreases pacemaker activity (and current) by reducing the inward movement of Ca^{++} and Na^+ into the cell and encouraging the exit of K^+ from the cell. Consequently, heart rate declines and eventually returns to its normal or 'resting' rate. A student of mine once commented regarding this scenario that increasing the amount of glucose in the runner's blood might be counterproductive since it would make the person 'sweeter' and therefore more 'delicious' to the bear. I didn't have the energy to discuss why this was wrong at the time and simply congratulated him on his original analysis and encouraged him to complete an ethics application for a study as soon as possible. Of course

it is not just exercise that influences sinoatrial node (pacemaker) activity and many other physiological factors increase/decrease heart rate. For example, raised hormone levels (e.g. adrenaline and thyroxin) and changes in the serum concentration of calcium, potassium and other ions can all have potentially serious consequences if left untreated. This also helps to explain how some medications are able to reduce heart rate for therapeutic effect. For example, beta-blocker drugs prevent ('block') adrenaline and nor adrenaline from stimulating the beta receptors of the heart in order to slow and steady heart rate. Similarly, calcium channel blockers prevent calcium from entering the cell which (amongst other things) reduces the force with which the cardiac muscle contracts. Both drugs reduce the force produced during cardiac contraction (contractility) and are used to treat high blood pressure (hypertension).

CHAPTER 7: TEST YOURSELF

Q. What is meant by the term cardiovascular?
A. Cardiovascular refers to the relationship between the heart and the blood vessels.

Q. How many litres of blood does an average adult possess?
A. Five litres.

Q. Arteries and veins both have a fibrous outer layer (tunica externa), muscular middle layer (tunica media) and a smooth inner lining (tunica intima). Explain how they differ.
A. Arteries always travel away from the heart and veins travel towards it. Arterial walls are thicker than veins since they contain more smooth muscle (in the tunica media) to withstand greater pressure. Since veins return blood to the heart (at low pressure), many also contain valves to prevent backflow.

Q. List two places where you could (easily) palpate a pulse.
A. The radial artery (wrist) and the carotid artery (neck).

Q. Describe the structure and function of capillaries.
A. Capillaries consist of a single layer of endothelial cells through which water and other small molecules can pass (e.g. nutrients and waste products). They connect small arteries (arterioles) to small veins (venules) via a network of vessels known as a capillary bed.

Q. What is the principle function of the heart?
A. The heart is a muscular pump that propels blood through the circulatory system in order to deliver nutrients (including O_2) to the body and remove waste products.

(Continued)

(Continued)

Q. What are the three layers of heart called (from the outside in)?
A. Pericardium, myocardium and endocardium.

Q. What is the name of the structure that divides the heart into the right and left sides?
A. The ventricular septum.

Q. The heart has four chambers: right/left atria and right/left ventricles. How do atria and ventricles differ in structure and purpose?
A. The atria are receiving chambers for venous blood and have relatively thin myocardial walls since only a small amount of muscular contraction is necessary to push the blood into the ventricles below. The ventricles have much thicker muscular walls since they have to pump blood against gravity into the arteries.

Q. Name the veins that deliver blood to the heart and whether or not the blood is oxygenated or deoxygenated.
A. The superior and inferior vena cava deliver deoxygenated blood to the right atrium. The pulmonary veins deliver oxygenated blood to the left atrium (from the lungs).

Q. Name the arteries that transport blood away from the heart and whether the blood is oxygenated or deoxygenated.
A. The pulmonary artery transports deoxygenated blood from the right ventricle to the lungs. The aorta transports oxygenated blood from the left ventricle to the body as a whole.

Q. Describe the function and location of the four heart valves.
A. All four valves prevent back flow of blood into the preceding chamber. The tricuspid valve is located between the right atrium and ventricle. The bicuspid (or mitral) valve is located between the left atrium and ventricle. The pulmonary semilunar valve is located at the entrance to the pulmonary artery (to prevent back flow into the right ventricle). The aortic semilunar valve is located at the entrance to the aorta (to prevent back flow into the left ventricle).

Q. What is meant by ventricular systole and diastole in relation to the cardiac cycle?
A. Ventricular systole refers to the contraction of the ventricles to push blood into the arteries. Ventricular diastole refers to relaxation period where blood fills the ventricles ready for the next contraction.

Q. Cardiac output is the total amount of blood (in ml) pumped from each ventricle in one minute. It is calculated by multiplying stroke volume (SV) by how many times the heart contracts per minute (heart rate/HR). What is meant by stroke volume?
A. Stroke volume is defined as the amount of blood (in ml) pumped from each ventricle in one contraction or heartbeat.

Q. If a healthy adult has as heart rate of 75 beats per minute, and a stroke volume of 72 ml, what will their cardiac output be?
A. $75 \times 72 = 5,400$ ml per minute (or 5.4 litres per min).

Q. What is the function of the sinoatrial node (SAN) and where is it located?
A. The SAN is located in the wall of the right atrium and generates nerve impulses that set the pace and rhythm for the heart. It is often referred to as the 'pacemaker'.

Q. What is the function of the atrioventricular (AV) node and where is it located?
A. The AV node is located between the right atrium and right ventricle and functions as a distribution centre for the nerve impulses it receives from the SAN. After a brief delay, to allow the atria to finish contracting, it dispatches the impulse towards the next stage of the conduction system.

Q. What effect does the sympathetic nervous system have on heart rate?
A. The sympathetic nervous system increases heart rate by stimulating beta-1 receptors on the SAN (pacemaker).

Q. What effect does the parasympathetic nervous system have on heart rate?
A. The vagus nerve of the parasympathetic nervous system inhibits pacemaker activity and reduces heart rate.

Contents

CHAPTER 8

BLOOD PRESSURE

BLOOD PRESSURE

Blood pressure (BP) simply refers to the pressure exerted on the on the walls of the blood vessels each time the heart contracts. Whenever any substance is held in a container it exerts some kind of pressure on the walls of that container. For example, if we attach a garden hose to a kitchen tap (essentially a pump) the water pressure on the walls of the hose gradually decreases the further it gets from the tap – resulting in a low pressure dribble at the very end. However, if we increase the volume of water entering the hose at the tap, we also increase the pressure within the tube and the rate at which water

passes through it. Similarly, if we squeeze the hose where the water exits, we further increase the water pressure exerted against the walls of the hose (because we have created a partial blockage) which allows the water to spray further into the garden. Every child intuitively discovers this basic principle when attempting to soak their friend/sibling/parent as they run away from the freezing jet of water aimed at them. In much the same way, blood exerts pressure on the walls of the vessels as it passes through them. The closer to the pump (ventricles) the vessels are, the greater the pressure exerted by the blood within them and in Chapter 7 we noted that arteries have a greater proportion

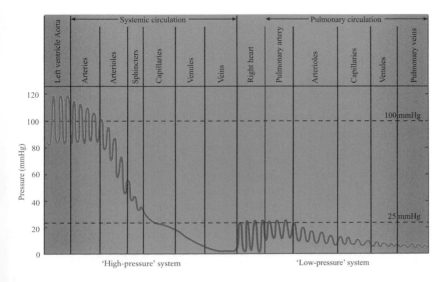

Figure 8.1 Blood pressure changes within the circulatory system.

of muscle than veins and capillaries in order to accommodate greater pressure. Consequently, systemic blood pressure is highest in the aorta (leaving the left ventricle) and lowest in the vena cava as it returns to the right atrium (Figure 8.1).

SYSTOLIC AND DIASTOLIC PRESSURE

Like the cardiac cycle discussed in Chapter 7, blood pressure is divided into systolic and diastolic measurements which reflect the difference in pressure when the heart is and isn't contracting (i.e. the heart at work and the heart at rest). When the left ventricle contracts, it pushes blood through the aortic semilunar valve into the aorta. Blood moves forwards because the pressure exerted by the contracting ventricle is greater than that in the arteries and distal vessels. The systolic pressure represents the pressure exerted by the blood against the walls of the arteries and, in a healthy adult, averages about 120 mmHg. The fact that blood is under relatively high pressure in the arteries (as a result of ventricular contraction) explains why, when an artery is cut, blood pumps rhythmically and copiously from the vessel. The actual distance a punctured artery can 'squirt' depends on whether the artery is completely or partially severed and whether it is squirting vertically or horizontally. The diastolic pressure, on the other hand, represents the lowest pressure in the arteries as the ventricles relax following contraction and averages about 80 mmHg in a healthy adult (Figure 8.1). The difference between systolic and diastolic pressure is known as pulse pressure (PP) and represents the force that the heart generates each time it contracts. For example, the pulse pressure for somebody with a BP of 120/80 mmHg is 40 mmHg (120–80 = 40).

MEAN ARTERIAL PRESSURE

Another important measurement is the mean arterial pressure (MAP). This is the average arterial pressure during a single cardiac cycle or the pressure that propels blood to the tissues. However, because diastole (filling) typically lasts twice as long as systole (pumping), MAP is not simply a 'central' value between the two pressures. Instead, it is calculated by adding x2 diastolic to x1 systolic pressure and then dividing by 3.

$$MAP = [(2 \times diastolic) + systolic] \div 3$$

Consequently, the MAP for a man with a blood pressure of 120/80 is 93 mmHg.

$$(80 + 80 + 120) \div 3 = 93.3$$

Or, if you prefer, you can calculate MAP by adding the diastolic value to the pulse pressure divided by 3.

$$80 + (40 \div 3) = 93.3$$

The reason it is important to measure/be aware of MAP, is that it reflects the perfusion pressure of the vital organs. A MAP of 60 mmHg or above is necessary to perfuse the tissues of the brain and kidneys and normal range is typically 70–110 mmHg.

VENOUS RETURN

Before we examine how the body controls blood pressure, it is important to discuss venous return (i.e. how blood returns to the right side of the heart and why it is important). Venous return is defined as the quantity of blood delivered to the right atrium each minute by the superior and inferior vena cavae. If venous return is poor or inadequate, it has a direct effect on the amount of blood the ventricles are able to pump from the heart each minute (cardiac output). However, by the time blood reaches the veins from the capillaries, pressure is low and it requires mechanical assistance to continue its journey from the peripheries to the heart. For example, in order to facilitate the passage of blood from the toes to the torso (against gravity), the veins of the lower leg contain one-way valves (Figure 7.2). As the veins are squeezed by the muscles of the calf during physical activity, blood is forced upwards through these valves. Back flow is not possible, because the weight of the blood compresses the valve's two membranous flaps and forces it shut in a similar fashion to the semilunar valves of the pulmonary artery and aorta. Over time, however, valves become less competent which can lead to the development of varicose (abnormally swollen) veins as gravity causes backflow and the blood pools in the lower vessels. This increases venous blood pressure which not only leads to their twisted and lumpy appearance but also contributes to the incidence of venous leg ulcers.

PRELOAD AND AFTERLOAD

Another mechanism that assists venous return is the respiratory muscle pump. As the respiratory muscles contract and relax during breathing (see Chapter 11), pressure changes in the thoracic and abdominal cavities squeeze the veins and propel or 'pull' blood back towards the heart. These (and other) mechanisms ensure that venous return is always equal to cardiac output (otherwise blood would accumulate in either the systemic or pulmonary circulations). Both venous return and cardiac output are regulated by what is known as Starling's law (or the Frank–Starling mechanism). This states that the strength of the heart's systolic contraction is directly proportional to its diastolic expansion. This sounds very 'sciency' but is really quite straightforward. Basically, the more blood that returns to the heart (venous return), the more ventricular filling that occurs. This is referred to as preload or end-diastolic volume (EDV) since it equates to how much blood fills the ventricle at the end of diastole. The word preload more accurately describes the force exerted by the blood on the walls of the ventricle before (pre) contraction. This extends or 'stretches' the ventricular myocardium (heart muscle) which results in a corresponding increase in force-generation when contraction occurs. This is often compared to stretching an elastic band since the further you extend it, the greater the recoil will be (and pain if it snaps back against your hand).

Any change in ventricular preload, therefore, must affect ventricular stroke volume. For example, if a person bleeds (haemorrhages) from an arterial wound, their blood quickly exits the circulatory system and overall circulatory volume declines. This leads to poor venous return and a corresponding decrease in cardiac output (possibly leading to acute cardiac failure and cardiac arrest if untreated). Stroke volume and cardiac output are also influenced by afterload. This refers to the force exerted by the blood on the walls of the ventricle following contraction. Only about two-thirds of the blood in the ventricle is pumped out with each beat and the remaining blood is known as the end systolic volume (ESV). Afterload also describes the pressure that the ventricle must generate in order to force open the aortic semilunar valve and eject blood into the systemic circulation. Any factor that restricts arterial blood flow (e.g. peripheral resistance or obstruction) causes an increase in afterload and end systolic volume, and a decrease in stroke volume.

EJECTION FRACTION

It is possible to calculate stroke volume by subtracting end systolic volume (afterload) from end-diastolic volume (preload). Put simply: the volume of blood in the ventricle after contraction divided by the volume of blood in the ventricle before contraction. If we then divide stroke volume by end-diastolic volume (preload) and multiply by 100 we can also calculate what is known as the ejection fraction (EF).

$$[SV \div EDV] \times 100 = EF$$

Ejection fraction is simply the percentage of blood pumped from the filled ventricle following one heartbeat. As stated above, only about two-thirds of the blood in the ventricle is ejected with each contraction and an ejection fraction of 55–70% is considered normal. For example, the stroke volume (SV) for an average 70 kg man is about 70 ml and the (left ventricular) end-diastolic volume (EDV) is about 120 ml. This provides an ejection fraction of 58%

$$[70 \div 120 = 0.58] \times 100 = 58\%$$

An ejection fraction of 40% or less is usually indicative of heart failure. An ejection fraction of more than 75% may indicate a heart condition where the heart muscle begins to thicken called hypertrophic cardiomyopathy (enlargement + heart + muscle + disease).

SHORT-TERM CONTROL OF BP

Although blood pressure is affected by a number of different factors (e.g. age, exercise, posture, medication etc.), the two principle determinants of blood pressure are cardiac output (CO) and total peripheral resistance (TPR). Cardiac output, as we know from Chapter 7, refers to the total amount of blood (ml) pumped from each ventricle in one minute (SV × HR = CO). In simple terms, this is a reflection of the 'work done' by the heart. Total peripheral resistance, on the other hand, is the total resistance to the flow of blood that is caused by the peripheral (small vessel) circulation. There are three factors that influence TPR: blood vessel diameter, total blood vessel length and blood viscosity. Viscosity refers to how 'thick' or 'sticky' a fluid is. A fluid with low viscosity such as water (viscosity = 1 centipoise/cP) is said to be 'thin'; whilst a fluid with high viscosity such as honey (viscosity = 2,000–3,000 cP) is said to be 'thick'. Blood is literally and metaphorically thicker than water (viscosity = 5 cP) because it contains erythrocytes, leucocytes, plasma proteins and a variety of solutes (Chapter 5). The more of these cells and solutes that blood contains, the more viscous it will become and the greater the resistance that will occur as it travels through the small vessels in particular. Other factors that influence blood viscosity include the amount of circulating fat and temperature (Chapter 3). The world's longest running experiment (started in 1927 at the University of Queensland, Australia) was established to investigate (amongst other things) the viscosity of pitch (tar). It has been estimated that it takes between 7 and 13 YEARS for one drop of pitch to form but only a tenth of a second for it to fall. Frustratingly, John Mainstone (who oversaw the experiment for more than 50 years) missed the drops fall on all three occasions during his 'watch'.

RESISTANCE

We have observed that the pumping action of the heart generates flow and when flow is opposed by resistance it results in pressure. This is not necessarily a bad thing, of course, and it is important to remember that maintaining adequate blood pressure is essential for cellular health. In order for blood to circulate to and from the heart and lungs it must frequently travel against gravity. This is nowhere more important than the passage of oxygenated blood from the left side of heart to the brain via the carotid and vertebral arteries. If blood pressure is inadequate for some reason (e.g. dehydration) it can result in cerebral hypoxia (low levels of oxygen reaching the brain tissue) and loss of consciousness. So how does the body prevent this from occurring? Well, since blood pressure is determined by cardiac output and total peripheral resistance, the cardiovascular centre of the brain can do two things more or less immediately: increase heart rate (HR × SV = CO) and selectively narrow blood vessels (vasoconstriction) in order to increase resistance. Alternatively, if blood pressure is too high (putting additional strain on the heart muscle and blood vessels) it can stimulate the heart to beat less forcefully and vasodilatation to take place. In order for this to occur, however, the body must detect that blood pressure is outside normal homeostatic parameters. This is achieved in exactly the same way as other homeostatic mechanisms – using a homeostatic feedback loop consisting of a detector, an integrator (control centre) and effector processes (influencing CO and TPR). In this instance, the detectors (or sensors) are called baroreceptors and are situated in the carotid arteries and aortic arch (Figure 8.2). This location makes perfect sense since these vessels experience the greatest pressure, as

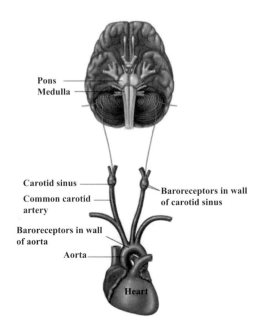

Pons
Medulla

Carotid sinus
Common carotid
artery
Baroreceptors in wall
of carotid sinus

Baroreceptors in wall
of aorta
Aorta
Heart

Figure 8.2 Baroreceptors.

blood is pumped out of the left ventricle, and provide blood to all of the organs of the cranial, thoracic and abdominal cavities. When arterial blood pressure increases, it stretches the baroreceptors and stimulates the transmission of nerve impulses (action potentials) towards the cardiovascular centre situated in the medulla of the brainstem (see Chapter 12).

CARDIOVASCULAR CENTRE (CVC)

The CVC consists of two complementary systems which help to regulate blood pressure: the vasomotor centre which adjusts the diameter of the blood vessels (vasoconstriction/dilation) to provide more or less resistance to flow, and the cardiac control centre which increases/decreases heart rate. The vasomotor centre is a cluster of neurons (nerves) that transmits action potentials at regular intervals along sympathetic motor nerves to the smooth muscle of blood vessels. The majority of these blood vessels are arterioles which remain in a state of moderate constriction called

vasomotor tone. In Chapter 7 we saw how the CVC utilises the cardio-acceleratory and cardio-inhibitory pathways of the sympathetic and parasympathetic nervous system to regulate heart rate and therefore cardiac output/blood pressure. However, to recap: following exertion (having escaped from the bear), blood pressure is still high. In order to return blood pressure (and heart rate) to normal, the cardiac control centre responds in two ways. Firstly, the cardio-acceleratory pathway is INHIBITED which results in fewer action potentials travelling down sympathetic motor nerves to the heart. This results in the secretion of less adrenaline and noradrenaline which inhibits sinoatrial node (pacemaker) activity. The cardio-inhibitory neurons of the parasympathetic nervous system, on the other hand, respond by generating more action potentials which also inhibit sinoatrial node activity and lessen heart rate/force of ventricular contraction. At the same time, fewer action potentials travel down the sympathetic motor neurons to the blood vessels. This results in the relaxation of the muscle (tunica media) and vasodilation occurs. All three of these responses combine to lower blood pressure (Figure 8.3). The opposite occurs to correct low blood pressure.

PROPRIOCEPTORS AND CHEMORECEPTORS

Two other types of sensory nerve also provide input to the CVC in order to manage blood pressure. The first, proprioceptors, are situated in muscles and joints and provide awareness of movement and position (Chapter 4). However, they also transmit action potentials to the CVC during exercise and account for the rapid increase in heart rate at the beginning of intense physical activity (such as sprinting from a bear). The other type of receptors that contribute to the regulation of blood pressure, monitor the concentration of carbon dioxide and pH in the blood. They are known as chemoreceptors (chemical receptors) and are situated in the aortic arch and carotid arteries (the same place as the baroreceptors) and in the medulla oblongata. Chemoreceptors are

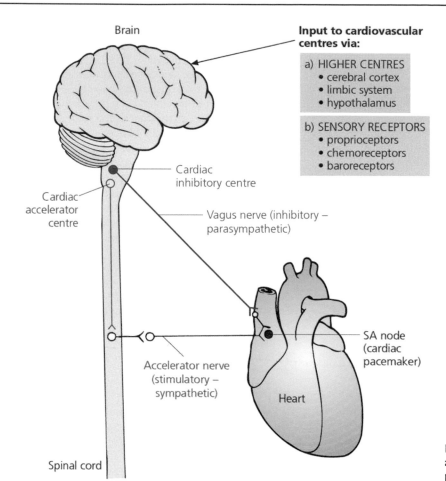

Figure 8.3 Cardio-acceleratory and inhibitory pathways.

more commonly associated with respiratory rate (see Chapter 9) and only influence blood pressure when there is severe disruption of respiratory function or when arterial blood pressure falls below about 80 mmHg.

LONG-TERM CONTROL OF BLOOD PRESSURE

Short-term control of blood pressure is principally regulated by the nervous system through adjustment and correction of cardiac output and peripheral resistance. Long-term control, on the other hand, is coordinated by the kidneys through the management of blood volume. This is because although baroreceptors are able to respond to sudden changes in blood pressure, they are relatively ineffective when changes are persistent or sustained. That is to say, over a period of time, they adjust or 'acclimatise' to high or low blood pressure. We have already observed that the average adult has approximately 5 litres of blood distributed throughout their cardiovascular system (of which about 3 litres is plasma). We also know that fluid exerts pressure on the walls of its container. Consequently, by increasing or decreasing the amount of fluid (plasma) in the cardiovascular system it is possible to regulate the pressure it exerts (blood pressure). The kidneys achieve this in a number of ways. Firstly, when blood volume and blood pressure rise (as an inevitable consequence of drinking) the rate at which plasma filters from the blood into the microtubules of the kidney also increases (see Chapter 10). This results in the production of more urine and a reduction in blood volume and pressure. Conversely, when blood volume/pressure is low, the kidneys secrete a hormone called renin that triggers a series of chemical and enzymatic reactions in order to increase blood volume and pressure (Figure 8.4). Firstly, the glycoprotein angiotensinogen (produced in the liver) is cleaved/broken-up by renin to produce angiotensin I. This in turn, is quickly converted into angiotensin II by angiotensin-converting enzyme (ACE). Angiotensin II has two very important functions. Firstly, it is a powerful vasoconstrictor. This increases blood pressure by increasing vascular resistance (i.e. TPR). Secondly, it stimulates the adrenal glands to secrete a steroid hormone called aldosterone. Aldosterone increases the amount of sodium (Na^+) reabsorbed from the 'early urine' (produced in the millions of renal tubules found in the kidney) back into the capillary circulation. In Chapter 1, we observed that the quantity of an ion (or other solute) dissolved in water will have an effect on the osmolality (osmotic concentration) of that solution. Consequently, the addition of Na^+ to the capillary blood serves to increase

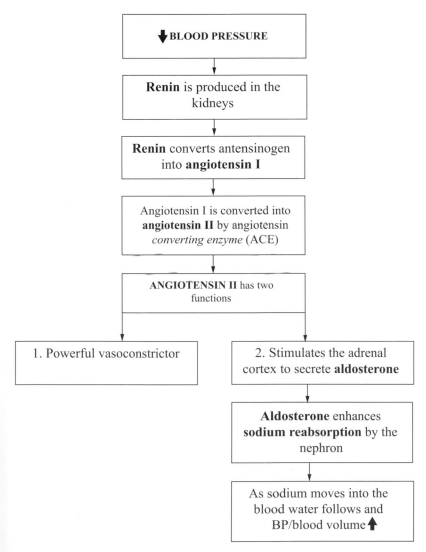

Figure 8.4 Renin – Angiotensin – Aldosterone System (RAAS).

its osmolality and 'pulls' fluid from the early urine, across the semi-permeable walls of the renal tubules into the bloodstream. Or, to put it another way, fluid is transported from a high concentration of water in the renal tubules, to a lower concentration of water in the capillary blood (via osmosis). The result is a decrease in urine output, an increase in blood volume and a corresponding increase in blood pressure (don't worry if you are struggling to follow this, it will be explained again in Chapter 10).

PREVENTING REABSORPTION

It is possible to 'interfere' with the mechanism described above in order to manage chronic high blood pressure (hypertension). For example, a group of drugs called ACE inhibitors hinder the action of angiotensin-converting enzyme (ACE). This reduces the production of angiotensin II which – in turn – reduces vasoconstriction and the secretion of aldosterone (which would normally result in sodium reabsorption in the kidney and fluid retention). Another group of drugs that also interfere with the action of aldosterone in order to treat high blood pressure are called aldosterone receptor antagonists (aldosterone blockers). These encourage urine production (diuresis) by inhibiting aldosterone sensitive sodium reabsorption at the distal (far) end of the renal tubules. This sounds more complicated than it is and essentially they make you wee more by preventing sodium transport from the renal tubules into the blood (see Chapter 10). The body also produces a number of hormones to manage and correct high blood pressure. For example, atrial natriuretic hormone (ANH) is a peptide (protein) hormone secreted by the atrial myocardiocytes in response to atrial distention (stretching) and high blood pressure. In simple terms, it performs the opposite function of aldosterone which is secreted in response to low blood pressure/hypotension. ANH is a powerful vasodilator and helps to reduce the reabsorption of sodium in the

renal tubules resulting in increased sodium loss/urine output (natriuresis) and decreased circulatory volume. Many of these hormones and mechanisms are discussed again in Chapters 10 and 13.

RECORDING BLOOD PRESSURE

We have observed that different blood vessels withstand different ranges of pressure depending on their type and position within the circulatory system (Figure 8.1). When recording blood pressure in practice, however, the clinician is seeking to measure arterial pressure and, more specifically, the highest pressure in the arteries when the ventricles contract (systole) and the lowest pressure in the arteries when the ventricles relax (diastole). This is expressed as the systolic value over the diastolic value (e.g. 120/80 mmHg) and is typically recorded using an automatic or manual sphygmomanometer. The word 'sphygmo' is from the Greek for 'pulse' and a manometer is an instrument that records pressure (i.e. the pressure of a pulse). When recording a manual blood pressure, the clinician secures the deflated cuff of the sphygmomanometer around the upper arm just above the elbow and over the brachial artery (Figure 8.5). They then palpate (feel) for the radial pulse located at the wrist. A pulse is simply a wave of distension (swelling from internal pressure) felt in an artery, as blood is propelled through it following ventricular contraction. It can be palpated at any point where a superficial artery can be pressed against a bone or solid prominence (a hard bit). For example, the radial artery is palpated against the distal radius of the wrist, whilst the carotid artery is palpated against the thyroid cartilage of the neck. Once the clinician can feel the radial pulse they inflate the cuff – watching the pressure dial/gauge at all times – until the pulse can no longer be detected. This indicates that the pressure in the cuff is greater than the systolic pressure in the brachial artery. The artery has essentially been flattened by the inflated cuff,

(a)

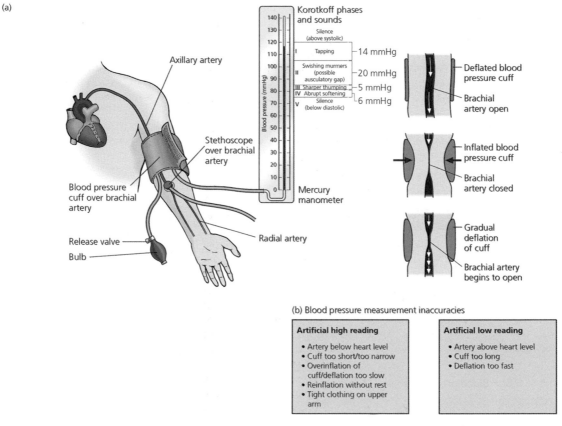

Figure 8.5 (a) Measuring blood pressure. (b) Common blood pressure measurement inaccuracies.

which prevents blood from flowing through the vessel. As soon as the radial pulse can no longer be felt, the pressure reading on the dial is noted (e.g. 120 mmHg) and the cuff is quickly deflated to allow blood to return to the lower arm. This 'number' provides a rough indication of the systolic pressure and a guide for future cuff inflation.

KOROTKOFF SOUNDS

When the clinician is ready to record the patient's blood pressure they place the diaphragm of their stethoscope over the brachial artery and inflate the cuff to approximately 30 mmHg above the estimated systolic pressure

(in this case 120 mmHg). The cuff once again flattens the artery and no sound can be heard via the stethoscope since blood flow has been interrupted. However, as the clinician slowly deflates the cuff, blood forces its way through the compressed vessel once the systolic pressure in the artery is equal to that of cuff. But how does this generate noise that can be heard and interpreted using a stethoscope? We know that blood pressure alternates between systolic and diastolic pressures as the heart contracts and relaxes (refills). During systole, therefore, blood pressure is great enough to force the artery walls open (beneath the cuff) and for blood to advance. As the pressure falls during diastole, however, the artery walls collapse and blood flow is once again interrupted. This process generates turbulence in the vessel that can be detected as a 'thudding' or 'swishing' sound. When these sounds are no longer audible, it demonstrates that the pressure in the artery is equal to the diastolic pressure (i.e. there is no sound because there is no turbulence). In summary: the first sound heard through the stethoscope represents the systolic value, and the cessation of all sound represents the diastolic value. This explains the look of pained concentration on the face of many clinicians when attempting to record a manual blood pressure. The sounds themselves are known as Korotkoff sounds after the Russian surgeon Nikolai Korotkoff (1874–1920), who first recognised that they were generated in the arteries and could be employed to measure blood pressure. They are typically divided into five phases characterised by volume and tonal quality (Table 8.1). Normal blood pressure is considered to be around 120/80 mmHg and Table 8.2 summarises normal and high (hypertensive) values.

TABLE 8.1 Korotkoff sounds

Phase	Korotkoff sounds	Typical cuff pressure (mmHg)
I	Tapping or thud	120
II	Swishing sound	110
III	Softer thud	100
IV	Softer blowing sound (that disappears)	90
V	Silence	80

TABLE 8.2 Blood pressure range

Range of blood pressure	Systole (mmHg)	Diastole (mmHg)
Optimal	<120	<80
Normal	120–129	80–84
High-normal	130–139	85–89
Grade 1: mild hypertension	140–159	90–99
Grade 2: moderate hypertension	160–179	100–109
Grade 3: severe hypertension	>180	>110

CHAPTER 8: TEST YOURSELF

Q. Provide a simple definition for blood pressure (BP)?
A. The pressure exerted on the circulatory system (blood vessels) each time the heart contracts.

Q. What are the two principle determinants of BP?
A. Cardiac output (CO) and total peripheral resistance (TPR).

Q. What is considered to be a 'normal' BP for an adult (remember to include the units)?
A. 120/80 mmHg.

Q. When recording a BP, the upper number refers to the systolic value and the lower number to the diastolic value. Describe what is meant by the terms systolic and diastolic pressure?

A. Systolic pressure represents the pressure exerted by the blood against the walls of the arteries following ventricular contraction. Diastolic pressure represents the lowest pressure in the arteries as the ventricles relax following contraction. This value is influenced by the diameter of blood vessels.

Q. What is meant by pulse pressure (PP) and mean arterial pressure (MAP)?

A. PP is the difference between systolic and diastolic pressure and represents the force that the heart generates each time it contracts. MAP is the average arterial pressure during a single cardiac cycle or the pressure that propels blood to the tissues. A MAP of ≥60 mmHg is necessary to perfuse the tissues of the brain and kidneys.

Q. Is BP the same in arteries and veins?

A. BP is significantly higher in arteries. The highest pressure is in the aorta (exiting the left ventricle) and the lowest is in the vena cavae as blood returns to the right atrium (typically 2–4 mmHg).

Q. The cardiovascular centre (CVC) of the brain controls BP. What are the principle mechanisms it employs to do this?

A. The vasomotor centre adjusts the diameter of the blood vessels (vasoconstriction/dilation) to provide more or less resistance to flow (TPR). The cardiac control centre uses the sympathetic and parasympathetic nervous systems to increase/decrease heart rate and therefore CO (since HR × SV = CO).

Q. What is the name of the sensory nerve receptors that detect when BP is too high/low and where are they located?

A. Baroreceptors transmit nerve impulses towards the CVC in response to an increase/decrease in arterial BP (stretch). They are located in the carotid arteries and aortic arch.

Q. Long-term control of BP is coordinated by the kidneys through the management of blood volume. What is the name of the hormone secreted by the kidneys in response to low BP and how does it bring about change (remember the acronym RAAS)?

A. When blood pressure/volume is low, the kidneys secrete a hormone called renin. Renin triggers the production of angiotensin I which is converted into angiotensin II by angiotensin-converting enzyme (ACE). Angiotensin II helps to increase BP in two ways: it is a powerful vasoconstrictor and it triggers the secretion of aldosterone from the adrenal glands. Aldosterone increases the amount of sodium (Na^+) reabsorbed from the distal convoluted tubule (DCT) of the nephron back into the capillary circulation. Water is transported by osmosis from a high concentration (in the DCT) to a lower concentration (in the capillary blood). The increase in blood volume produces a corresponding increase in BP (and decrease in urine output).

Q. What is the principle function of atrial natriuretic hormone (ANH) and where is it secreted?

A. ANH is secreted by heart muscle cells (myocardiocytes) in response to atrial distention and high BP. It is a powerful vasodilator and reduces the reabsorption of sodium in the renal tubules resulting in increased production of urine (diuresis). This decreases circulatory volume and helps to lower BP (the opposite effect of aldosterone).

Contents

LUNGS

The lungs are a pair of cone-shaped organs situated in the thoracic (chest) cavity on either side of the heart/mediastinum. Contrary to popular belief, they are not identical to one another and the right lung has three lobes whilst the left has only two in order to accommodate the heart (Figure 9.1). Unlike the heart, the apex (point) of each lung is located at the top (at the level of the clavicles) whilst the base rests upon the diaphragm below. The anterior, posterior and lateral surfaces of the lungs are situated in close contact to the ribs and form a continuous curving surface held in place by a thin membranous sheet called the parietal pleura. This membrane also covers the thoracic surface of the diaphragm and separates the pleural cavity from the mediastinum. Another membrane called the visceral (organ) pleura overlays the surface of the lungs and dips into the fissures. The two opposing membranes secrete serous fluid into the thin space or pleural cavity between them. This allows the lungs to expand and deflate in a frictionless environment similar to that produced by the parietal and visceral pericardium

of the heart (Chapter 7). Although the pleural membranes glide over one another during inspiration and expiration, the surface tension created by the lubricating fluid prevents them from separating. This is often compared to a thin film of water between two plates of glass, which allows them to slide over one another but also makes it difficult to separate them. The importance of these two membranes is painfully demonstrated when they become inflamed and produce less pleural fluid than normal as a result of the condition pleurisy. Pleuritic chest pain is often described as sharp, stabbing or burning and results when the two membranes scrape over one another during breathing, sneezing or laughing. Conversely, the pleura can also produce too much fluid which exerts pressure on the lungs and limits expansion. In health, however, the pleural membranes ensure that the exchange of air between the lungs and the atmosphere (ventilation) remains a passive and largely unconscious process (see below). Air enters and leaves the lungs via a series of large and small airways but before we look at these in detail, it is important to understand why and where respiration takes place – the lungs are only the beginning of the process.

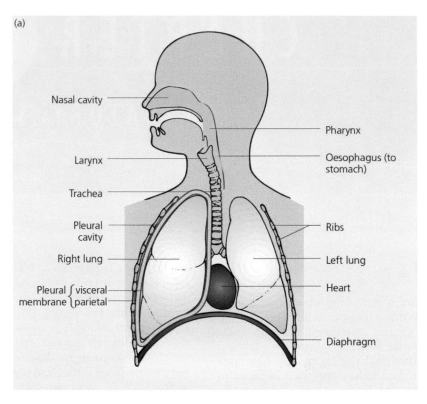

(a)

Nasal cavity

Pharynx

Larynx

Oesophagus (to stomach)

Trachea

Pleural cavity

Ribs

Right lung

Left lung

Pleural { visceral
membrane { parietal

Heart

Diaphragm

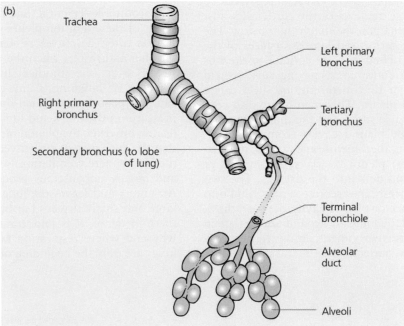

(b)

Trachea

Left primary bronchus

Right primary bronchus

Tertiary bronchus

Secondary bronchus (to lobe of lung)

Terminal bronchiole

Alveolar duct

Alveoli

Figure 9.1 (a) Upper respiratory tract and thoracic cavity. (b) Lower respiratory tract and alveoli.

RESPIRATION

Everybody knows that breathing is an essential requirement for good health and that failure to do so will, in a relatively short period of time, lead to asphyxia and death. However, it is important to recognise that there are three types of respiration occurring simultaneously at different locations within the human body: external, internal and cellular respiration. External respiration describes the process of gaseous exchange that takes place in the lungs. That is to say: oxygen (O_2) from the atmosphere is exchanged for carbon dioxide (CO_2) from the pulmonary blood supply (capillaries). Internal respiration refers to the process by which oxygen in the blood is made available to the cells and exchanged for carbon dioxide across the plasma membrane. Lastly, cellular respiration refers to the production of energy (ATP) within the cells (by oxidative metabolism) described in Chapter 2 (glucose + $O_2 \rightarrow$ ATP + CO_2 + H_2O). All three processes are absolutely essential for health and take place at the same time. In general terms, external and internal respiration ensure that the blood is provided with a constant supply of oxygen for cellular metabolism and provide a means for the excretion of carbon dioxide. However, before we look at how the respiratory tract facilitates this process, it is necessary to first consider the air that we breathe.

AIR AND ALTITUDE

In Chapter 1, we saw that air is a mixture of gases consisting of about 78% nitrogen (N) and 21% oxygen. To be more precise, dry air is composed of 78.06% nitrogen, 20.98% oxygen, 0.04% carbon dioxide and 0.92% other gases such as argon, helium, etc. It is important to consider that these molecules occupy space, have mass and weight, and collectively exert pressure upon us. For example, at sea level, the atmosphere is pressing against us with a force of 1 kilogram per square centimetre. This equates to a remarkable 1 ton of pressure per 1,000 square centimetres (a little larger than a square foot). Fortunately, the human body also contains gas molecules and our internal pressure is roughly the same as the air that surrounds us which prevents us from being squashed beneath an 'ocean' of compressed gas. Air is most compressed at sea level since, relatively speaking, it is at the bottom of the atmosphere. This sounds a bit odd but it is the same principle as water pressure. The deeper we dive, the more pressure we experience from the weight of compressed water above and around us. We are simply less aware of atmospheric (air) pressure since we are 'acclimatised' to our normal environment. However, as we climb above sea level, the air becomes 'thinner' as air pressure decreases. Although the PERCENTAGE of oxygen remains the same (21%), there is less air overall and, therefore, less oxygen is available for respiration. For example, let's imagine that following an ill-advised bet, you agree to climb Mount Everest. First you fly from the UK (sea level = 0 metres) to Kathmandu in Nepal (sea level +1,400 metres) and eventually find yourself at Lukla airport (sea level +2,860 metres) at the foot of the Himalayas. The air here is much thinner than someone from (insert your hometown here) is accustomed to and it is essential that would-be mountaineers acclimatise to the relatively low oxygen levels experienced at this altitude. Altitude sickness is common above 2,400 metres and occurs because of acute exposure to low partial pressure of oxygen (PO_2). This is before you have even left your hotel room! Everest Base Camp is a further 2,600 metres climb from the airport and the summit itself is approximately 8,850 metres above sea level. It is estimated that the available oxygen at this altitude is 33% of that at sea level and the vast majority of climbers require supplemental oxygen to safely complete their ascent. Even with oxygen, there have been many deaths from altitude sickness on Mount Everest (and elsewhere). Now that I have put you off climbing, why is it important to know about air pressure before considering the process of respiration and respiratory gases?

PARTIAL PRESSURE

All gas exerts pressure on the walls of its container. For example, the greater the volume of air you blow into a balloon, the greater the pressure it exerts against the walls of the balloon and the bigger it becomes. Gases which are dissolved in plasma also exert pressure on the walls of their container (measured in mmHg or kilopascals/kPa). Partial pressure describes the portion of total pressure exerted by a single gas in a mixture of gases. Put simply, partial pressure is a way of describing how much gas is present in solution. For example, atmospheric pressure at sea level is approximately 760 mmHg (101 kilopascals).

Nitrogen constitutes 79.03% of the atmosphere so its partial pressure is about 600 mmHg.

79.03% of 760 mmHg = 600.628 mmHg

or

[760 ÷ 100 = 7.6] × 79.03 = 600.628 mmHg

Oxygen constitutes 20.93% of the atmosphere so its partial pressure is about 159 mmHg.

20.93% of 760 mmHg = 159.068 mmHg

or

[760 ÷ 100 = 7.6] × 20.93 = 159.068 mmHg

Carbon dioxide constitutes only 0.04% of the atmosphere so its partial pressure is about 0.3 mmHg.

0.04% of 760 mmHg = 0.304 mmHg

or

[760 ÷ 100 = 7.6] × 0.04 = 0.304 mmHg

N + O2 + CO2 = total air pressure

600.628 + 159.068 + 0.304 = 760 mmHg

More importantly, partial pressure helps to explain how diffusion (the movement of a gas from a high concentration to a low concentration) of oxygen and carbon dioxide takes place during external and internal respiration. That is to say, there is diffusion in both directions but it is the difference between the two partial pressures that determines the net direction of diffusion. For example, the partial pressure of oxygen (PO_2) in the air sacs of the lungs (alveoli) is about 100 mmHg compared to about 40 mmHg in venous and pulmonary capillary blood (since oxygen has been 'used up' by the body's cells to produce energy/ATP). The net direction of diffusion for oxygen, therefore, is from the alveoli to the pulmonary capillaries (it moves from a high to a low concentration/pressure). However, we will return to this later in the chapter once we have discussed alveolar diffusion in more detail.

AIRWAYS

The respiratory system consists of the airways, the lungs, the muscles of respiration and the areas of the nervous system which control the rate and depth of ventilation. The airways are often divided into the upper and lower respiratory tract at the larynx (voice box). The upper respiratory tract consists of the nasal cavity, the mouth and the pharynx (Figure 9.1). Although we breathe using our nose *and* our mouth we are born nose breathers. Newborns are known as 'obligate nose breathers' since they demonstrate a strong preference to breathe through their nose rather than their mouth. This instinct is partly explained by differences in the anatomic proportions of their respiratory tract compared to an adult and the fact that they have not yet achieved control of the muscles in their mouths (or anywhere else for that matter). This can be problematic if the child has nasal congestion, as they frequently do, and most parents have looked on with a degree of alarm as their child's nostrils flair with the effort of breathing with a blocked up nose. However, even as an adult, the nasal cavity is a much better channel for respiration than the mouth since it is lined with a ciliated mucous membrane which contains mucus-producing goblet cells. At first glance this seems a little counter intuitive – how are cilia (hair-like projections) and mucus of benefit when breathing? Firstly, as we noted in Chapter 6, nasal secretions contain an enzyme called lysozyme that destroy the cell walls of some bacteria. It is also very 'sticky' which helps to trap airborne particles (including irritants and pathogens). Once trapped, this material is either swept forwards by the cilia out of the nostrils or swept backwards towards the throat where it is swallowed. This sounds unpleasant but, once in the stomach, most trapped material is quickly destroyed by hydrochloric acid (pH 1.5–3.5). In addition to this, as air flows over the moist surfaces of the nasal epithelium it is humidified as it becomes saturated with water vapour. For example, inspired air contains about 0.5% water vapour whilst expired air contains about 6%. This allows you to breath (or 'huff') onto the surface of a mirror/pain of glass and write a short message in the condensation you have produced. The air is also warmed in the nose by the numerous blood vessels situated in the nasal mucosa, and heat radiates from these vessels in much the same way that it does from the cutaneous (skin) circulation. In childhood and adolescence, these vessels are often quite fragile and nosebleeds (epistaxis) are common. In both children and adults, it is often difficult to establish the underlying cause of epistaxis but it can occur as a result of sneezing, temperature, altitude, hypertension, haematological disorders, excessive alcohol consumption and – of course – trauma (often self-inflicted by nose-picking).

NASAL CAVITY

The nasal cavity itself it much larger than it appears from the outside and is divided into four air passages by a series of thin, scroll-shaped bones collectively known as nasal conchae or turbinates (Figure 9.2). These increase surface area and facilitate rapid warming and humidification of the air as it passes through the nasal cavity. We tend to refer to 'things' going up the nose (e.g. an inquisitive finger). Whilst this is correct from the point of view of the nostrils (nares), if you really want to push an object (e.g. an airway or nasogastric tube) into/through the nasal cavity you need to insert it horizontally. Think of a classic Halloween pumpkin: the 'nose' is a simple triangular cavity situated in the middle of the face. This is a fairly accurate representation of the human nasal cavity as viewed from the outside. The nasal bone itself is quite short and the shape of the nose is largely determined by the septal and upper/lower lateral cartilages. This is why boxers often suffer from what is known as saddle-nose deformity or boxer's nose. It occurs when the cartilaginous portion of the nasal bridge collapses as a result of repeated trauma. The nasal bone may or may not be affected but the cartilage is permanently misshapen over time. Anyway, the point is this, if you push something 'up' your nose it won't go very far.

WARMING AND HUMIDIFYING

Air is inhaled through the nose and is filtered, warmed (almost to body temperature) and

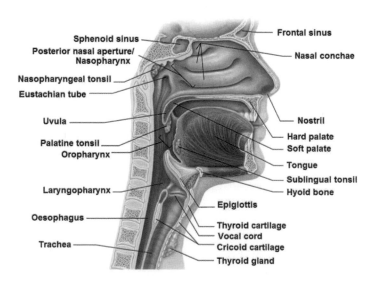

Figure 9.2 Upper respiratory tract.

humidified as it passes through the nasal conchae and makes its way to the posterior chamber of the nasal cavity and the upper part of the pharynx – the nasopharynx. This protects the more delicate respiratory surfaces (lower down) from getting cold and drying out, and helps to minimise heat and moisture loss during exhalation. Over the years I have removed an interesting assortment of items from adults and children's nasal cavities including a pencil-top eraser shaped like an owl, a surprisingly large piece of (very wet) folded-up paper and many raisins. In fairness to those who find themselves in this situation, the mechanism is often purely accidental. For example, I remember as a child sneezing violently whilst eating cheese-and-onion crisps. I forced my mouth shut to avoid spitting the contents across the room (only partially successfully). This had the unexpected and undesired effect of firing the partially chewed crisps from my mouth, up the back of throat, into my nasal cavity. I can vividly recall the unpleasant sensation of monosodium glutamate and a variety of other 'flavour enhancers' stinging the mucous membranes of my nasal conchae. That was the easy bit, getting it out again was much more difficult.

PHARYNX

The pharynx (from the Greek word for 'throat') is a musculomembranous tube that extends from the back of the nasal cavity to the level of the sixth cervical vertebrae where it becomes continuous with the oesophagus (Figure 9.2). Consequently, it is a common pathway for food/drink and inhaled/exhaled gases and there are a number of mechanisms in place to ensure that the former does not compromise delivery of the latter. For example, the walls of the pharynx contain both circular and longitudinal muscles. The circular muscles help to propel food into the oesophagus (digestive tract) and prevent air from being swallowed. At the same time, the longitudinal muscles lift the walls of the pharynx to prevent food and/or drink passing into the lower respiratory tract via the larynx. For convenience, the pharynx is subdivided into three sections:

the nasopharynx, oropharynx and laryngopharynx. The first section, the nasopharynx, is situated behind the nasal cavity just above the level of the soft palate. In each of its lateral walls there is a small opening which leads to the middle part of each ear. These auditory or Eustachian tubes (named after Bartolomeo Eustachio) help to ensure air pressure in the middle ear remains the same as that in the throat (i.e. atmospheric pressure). Under normal circumstances, the tubes remain closed but they can open to allow a small amount of air to enter if the pressure changes. For example, during take-off in an aircraft, the air pressure in the middle ear quickly becomes higher than that in the cabin since air pressure decreases as we ascend (as noted above – air becomes 'thinner'). As a result, the greater pressure in the middle ear compresses or pushes against the tympanic membrane (eardrum) from the inside and results in discomfort and temporary hearing loss. Yawning, swallowing or blowing against a closed mouth and pinched nose (the Valsalva manoeuvre) help to reverse this process by forcing air into the Eustachian tubes in order to 'equalise' the pressure on either side of the eardrum. People often experience a popping or clicking sensation when this occurs, followed by gradual improvement in the quality of their hearing. Others, however, struggle to equalise the pressure in their ears and experience hearing loss and pain for some time after landing. This may be because their Eustachian tubes are narrow, blocked, inflamed or simply because their equalisation technique is poor. I remember struggling to equalise the pressure in both ears the first time I flew. As the plane began its ascent, I performed the Valsalva manoeuvre and was surprised to feel air passing over my eyes. At the time, I was genuinely concerned that my eyeballs didn't fit properly and it was only years later that I realised, much to my embarrassment, that I was forcing air out of my nasolacrimal (tear) ducts and over my eyes!

EUSTACHIAN DRAINAGE

In health, the Eustachian tubes also drain mucus from the middle ear into the throat where it is swallowed. If the tubes become blocked or inflamed (e.g. secondary to upper respiratory tract infection) the mucus remains in situ and a middle ear infection (otitis media) may occur. Children are particularly susceptible to this process since their Eustachian tubes are often shorter and more horizontal than adults. Middle ear infections with large quantities of mucus are known as otitis media with effusion (glue ear) and can be particularly painful since the fluid compresses the inner surface of the tympanic membrane (eardrum). If pressure becomes too great, it can result in the perforation of the membrane and partial/total hearing loss in the affected ear. However, the perforation usually heals within about 4–6 weeks with no permanent damage. Another feature of the nasopharynx is the nasopharyngeal tonsils or adenoids discussed at the very end of Chapter 6. These are situated on the posterior wall of the nasopharynx and are most prominent in children up to about 7 years old.

OROPHARYNX

The next section of the pharynx is the oropharynx situated at the back of the oral cavity between the soft palate and the base of the tongue (at the level of the hyoid bone/third cervical vertebrae). At the border of the nasopharynx and oropharynx, the epithelial cells that line the throat change from columnar to squamous epithelium. The soft palate (or velum) is a muscular flap of tissue situated at the back of the roof of the mouth. It forms a barrier between the oral and nasal cavity when swallowing or sucking occurs. Another flap of elastic cartilage, the epiglottis, prevents the aspiration (inhalation) of food and drink into the lower respiratory tract during swallowing (Figure 9.2). The epiglottis projects upwards from the base of the tongue and hyoid bone and flaps over the opening of the larynx (the glottis) when swallowing occurs. At the same time, as noted above, longitudinal muscle fibres in the walls of the pharynx, lift the walls of the pharynx to prevent food or drink passing into the lower respiratory tract. However, these mechanisms are not always

successful as demonstrated by my cheese-and-onion sneeze example. Most people have witnessed their own/other people's children laughing at exactly the wrong moment when drinking juice. This results in either a violent cough reflex (spraying juice across the room) or the spectacle of 'nose-juice', where it runs out of one or both nostrils to the amazement and hilarity of the child concerned. Coughing and sneezing are both protective reflexes initiated by irritant receptors situated in the pharynx, larynx, trachea, bronchi and nasal cavity. When activated, the result is forced, involuntary expiration of air from the mouth and/or nose at a velocity of over 100 mile-per-hour in some instances (see Chapter 6). The final section of the pharynx is the laryngopharynx which is situated between the third and sixth cervical vertebrae. Below this point, it continues to the stomach as the oesophagus (see Chapter 11) which passes behind the larynx and trachea (Figure 9.2).

LARYNX

The larynx is essentially a cartilaginous box, open at both ends, that contains the vocal cords (Figure 9.2). It is often referred to as the voice box and is constructed from nine irregularly shaped cartilages attached by a series of ligaments and membranes. At the top, it is secured to the hyoid bone (see Chapter 4) and extends for about 5 cm between the level of the fourth and sixth cervical vertebrae. The largest of the laryngeal cartilages is the thyroid cartilage (from the Greek word *thyreoiedes* for 'shield-shaped') situated at the front and sides. This provides the prominent bulge visible in the middle of the throat known as the Adam's apple (typically larger in men than women). Air enters the larynx through the epiglottis which protects the glottis and lower respiratory tract when swallowing occurs. The 'stem' of the epiglottis is attached to the anterior (front) rim of the thyroid cartilage whilst the larger 'leaf' section is free to move up and down like a trap door (Figure 9.2). The glottis consists of a pair of mucous membranes attached to the vocal folds or vocal cords as they are more commonly known. The mucous membranes help to protect the lower respiratory tract from aspirating fluid or food into the airway but do not contribute to sound production (phonation). When the glottis is open, expired air passes over the vocal cords and causes them to vibrate. This produces sound waves that can be controlled by the contraction of voluntary muscle attached to the arytenoid cartilages. Pitch is regulated by the tension in the vocal cords and when they are stretched they vibrate more rapidly at a higher frequency. The same principle can be observed in stringed instruments where the tighter the strings are tuned, the higher the pitch. Pitch is also influenced by the length and thickness of the vocal folds and, in men, testosterone stimulates additional growth of the larynx and thickening of the vocal cords. From puberty, these changes cause a gradual deepening of the voice (see Chapter 14). Again, this principle can be observed in stringed instruments where the thicker 'base' strings vibrate more slowly to produce notes at a lower pitch.

SPEECH

Although sound originates from the vibration of the vocal folds in the glottis, clear speech requires articulation and modification of these vibrations by other structures such as the tongue, teeth and lips. The pharynx, oral cavity and nasal cavity also act as a resonating chamber that helps to provide the distinctive sound quality (timbre) of the voice. For example, when making the 'mmmmm' sound the mouth is closed and the air is released from nose only. If you squeeze your nose you cannot produce this sound with open or closed mouth (I can't at any rate). Some people are described as having a nasal quality to their voice. This may be hyponasal, such as when someone has nasal congestion, or hypernasal when airflow through the nose is increased during speech. Some languages use 'ingressive sounds' that are made when the airstream flows inward through the mouth or nose. An instantly recognisable example

of an ingressive sound is Scooby Doo's 'gulp' which can only be made whilst swallowing. One of the most common causes of dysphonia (impairment in the ability to produce vocal sounds) is viral laryngitis. This occurs when the mucous membrane lining the larynx and the vocal cords become infected and inflamed, resulting in hoarseness and temporary loss of voice. Children often develop croup because their larynx is small and therefore more susceptible to spasm and obstruction. This produces a distinctive barking cough and a loud, high-pitched sound made during inspiration called stridor. Although croup sounds awful (and is frequently distressing for both child and parents) most cases are mild and are easily treated at home with anti-inflammatory medication.

TRACHEA

The next part of the lower respiratory tract is the trachea or windpipe. This large airway has a diameter of about 2.5 cm and is composed of between 15 and 20 incomplete (C-shaped) rings of hyaline cartilage connected to one another by fibrous and muscular tissue (Figure 9.1). The cartilage forms the anterior (front) and lateral (side) walls of the trachea and ensures that it does not collapse when internal air pressure is less than inter-thoracic pressure (e.g. during inspiration). The non-cartilaginous (posterior) section is situated directly in front of the oesophagus (food pipe) and allows expansion to occur when food travels down the oesophagus into the stomach (see Chapter 11). The trachea is typically between 10 and 12 cm in length and extends downwards to about the level of the fifth thoracic vertebrae where it divides (bifurcates), at the carina (lowest tracheal cartilage), into the left and right primary bronchus. The trachea is lined with ciliated epithelium and mucus-producing goblet cells that trap irritants and pathogens in the same way as the lining of the nasal cavity. The cilia beat constantly in the same direction, at a rate of about 12 beats per second, in order to propel mucus and trapped material upwards towards the pharynx where it is swallowed and eliminated by the digestive system. This mechanism is often compared to a conveyer belt and is known as the mucociliary escalator. It is estimated that, each day, we can swallow up to 900 ml of mucus from our nasal cavity and respiratory tract. Fortunately, we are largely unaware of this since the mucus passes directly into the pharynx and oesophagus and does not come into contact with the taste buds of the tongue. If the upper respiratory tract becomes obstructed (e.g. because of swelling following an allergic reaction) it is possible to make a surgical incision into the trachea at the level of the second or third cartilaginous rings and insert a temporary airway. This procedure is called a tracheotomy and the surgical opening a tracheostomy (the Greek word *stoma* means 'mouth').

BRONCHIAL TREE

The left and right primary bronchus are also constructed from C-shaped cartilaginous rings and are lined with ciliated columnar epithelium. The left bronchus is slightly narrower,

longer and less vertical then the right since the left side of the thoracic cavity has to accommodate the mediastinum and heart as well as the left lung. Both primary bronchi subdivide or branch into progressively smaller and narrower airways. For example, the right lung has three secondary bronchi (one for each lobe) whilst the smaller left lung has two. These subdivide into tertiary bronchi whose walls are supported by small irregular cartilage plates rather than C-shaped rings. Each tertiary bronchus branches several more times to form bronchioles (small airways) which themselves subdivide to produce terminal (end) and respiratory bronchioles serving several alveolar ducts. It is estimated that the airways, from the trachea to the alveolar ducts, contain about 25 orders of subdivision. This arrangement resembles the branches of an upturned tree and is often referred to as the bronchial tree (Figure 9.1). The bronchioles are lined with non-ciliated and non-mucus-producing cuboidal epithelium and any inhaled irritants and pathogens must be removed by macrophages (big eaters). The walls of the bronchioles also contain no cartilage and are supported by spiral bands of smooth muscle which encircle the airways (Figure 9.3). Resting tension in the smooth

Normal Bronchiole

Asthmatic Bronchiole

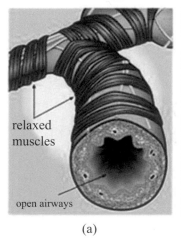
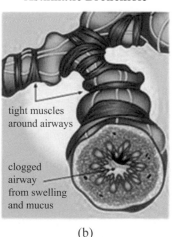

relaxed muscles

open airways

(a)

tight muscles around airways

clogged airway from swelling and mucus

(b)

Figure 9.3 (a) Normal bronchiole (smooth muscle relaxed). (b) Asthmatic bronchiole (smooth muscle constricted).

muscle leads to folding or corrugation of the bronchiole mucosa. It also enables the bronchioles to alter their diameter and is the principal determinant of resistance to air flow. For example, during exercise (or whenever ventilation needs to increase) the bronchial smooth muscle relaxes in response to sympathetic nervous system stimulation (flight-or-fight). Adrenaline and noradrenaline stimulate beta-2 receptors of the bronchial smooth muscle which results in bronchodilation and a reduction in resistance to air flow during breathing. The parasympathetic nervous system, on the other hand, stimulates contraction of bronchial smooth muscle which results in bronconstriction and increased resistance during breathing. Bronchoconstriction may occur during allergic or hypersensitivity reactions, such as asthma, or as a result of lower respiratory tract infection.

ASTHMA

Asthma (Greek for 'panting') is a chronic respiratory condition that affects the small airways (bronchioles) and is often triggered by the inhalation of an allergen. An allergen is simply a foreign substance that produces a disproportionate immune response in sensitive individuals. Common allergens include pollen, animal fur, fungal spores, dust and dust mite (a microscopic, eight-legged 'acari' living in your mattress with several million friends – sweet dreams). When an allergen is inhaled by an asthmatic, their immune system releases immunoglobulin E (IgE) which attaches to special binding receptors on mast cells (see Chapter 6). This attracts an allergen which, in turn, attaches itself to the adjacent stems of two immunoglobulins (sticking up from surface of the mast cell) like a tiny bridge. This process is known as cross-linking and when a sufficient number of allergens cross-link with immunoglobulins attached to mast cells, it causes the cell to burst open (degranulate), spilling inflammatory chemicals such as histamine into the surrounding tissue. This produces a large and disproportionate inflammatory response and encourages eosinophil migration (which release toxins). It also triggers constriction of the bronchial smooth muscle which further

narrows the airways leading to symptoms such as breathlessness and expiratory wheeze (Figure 9.3).

REVERSING BRONCHOCONSTRICTION

Asthma is one of a number of respiratory diseases that are characterised by increased airway resistance and are known collectively as chronic obstructive pulmonary disease (COPD). However, unlike other types of COPD (e.g. chronic bronchitis and emphysema), asthma is reversible when treated quickly. One type of drugs commonly used to treat asthma are short acting beta-2 agonists (stimulants) such as salbutamol. These drugs are usually delivered directly into the airways via a metred dose inhaler (puffer) and act upon the beta-2 receptors of the sympathetic nervous system located in bronchial smooth muscle (and elsewhere). When stimulated, as noted above, these receptors trigger relaxation of bronchial smooth muscle and allow the lumen of the airway to increase in size (bronchodilation). Anticholinergic drugs, such as ipratropium bromide, are also bronchodilators but rather than stimulate the sympathetic nervous system, they inhibit the parasympathetic nervous system. They accomplish this by blocking cholinergic receptors present in bronchial smooth muscle, which prevent parasympathetic stimulation and therefore bronchoconstriction from taking place. Consequently, beta-2 agonists and anticholinergics are often used together because they bring about bronchodilation in different but complementary ways.

ALVEOLI

The walls of the bronchioles gradually become thinner and thinner until muscle and connective tissue disappear altogether leaving only a single layer of simple squamous epithelial cells (type I pneumocytes) in the alveolar ducts and alveoli (air sacs). It is estimated that each lung contains about 150 million alveoli surrounded

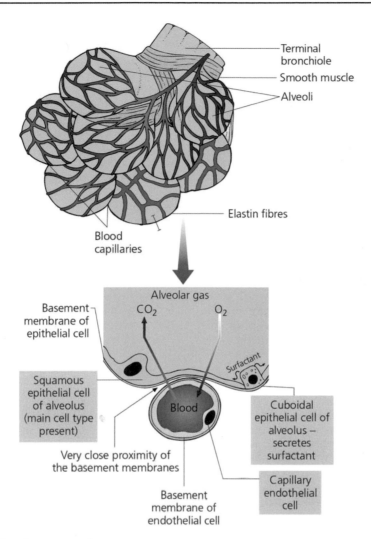

Terminal bronchiole

Smooth muscle

Alveoli

Elastin fibres

Blood capillaries

Alveolar gas

CO_2 O_2

Basement membrane of epithelial cell

Surfactant

Squamous epithelial cell of alveolus (main cell type present)

Blood

Cuboidal epithelial cell of alveolus – secretes surfactant

Very close proximity of the basement membranes

Basement membrane of endothelial cell

Capillary endothelial cell

Figure 9.4 Alveoli and gaseous exchange.

by an extensive network of pulmonary capillaries (Figure 9.4). They are also supported by an intricate network of elastic fibres that provide natural recoil during expiration. Alveoli are arranged in 'bunches' around an alveolar sac at the end of the alveolar duct. This arrangement greatly increases the surface area available for gaseous exchange in the lung (estimated to be about 70 m²). The thin, type I, pneumocytes are the main site of gas exchange but interspaced between them are, less numerous, type II pneumocytes.

These are cuboidal epithelial cells that secrete alveolar fluid in order to ensure the surface between the cells and the air remains moist. They also produce an oily secretion (a mixture of phospholipids and proteins) called surfactant that lowers the surface tension of alveolar fluid and reduces the likelihood of alveolar collapse during expiration (i.e. it stops them from sticking together). This also helps to maximise the available surface area for gaseous exchange. Babies born before 35 weeks are often unable to breathe normally at birth since they have not had enough time to produce a sufficient quantity of surfactant in utero. In order to prevent alveolar collapse and respiratory exhaustion after birth, they are immediately given surfactant replacement therapy directly into their lungs via an endotracheal tube. Repeated doses are usually necessary and the baby may also require artificial ventilation. Another feature of the epithelial surface of the alveoli are dust cells or alveolar macrophages. These phagocytic (devouring) cells remove fine particles and other material that has eluded the bronchial macrophages and sticky mucus above.

GASEOUS EXCHANGE

We observed at the very beginning of the chapter, that oxygen from the atmosphere diffuses from a high concentration in the alveoli to a lower concentration in pulmonary circulation. The partial pressure of oxygen in alveolar air is about 100 mmHg whilst the partial pressure of oxygen in the blood entering the pulmonary capillaries (at rest) is about 40 mmHg. Once diffusion has taken place, however, the partial pressure of the blood entering the pulmonary veins (and returning to the left side of the heart) is about 100 mmHg. At the same time, carbon dioxide diffuses from a high partial pressure in the pulmonary capillaries to a lower partial pressure in the alveoli. It is then expelled back into the atmosphere and made available to grateful trees for photosynthesis. The walls of the alveoli and pulmonary capillaries are collectively known as the respiratory membrane and, although they consist of a number of layers, it is incredibly thin (one-sixteenth the diameter of an erythrocyte).

OXYGEN TRANSPORT

Once oxygen has diffused into the pulmonary capillaries, it is transported in two ways. In Chapter 5 we observed that approximately 98.5% of oxygen is bound to haemoglobin as oxyhaemoglobin (HbO_2). Each haemoglobin molecule contains four heme units (capable of binding with oxygen) and each erythrocyte contains about 280 million haemoglobin molecules. This means that a healthy erythrocyte is capable of carrying over a billion oxygen molecules at any one time ($4 \times 280,000,000 = 1,120,000,000$). Oxygen does not easily dissolve in water which explains why only 1.5% is carried in plasma. It is estimated that for someone with a haemoglobin (Hb) concentration of 15g per 100ml, each 100ml of oxygenated blood contains the equivalent of 20ml of gaseous oxygen (of which 19.7ml is bound to haemoglobin). It is important to note that deoxygenated blood also carries oxygen (about 15ml/100ml). The difference in oxygen content is about 25% (hence deoxygenated) which results in a less red appearance because of the colour difference between the two forms of haemoglobin. Loading and unloading of oxygen is summarised in the (reversible) equation below:

$$Hb + O_2 \leftrightharpoons HbO_2$$

The four polypeptides of the haemoglobin molecule exhibit a kind of cooperative relationship and after an oxygen molecule attaches itself to the first polypeptide, haemoglobin changes shape. This encourages uptake of the next two oxygen molecules and the uptake of the fourth is easier still. When all four heme molecules are bound to oxygen, haemoglobin is said to be fully saturated (as opposed to partially saturated when one, two or three molecules are attached). Unloading of oxygen from haemoglobin takes place in a similar fashion, and once one oxygen molecule has dissociated, it facilitates the next (and so on). As a result, the affinity of haemoglobin for oxygen changes in relation to its state of saturation.

OXYGEN SATURATION

In a healthy person, who is breathing air at normal altitude, arterial blood is almost completely saturated with oxygen (98% saturation or above). Percentage saturation levels are an important measurement in clinical

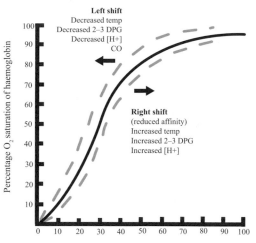

pO₂ (mmHg)	% saturation of Hb
10	13.5
20	35.0
30	57.0
40	75.0
50	83.5
60	89.0
70	92.7
80	94.5
90	96.5
100	97.5

Figure 9.5 Oxygen-haemoglobin dissociation curve.

practice and pulse oximetry works by passing a beam of red and infrared light through a capillary bed (usually under the finger nail). Haemoglobin that is fully saturated with oxygen, absorbs light differently from partially or de-saturated haemoglobin (which allows a percentage reading to be provided). A number of factors influence the rate at which haemoglobin binds to/releases from oxygen including the partial pressure of oxygen (PO_2) and carbon dioxide (PCO_2), temperature, hydrogen ion level (H^+) and the concentration of a chemical produced by erythrocytes called 2,3-BPG (2,3-biphosphoglycerate). However, the most important factor for oxygen saturation is PO_2: the higher the PO_2, the more oxygen that combines with haemoglobin. The oxygen-haemoglobin dissociation curve (Figure 9.5) demonstrates this relationship between haemoglobin saturation and PO_2 at normal body temperature. In general terms, an increase in temperature, PCO_2, 2,3-BPG and/or H^+ concentration will decrease the affinity of haemoglobin for oxygen. This enhances oxygen unloading from the blood and causes a shift in the oxygen-haemoglobin dissociation curve to the right (Figure 9.5). Conversely, a decrease in temperature, PCO_2, 2,3-BPG and H^+ concentration, increases the affinity of haemoglobin for oxygen and causes the dissociation curve to shift to the left.

CARBON DIOXIDE TRANSPORT

Carbon dioxide is produced as a result of cellular metabolism (i.e. glucose + O_2 → ATP + CO_2 + H_2O) and it is estimated that, at rest, our cells produce about 200 ml of carbon dioxide each minute. Each 100 ml of deoxygenated blood contains the equivalent of 52 ml of gaseous carbon dioxide and it is transported from the tissue to the lungs in three ways. The first way is directly dissolved in the plasma and although carbon dioxide is 20 times more soluble than oxygen, only 7% is transported like this. The remaining 93% diffuses from the plasma into available erythrocytes (Figure 9.6). About 23% of this is transported attached to haemoglobin as carbaminohaemoglobin ($HbCO_2$). Since carbon dioxide binds to the amino acids of globulin (rather than to heme) it does not interfere or compete with the oxyhaemoglobin mechanism described above.

$$Hb + H_2O \leftrightharpoons HbCO_2$$

However, the vast majority of carbon dioxide (about 70%) is transported in the form of bicarbonate ions (HCO_3). Once carbon

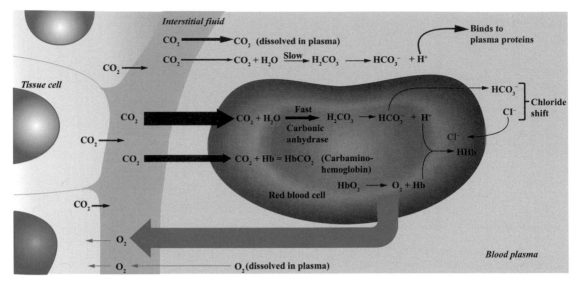

Figure 9.6 Oxygen (O_2) release and carbon dioxide (CO_2) uptake by an erythrocyte.

dioxide diffuses into an erythrocyte, it reacts with water (in the presence of the enzyme carbonic anhydrase) to form carbonic acid (H_2CO_3). However, because carbonic acid is unstable, it quickly dissociates into hydrogen ions (H^+) and bicarbonate ions (HCO_3^-):

$$CO_2 + H_2O \leftrightharpoons H_2CO_3 \leftrightharpoons H^+ + HCO_3^-$$

Most of the hydrogen ions bind to haemoglobin as HbH^+. This is an important buffering mechanism since it prevents hydrogen ions from leaving the erythrocytes and lowering plasma pH (Chapter 1). Bicarbonate ions, on the other hand, quickly diffuse out of the erythrocytes into the plasma where they are carried to the lungs. In order to compensate for this rapid loss of negative ions (HCO_3^-) there is a corresponding influx of chloride ions (Cl^-) from the plasma. This exchange process is known as chloride shift (Figure 9.6). Finally, it is important to note that carbon dioxide is also converted into carbonic acid in the plasma (when it dissolves) but since there is little carbonic anhydrase available, it is a much slower process. The outcome is much the same as within the erythrocytes (dissociation of H_2CO_3 into H^+ and HCO_3^-) but

rather than attaching to haemoglobin, hydrogen ions bond with (and are buffered by) plasma proteins. The overall effect of these processes is that carbon dioxide is removed from the tissues and transported to the lungs as HCO_3^-. As blood flows through the pulmonary capillaries, all these reactions reverse as carbon dioxide diffuses into the alveoli and is exhaled.

RESPIRATORY DRIVE

The rate and depth at which we breathe is set and controlled by the respiratory centres of the brain. The inspiratory and expiratory centres are located in the medulla oblongata and are assisted by the pneumotaxic and apneustic centres situated in the pons (see Chapter 12). In order to regulate respiratory activity, these centres require a constant source of information about the chemical composition of arterial blood. This information is provided by specialised nerve endings called chemoreceptors located in the medulla oblongata (central chemoreceptors) and in the aortic arch and carotid arteries (peripheral chemoreceptors, Figure 9.7). The most important chemicals monitored by

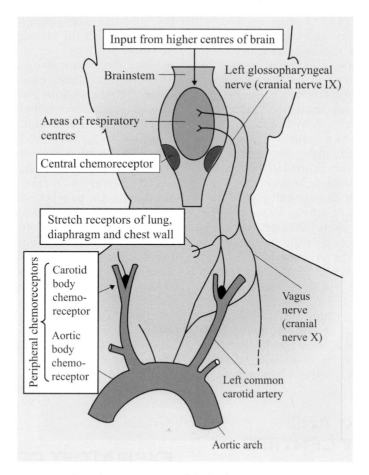

Figure 9.7 Chemoreceptors and respiratory centres of the brain.

these nerve endings are carbon dioxide, oxygen and hydrogen ions (H^+). In simple terms, if the concentration of carbon dioxide or H^+ rise, the chemoreceptors transmit nerve impulses to the medulla which increases respiratory effort to correct the imbalance. Respiratory rate is also influenced by the quantity of oxygen in the blood (hypoxic drive) but it is not as influential as carbon dioxide or H^+ concentration (see below).

CARBONIC ACID

Although the body is continually producing carbon dioxide as a result of cellular metabolism, the quantity of carbon dioxide in blood remains well regulated in health. For example, the partial pressure of carbon dioxide in arterial blood is maintained between 35 and 45 mmHg. Similarly, the concentration of hydrogen ions (H^+) in arterial blood is maintained between 40 and 45 nanomoles per litre (nmol/l) which corresponds to a pH of between 7.35–7.45 (see Chapter 1). Peripheral chemoreceptors respond to changes in carbon dioxide and H^+ concentration in arterial blood whereas central chemoreceptors respond to chemical changes in the cerebrospinal fluid (CSF). This is because carbon dioxide is lipid soluble and diffuses easily across the blood-cerebrospinal fluid barrier into the cerebrospinal fluid that circulates between the meninges of the brain and spinal cord (see Chapter 12). Carbon dioxide then combines with water to form carbonic acid (H_2CO_3) which quickly dissociates into hydrogen and bicarbonate ions. This process is very similar to that described above where carbon dioxide diffuses into erythrocytes and dissolves in plasma. Unlike erythrocytes and plasma, however, cerebrospinal fluid contains very few proteins that can buffer the newly liberated hydrogen ions and pH rapidly declines as a result (i.e. it becomes more acidic). This stimulates the central chemoreceptors/respiratory centres to increase the rate and depth of breathing (hyperventilation) to 'blow off' carbon dioxide and restore normal partial pressure of arterial blood (PCO_2). As carbon dioxide levels decrease, there is a corresponding reduction in the concentration of hydrogen ions in the cerebrospinal fluid and arterial blood. As a result, pH and respiratory rate return to normal. It is estimated that an increase of as little as 5 mmHg in the partial pressure of arterial carbon dioxide can result in a 100% increase in alveolar ventilation. This corrective mechanism is another example of the use of a negative feedback loop to maintain homeostasis discussed in Chapter 3.

INSPIRATORY AND EXPIRATORY CENTRES

We have observed that excess carbon dioxide in the blood (hypercapnia), and excess H^+ concentration in the cerebrospinal fluid and blood, stimulates the respiratory centres of the brain to increase nerve transmission to the respiratory muscles in order to intensify the rate and depth of breathing. We now need to discuss how the inspiratory and expiratory centres control the mechanics of breathing. The inspiratory centre contains a pace-setting nucleus (collection of nerves/neurons) that transmit nerve impulses along the phrenic and intercostal nerves to stimulate the diaphragm and external intercostal muscles respectively. The intercostal muscles contract, pulling the ribs upwards and outwards, whilst the diaphragm flattens and descends. This enlarges and expands the chest (thoracic) cavity which decreases the air pressure in the lungs to below atmospheric pressure. As a result, air from outside rushes into the lungs from high to low pressure. The Hering–Breuer reflex (discovered by Ewald Hering and Josef Breuer in 1868) prevents over-inflation of the lungs through the transmission of inhibitory nerve impulses towards the brain. Stretch receptors, situated in the smooth muscle of the bronchioles, generate nerve impulses when the lungs have inflated to a certain point. These travel along the vagus nerve and directly inhibit the action of the inspiratory centre of the medulla and the apneustic centre of pons. This not only allows expiration to take place (by allowing the diaphragm to relax and the ribs to return to their original position), it contributes to the rhythmicity of breathing and prevents excessive changes in lung volume. The natural elastic recoil of the lungs also provides an additional driving force to expel air from the thoracic cavity. It is impossible to expel all of the air from the airways and a small quantity always remains (residual volume). The inspiratory phase of respiration lasts for about two seconds and the expiratory phase for about three seconds. This on/off innervation of the respiratory muscles results in a normal respiratory rate of between 12 and 20 breaths per minute.

EXPIRATORY CENTRE

The expiratory centre of the medulla does not promote expiration during normal 'quiet' breathing and is only activated by nerve impulses from the inspiratory centre during exercise (or when dynamic expiration is required). When this occurs, the expiratory centre promotes vigorous contraction of the internal intercostal and abdominal muscles resulting in forced expiration. This stimulates faster expiration than simply relaxing the inspiratory muscles and allows inspiration to recommence sooner. If you pretend to blow out a candle (don't be embarrassed; no one is watching) you can feel your abdominal muscles contract as air is forced from the lungs. Although the inspiratory centre of the medulla generates the rhythm of inspiration, the pneumotaxic and apneustic centres of the pons also contribute to this process. They help to coordinate the transition between expiration and inspiration by exerting opposing effects on the inspiratory centre. For example, the pneumotaxic centre transmits a continuous series of inhibitory impulses to the inspiratory centre of the medulla which help to ensure that the lungs do not over-inflate and assist expiration. During exercise, impulses from the pneumotaxic centre also shorten the duration of inspiration and breathing becomes more rapid. The apneustic centre, on the other hand, transmits stimulatory impulses to the inspiratory centre that help to prolong inspiration and inhibit expiration (the term 'apneusis' refers to abnormally deep or sustained inspiratory effort). In normal circumstances, however, the apneustic centre is inhibited by impulses transmitted by the vagus nerves and the pneumotaxic centre. The role of the pneumotaxic and apneustic centres is not fully understood and the two are often collectively referred to as the pontine respiratory centre. In general terms, however, they smooth the transition from inhalation to expiration and 'fine-tune' respiratory rhythm during activities such as speaking, sleeping and exercising.

INVOLUNTARY CONTROL OF BREATHING

Respiration is largely an involuntary act resulting from the stimulation of the respiratory centres of the brain by carbon dioxide and H^+ levels in the blood/cerebrospinal fluid. However, non-chemical stimulation can also influence respiratory rate and rhythm. For example, we have already observed how stretch receptors (in the bronchial smooth muscle) transmit inhibitory nerve impulses to the medulla to prevent over-inflation of the lungs. In Chapter 8, we also saw how proprioceptors (situated in skeletal muscles and joints) transmit nerve impulses to the cardiovascular centre of the medulla during exercise to increase heart rate and cardiac output. The same is true of respiratory rate and, as soon as strenuous exercise commences, proprioceptors transmit nerve impulses to the inspiratory centre to increase the rate and depth of breathing well before arterial carbon dioxide and H^+ concentrations have begun to rise. Nerve impulses generated

in the hypothalamus and limbic area of the brain, in response to pain and strong emotion, can also alter the rate and rhythm of respiration (see Chapter 12). For example, sudden pain often results in temporary cessation of breathing (apnoea) whilst prolonged pain can increase respiratory rate and depth. Changes in temperature activate receptors in the hypothalamus and we observed in Chapter 3 that exposure to a cold stimulus (such as plunging into icy water) can result in temporary cessation of breathing (or an involuntary gasp) followed by uncontrolled hyperventilation. An increase in body temperature, on the other hand, typically causes respiratory rate to rise as cellular metabolism speeds up and more carbon dioxide is produced. Another interruption to normal breathing that you have experienced is produced by coughing and sneezing. Both begin with prolonged inspiration followed by sudden and forceful expiration (ejecting irritants and pathogens in the process). Although sneezing is undoubtedly an involuntary activity, coughing can be voluntary or involuntary.

VOLUNTARY CONTROL OF BREATHING

In Chapter 2, we saw that the muscles of respiration behave like involuntary (smooth) muscle but are actually voluntary (skeletal) muscle. This allows us to consciously determine the rate and depth of respiration. For example, the average person can hold their breath under water (static apnoea) for between 30–60 seconds. If you train yourself, it is possible to extend this time considerably and the illusionist Harry Houdini was famously able to hold his breath for over 3 minutes whilst suspended upside-down in a locked cabinet full of water. Impressive as this is (particularly given the circumstances), the current record for static apnoea, using a single lung full of air at normal atmospheric pressure, stands at over 11 minutes. However, there are techniques that allow humans to hold their breath for even longer periods of time. For example, breathing pure oxygen (100%) for a prolonged period of time before a dive, has allowed a number of determined individuals to hold their breath for up to 22 minutes! It is important to note, however, that repeated episodes of extended apnoea can be extremely dangerous and deaths have occurred during and after these attempts. A somewhat safer, but no less impressive, example of voluntary control of expiration is the world record for longest continual vocal note (103 seconds) and the world record for the longest sustained note on a wind instrument (73 seconds). Once again, it is possible to improve on the latter but only by employing a technique known as circular breathing. This involves breathing in through the nose while simultaneously pushing out the last of the previously inhaled air through the mouth (using air stored in the cheeks). The longest continuous note achieved using this method was over 47 minutes long but would have been incredibly boring to listen to. The reason the record for the longest continual vocal note is significantly longer than the record for the longest sustained note on a wind instrument is because of airway resistance. Blowing into a narrow mouthpiece or reed requires considerably more pressure and effort than holding a vocal note. Voluntary control of breathing is made possible by descending pathways from the cerebral cortex of the brain (see Chapter 12) which bypass the respiratory centres of the medulla and act directly on the spinal respiratory nerves. Although this is extremely useful and, in certain circumstances, potentially life-saving, it is also temporary and limited by the accumulation of carbon dioxide and hydrogen ions. For example, it is impossible to kill yourself by holding your breath – a threat uttered by many children when in a bad mood. Even if they were stubborn enough to hold their breath until they passed out (imagine the look of determined concentration on their small reddening face) the medullary respiratory centres would reassert control the moment consciousness was lost.

HYPOXIC DRIVE

We noted earlier in the chapter that respiratory rate is also influenced, in a very limited way, by the quantity of oxygen in the blood.

This is known as hypoxic drive and is thought to account for about 10–15% of the stimulus to breathe (principally regulated by the peripheral chemoreceptors). The normal range for the partial pressure of oxygen in arterial blood is 75–100 mmHg and it would have to fall to below 60 mmHg (hypoxaemia) before hypoxic drive became a major stimulus for ventilation. It seems odd that oxygen plays such a minor role in determining respiratory rate when it is so important for cellular metabolism and health. However, hypoxic drive is actually quite a cunning adaptation. For example, if arterial oxygen levels significantly decrease, it weakens the activity of central chemoreceptors even if carbon dioxide levels remain normal. This results in a reduction in the number of nerve impulses sent to the respiratory muscles and a corresponding reduction in ventilation (leading to respiratory arrest if uncorrected). Fortunately for us, hypoxaemia stimulates the peripheral chemoreceptors to signal the respiratory centres to increase ventilation and restore oxygen levels. Although this remains a weak stimulus (loss of consciousness may already have occurred) it is certainly better than nothing! Hypoxic drive is also thought to be an important respiratory mechanism for a small number of people who suffer from some forms of chronic obstructive pulmonary disease (COPD). For example, if the lower respiratory tract is damaged and obstructed, it makes it difficult for gaseous exchange to take place and can result in poor carbon dioxide clearance. If this occurs the central chemoreceptors gradually 'adjust' to the consistently elevated PCO_2 levels (hypercapnia) and their tolerance decreases. As a result, it is increasingly difficult for the respiratory centres to maintain homeostatic control using normal PCO_2 parameters and hypoxic drive becomes more influential. This is important to recognise (e.g. via arterial blood gases) since providing high-dose oxygen to these carbon dioxide retainers can result in a reduction in their respiratory drive as arterial oxygen tension increases. In very simple terms, the respiratory centre is confused by the high concentration of oxygen in the blood and breathing can stop. However, it is important to emphasise that only a small proportion of those suffering from COPD become carbon dioxide retainers and most maintain respiratory drive via the medullary centres (albeit less effectively and with a high degree of compensation). This is important since most hypoxaemic COPD patients benefit from titrated oxygen therapy during an acute exacerbation of the disease.

HYPERVENTILATION

Throughout this chapter we have discussed respiratory drive in relation to normal and elevated carbon dioxide levels but what happens when PCO_2 falls below normal parameters? Earlier in the chapter we observed that when CO_2 levels rise, central chemoreceptors and the medullary centres respond by increasing respiratory rate to 'blow off' the gas and restore normal PCO_2. In these circumstances, hyperventilation is an effective compensatory mechanism in order to quickly reduce carbon dioxide levels in the blood. Hyperventilation in the absence of raised PCO_2, however, can drive down carbon dioxide levels to the point where unwelcome changes begin to occur. For example, low PCO_2 causes the blood vessels in the brain to constrict resulting in reduced blood flow (cerebral hypoperfusion) and a feeling of light-headedness. If hyperventilation is the result of panic or anxiety this 'dizzy' sensation intensifies the sense of apprehension and may trigger a further increase in respiratory rate. As more carbon dioxide is drawn out of the blood and expelled via the lungs, the more alkaline the blood becomes. This increases the binding affinity of albumin for calcium (Ca^{++}) which makes it more difficult for calcium to dissociate from its carrier protein. Consequently, there is less calcium available for nerve conduction which results in further vasoconstriction, dizziness and a tingling sensation in the fingertips and around the mouth (paraesthesia). The simplest way to treat this PCO_2 imbalance is to rebreathe carbon dioxide from a paper bag. Although the person looks a little like a glue-sniffer, this simple intervention is a quick and effective way to return plasma pH to normal.

CHAPTER 9: TEST YOURSELF

Q. How many lobes do the right and left lung have, and why is there a difference between the two?

A. The right lung has three lobes and the left lung has two. This is because the left lung must accommodate the heart (and mediastinum).

Q. The lungs are surrounded by a double membrane: the parietal pleura and the visceral pleura. What is the principle function of these membranes?

A. The opposing membranes secrete fluid into the pleural cavity between them. This allows the lungs to expand and deflate in a frictionless manner.

Q. There are three types of respiration: external, internal and cellular. Briefly explain how they differ.

A. External respiration describes the process of gaseous exchange (O_2 and CO_2) that takes place between the alveoli and capillary blood. Internal respiration refers to the process by which O_2 in the blood is made available to the cells and exchanged for CO_2 across the plasma membrane. Cellular respiration refers to the production of energy (ATP) within the cells (glucose + $O_2 \rightarrow$ ATP + CO_2 + H_2O).

Q. What percentage of air is oxygen?

A. 21%

(Continued)

(Continued)

Q. What is meant by the term partial pressure?

A. Partial pressure describes the portion of total pressure exerted by a single gas in a mixture of gases. For example, the partial pressure of oxygen (PO_2) in air is 159 mmHg, in the alveoli it is about 100 mmHg, and in venous blood it is about 40 mmHg (since it has been used for cellular respiration).

Q. List the four main parts of the upper respiratory tract.

A. Nasal cavity, nasopharynx, oropharynx and laryngopharynx.

Q. What is the name for the flap of elastic cartilage (attached to the larynx) that prevents aspiration of food and drink into the lower respiratory tract during swallowing?

A. The epiglottis.

Q. What is the name for the mucus-producing cells and tiny hair-like projections that line the trachea and what is their principle function?

A. The trachea is lined with ciliated epithelium and mucus-producing goblet cells that trap irritants and pathogens. The cilia beat constantly in the same direction in order to propel mucus (and trapped material) towards the pharynx where it is swallowed.

Q. The small airways (bronchioles) are surrounded by smooth muscle. How does this control resistance to air flow?

A. Sympathetic stimulation of bronchial smooth muscles results in bronchodilation (widening) which reduces resistance to air flow. Parasympathetic stimulation of bronchial smooth muscles results in bronchoconstriction (narrowing) which increases resistance to air flow.

Q. Where in the lungs does gaseous exchange take place?

A. The alveoli.

Q. What is alveolar surfactant?

A. Surfactant is an oily secretion that lowers the surface tension of the fluid that lines the alveoli and reduces the likelihood of alveolar collapse during expiration. Surfactant also helps to maximise the available surface area for gaseous exchange.

Q. What percentage of oxygen is bound to haemoglobin and what percentage is carried in plasma?

A. 98.5% of oxygen is bound to haemoglobin as oxyhaemoglobin and 1.5% is carried in plasma.

Q. What is considered to be normal arterial oxygen saturation for a healthy person?

A. Arterial blood should be almost completely saturated with oxygen – 98% or above.

Q. How is carbon dioxide (CO_2) transported in the blood?

A. About 70% of CO_2 is transported in the plasma (having diffused in/out of erythrocytes first) in the form of bicarbonate ions (HCO_3). About 23% is transported attached to haemoglobin as carbaminohaemoglobin ($HbCO_2$). The remaining 7% is directly dissolved in plasma.

Q. What part of the brain controls the rate and depth of breathing (respiratory drive)?

A. The inspiratory and expiratory centres located in the medulla oblongata.

Q. In order to regulate respiratory activity, these centres require a constant source of information about the chemical composition of arterial blood and cerebrospinal fluid. What is the name of these sensors and where are the located?

A. Central chemoreceptors are located in the medulla oblongata. Peripheral chemoreceptors are located in the aortic arch and carotid arteries.

Q. What are the most important chemicals monitored by these nerve endings in relation to respiratory drive?

A. Carbon dioxide, hydrogen ions and (to a lesser degree) oxygen.

Q. Will an increase of CO_2 in the blood, lead to an increase or decrease in respiratory rate and why?

A. It will increase the rate and depth of breathing to 'blow off' CO_2 and restore normal PCO_2.

Contents

CHAPTER 10

RENAL SYSTEM

URINARY TRACT

The urinary tract is essentially a plumbing system that allows excess water and waste products to be removed from the blood via the urine. It consists of two kidneys, two ureters, one urinary bladder and one urethra (Figure 10.1). The ureters are thin muscular tubes about 30 cm in length and about 0.5 cm in diameter. They drain urine from the left and right kidney into the urinary bladder via a combination of gravity and smooth muscle contraction (peristalsis). In order to prevent backflow, the ureters enter the bladder at an oblique (slanting) angle through two slit-like openings. Both the ureters and the bladder are lined with transitional epithelium (urothelium) that is able to withstand the hypertonicity of

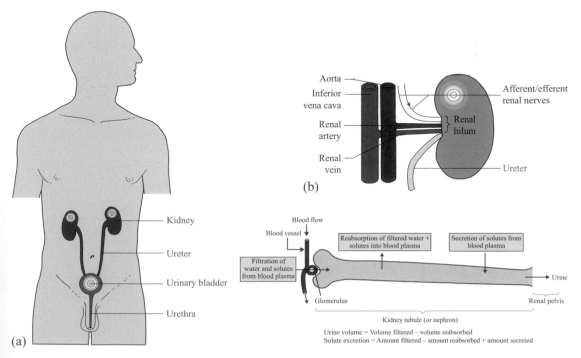

Figure 10.1 (a) Urinary tract. (b) Renal vessels and nerves.

urine (see below and Chapter 1) and allow the bladder to stretch and expand. They also produce a gel-like secretion known as mucin that forms a protective chemical barrier over the lining of the bladder. The bladder itself is essentially a hollow muscular organ which can accommodate 500–1,000 ml of urine prior to elimination. However, about 250 ml of fluid is usually enough to stimulate stretch receptors that alert us to the fact we probably need to go to the toilet at some point soon. At the base of the bladder, smooth muscle fibres form an internal sphincter which surrounds the urethra and opens in response to increased pressure within the bladder. The external urethral sphincter, on the other hand, is composed of a circular band of skeletal muscle and, from the age of two(ish), is under conscious control. At an appropriate time, therefore, we voluntarily relax the external sphincter and urine is driven into the urethra by the contraction of the smooth muscle in the bladder walls. The urethra extends from the neck of the bladder to the external urethral opening and is also lined with transitional epithelium (urothelium). The male urethra functions as both a urinary canal and the passageway for semen. It is approximately 20 cm in length and can be divided into three sections: the prostatic urethra, the membranous urethra and the penile urethra. The female urethra is only about 3–5 cm long and opens in front of the vaginal orifice (see Chapter 14). The relatively short length of the female urethra explains why women are more susceptible to urinary tract infection than men (i.e. it is easier for bacteria to migrate into the bladder).

KIDNEYS

The kidneys sit on either side of the spinal column between thoracic vertebra 12 and lumbar vertebra 3. The lower (floating) ribs provide a degree of protection at the back, and the upper abdominal organs and muscles protect them at the front. The right kidney is slightly lower than the left because it is situated beneath the larger right lobe of the liver (see Chapter 11). An adult kidney is about 12 cm long, 6 cm wide and 3 cm thick and is often described as resembling a bar of soap. Perched on top of each kidney (like a beret) is an adrenal gland that secretes a number of hormones including adrenaline, cortisol and aldosterone (see Chapter 13). The kidneys are secured in place by a dense layer of fibrous tissue known as the renal capsule, enclosed by a protective layer of adipose tissue (fat). Immediately below this is a reddish-brown layer of tissue called the renal cortex outer layer). The inner portion of the kidney is known as the renal medulla (inner layer) and is divided into a number of cone-shaped renal pyramids (Figure 10.2). Together, these layers represent the functional portion (parenchyma) of each kidney and contain about 1 million microscopic structures called nephrons (Figure 10.3). There are actually two types of nephron: cortical nephrons (located almost entirely within the renal cortex) and juxtamedullary nephrons (located in the renal cortex and medulla). Cortical nephrons are more abundant and account for about 85% of the total. However, despite their fewer numbers, juxtamedullary

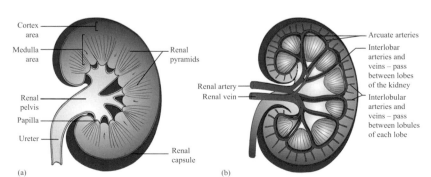

Cortex area
Medulla area
Renal pyramids
Renal artery
Renal vein
Renal pelvis
Papilla
Ureter
Renal capsule
Arcuate arteries
Interlobar arteries and veins – pass between lobes of the kidney
Interlobular arteries and veins – pass between lobules of each lobe

(a)   (b)

Figure 10.2 (a) Anatomy of the kidney. (b) Renal blood supply.

nephrons play an important role in the concentration of urine (see below).

DRAINAGE

Both types of nephron produce urine by three precisely regulated processes: filtration, reabsorption, secretion. Once this has taken place, urine drains from the nephron into a collecting duct (tubule) which transports it through the renal pyramids to the papilla ('nipple') and gives them their striped (striated) appearance (Figure 10.3). Urine eventually drains from the papilla into a number of cup-shaped structures known as calyces (singular: calyx). These form the distal part of a larger funnel-shaped structure known as the renal pelvis. The walls of the renal pelvis are lined with transitional epithelium (urothelium) and contain smooth muscle. This allows it to propel the urine into the ureters using peristaltic waves of muscular contraction. The final part of the kidney is known as the hilus (or hilum) and describes the area where the ureter, nerves and blood enter and exit the organ. It comes as a surprise to many people that urine is essentially filtered blood plasma that contains variable quantities of waste material depending on the time of day and environmental conditions. Consequently, without an adequate supply of blood (and blood pressure) the kidneys cannot produce urine and the body is unable to maintain chemical or fluid balance (homeostasis).

NEPHRON

As blood flows through the body, it collects and transports waste products that result from cellular metabolism and unavoidable wear and tear. If these waste products continue to accumulate in the blood they quickly become toxic and begin to exert a harmful effect on the body. For example, urea is normally synthesised in the liver as a result of protein metabolism and the breakdown of more toxic ammonia. If urea levels continue to rise (uraemia), it can result in fatigue, nausea, anorexia, peripheral nerve damage (neuropathy), decreased mental acuity and

possibly coma. It is absolutely essential, therefore, that the blood is continually 'cleaned' by the kidneys in order to prevent the toxic accumulation of urea and other potentially dangerous substances. Normally, about 20% of the total blood pumped by the heart each minute, will enter the kidneys via the renal artery to undergo filtration by the nephrons.

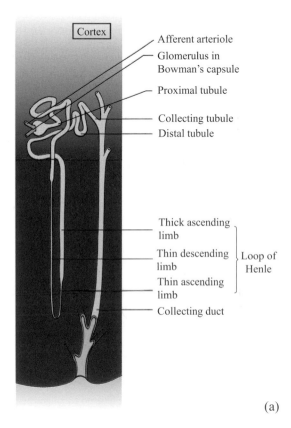

(a)

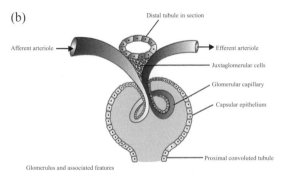

Figure 10.3 (a) Nephron. (b) Glomerulus.

Each nephron consists of two main portions: the renal corpuscle (Latin for: 'little body') where plasma is filtered, and the renal tubule into which the filtered fluid passes before undergoing a number of other processes. The renal corpuscle is further divided into the glomerulus and the glomerular or Bowman's capsule (named after Sir William Bowman who identified it in 1842). The renal tubule consists of the proximal convoluted tubule (PCT), the loop of Henle (named after Friedrich Henle) and the distal convoluted tubule (DCT) (Figure 10.3). The distal convoluted tubule eventually empties into a collecting duct which drains urine into the papilla and minor calyces mentioned above. The PCT, loop of Henle and DCT are often collectively referred to as the renal tubule. Renal tubules are surrounded by an intricate network of peritubular capillaries that enable water, ions and other molecules to be added and removed from the glomerular filtrate as required.

FILTRATION

Filtration is a non-selective (passive) process that takes place through the semi-permeable walls of the glomerulus and Bowman's capsule. The glomerulus (Latin for 'ball of thread') is a ball-shaped structure composed of capillary blood vessels. The afferent arteriole carries blood into the glomerulus whilst the efferent arteriole carries it out again (Figure 10.3).

In actual fact, the glomerulus, afferent and efferent arteriole are one continuous structure – imagine a ball of thread (glomerulus) with one end leading in (afferent arteriole) and the other end leading out (efferent arteriole). The glomerulus is lined with a thin layer of endothelial cells that contain numerous pores (fenestrations) which allow solute-rich plasma to pass through the glomerulus into the Bowman's capsule. In very simple terms, this membrane is a little like a teabag. The filtration process is assisted by the difference in pressure in the glomerulus (high) and the Bowman's capsule (lower). One of the reasons for this pressure gradient is that the diameter of the afferent arteriole (into the glomerulus) is wider than that of the efferent arteriole (out of the glomerulus). This creates a bottleneck situation which increases pressure in the glomerulus (ball) as blood tries to escape through the narrow lumen of the efferent arteriole. Plasma (and anything dissolved in plasma) is forced through the semi-permeable membrane (teabag) of the glomerulus towards the Bowman's capsule (Figure 10.3). On the other side of the glomerular membrane is a layer of podocytes ('foot cells') which form part of the Bowman's capsule. These terminate in a series of long processes called pedicels ('little feet') that wrap around the capillaries and provide openings called filtration slits or slit pores. These slits allow water and dissolved substances to pass into the Bowman's capsule but prevent larger structures, such as erythrocytes, leukocytes

TABLE 10.1 Blood constituent filtered through the glomerulus

Blood constituents filtered through the glomerulus	Blood constituents NOT filtered through the glomerulus
Water	Erythrocytes (red blood cells)
Ions	Leukocytes (white blood cells)
Glucose	Thrombocytes (platelets)
Amino acids	Plasma proteins
Urea	Some drugs
Uric acid	—
Creatinine	—

and thrombocytes, from getting through. The glomerulus and Bowman's capsule are often compared to a double sieve with the size of the 'holes' determining which constituents of the blood are filtered and which are not. The water, waste products, electrolytes, glucose and other molecules that have been filtered out of the blood are known collectively as glomerular filtrate or 'early urine'. This filtrate, as mentioned above, is essentially blood plasma without plasma proteins and Table 10.1 provides a summary of what should and shouldn't be present. Glomerular filtration rate (GFR) is about 120 ml/min which means that if all the glomerular filtrate was excreted as urine we would produce about 180 litres of urine each day! Clearly this does not happen and the actual amount of urine produced is typically between one and two litres. So what prevents us from spending our lives in a constant cycle of drinking and urinating?

REABSORPTION

The next phase of urine production is known as reabsorption and simply describes the movement of water and other substances from the renal tubule back into the peritubular capillaries that surround it. Much of this process occurs immediately after filtration in the proximal convoluted tubule (PCT). The walls of the PCT consist of a layer of cuboidal epithelial cells covered on their apical (facing) side by finger-like projections called microvilli (Figure 10.4). This 'brush border'

greatly increases the surface area available for reabsorption of water and other dissolved substances. For example, about 70% of the sodium ions (Na^+) present in the glomerular filtrate are reabsorbed from the PCT via a combination of passive and active transport mechanisms (Chapters 1 and 2). Some of the ions are reabsorbed into the cytoplasm of the epithelial cells via diffusion (from a high to a low concentration) through ion channels (transcellular reabsorption). In order to maintain a sufficient concentration gradient to allow diffusion to take place, it is essential that sodium is not allowed to build up in the cell and it is actively transported across the basolateral membrane into the interstitial fluid by Na^+/K^+ ATPase pumps (Figure 10.4). From here, it quickly diffuses into the adjacent peritubular capillaries and returns to the circulation. The absence of sodium pumps in the apical (facing) membrane ensures that this process is one way only.

SECONDARY ACTIVE TRANSPORT

Sodium is also reabsorbed from the PCT by a process known as secondary active transport. This occurs when a protein carrier (or co-transporter) binds with two molecules (e.g. sodium and glucose) and transports them across the cell membrane either in the same direction (symporters) or in opposite directions (antiporters). Both types of transporter have an upper limit on how fast they

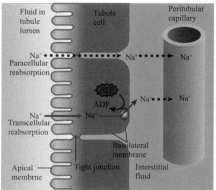

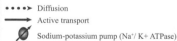

•••• ▸ Diffusion

⟶ Active transport

⊘ Sodium-potassium pump ($Na^+/K+$ ATPase)

Figure 10.4 Sodium (Na^+) transport across the brush border of the proximal convoluted tubule/PCT.

can work, much like an elevator has a limit on how many people it can carry up and down in a given period of time. The movement of positively charged sodium ions (Na^+) through the epithelial cells into the peritubular capillaries also helps to establish an electrical gradient that encourages passive reabsorption of anions (e.g. Cl^- and HCO_3^-) to restore electrical neutrality in the glomerular filtrate and plasma. Finally, some sodium ions diffuse directly across the junctions between the cells into the interstitial fluid (paracellular reabsorption). Although the majority of sodium is reabsorbed in the PCT, about 20% is reabsorbed in the loop of Henle, about 5% in the DCT and 1–4% in the collecting duct (see below). The quantity of cellular energy (ATP) used by the sodium pumps in the renal tubules during this process is surprisingly high – about 6% of total ATP consumption at rest! This is roughly equivalent to the same level of energy used by the diaphragm as it contracts during normal (quiet) breathing. The actual quantity of Na^+ reabsorbed each day is variable and depends upon a number of factors including hydration status and the amount of salt in our diet. Typically, however, it is estimated that we reabsorb about 575 g of Na^+ each day and excrete 2–4 g.

WATER AND GLUCOSE TRANSPORT

Reabsorption of sodium, chloride and other molecules in the PCT also establishes a strong osmotic gradient which 'pulls' water after it. This process is known as obligatory water reabsorption and normally recovers about 85% of the total volume of filtrate produced by the glomerulus and Bowman's capsule (renal corpuscle). About 65–70% of this is reabsorbed in the PCT and 20–25% in the descending limb of the loop of Henle (water reabsorption does not occur in the ascending limb since it is impermeable to water). The remaining 15% (about 20 litres of water per day) is selectively reabsorbed in the DCT and collecting duct in response to the secretion of antidiuretic hormone (ADH). This process is known as facultative water reabsorption since

it occurs 'optionally' in response to hydration status and determines how much urine we actually produce each day (see below). In normal circumstances, about 99% of the 180 litres of water filtered from the blood returns to the circulation via passive reabsorption (osmosis) and 100% of glucose from the glomerular filtrate is reabsorbed in health. We noted earlier that glucose is co-transported with sodium ions into the epithelial cells of the PCT (against a concentration gradient). Other sugars (e.g. fructose and galactose) are also transported in this manner but glucose is 'preferentially' bound to carrier molecules when levels are high. This is important since, as we saw in Chapter 2, glucose is essential for cellular metabolism/ATP production and it would be physiologically wasteful to excrete such an important resource. Having said that, glucose transport of this nature can only be sustained at a certain level known as the transport maximum. For example, symporters (protein carriers) in the PCT are able to reabsorb 100% of filtered glucose for healthy individuals with plasma glucose levels of 4–7 mmol/l. However, if plasma glucose levels exceed 10 mmol/l, the symporters become saturated and are unable to work fast enough to reabsorb all of the glucose from the glomerular filtrate (remember the lift analogy). If this occurs, glucose is conveyed through the renal tubule and collecting duct and is lost via the urine. This is known as glycosuria and typically occurs as a result of type I diabetes mellitus (see Chapter 13).

SECRETION AND HYDROGEN IONS

The final process or phase of urine production is tubular secretion and is essentially reabsorption in reverse. That is to say, whereas reabsorption moves substances out of the renal tubules and into the blood, secretion moves substances out of the blood and into the renal tubules where they mix with water and other waste material in order to produce urine. For example, hydrogen ions (H^+), potassium ions (K^+), creatinine and a number of drugs are secreted from the peritubular capillaries into

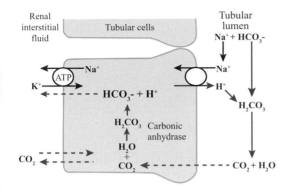

Figure 10.5 Secretion of hydrogen ions (H$^+$).

the filtrate of the PCT, DCT and collecting duct by a combination of passive and active transport (Figure 10.3). Secretion is particularly important for removing substances and drugs that are too large to pass through the glomerulus and Bowman's capsule (e.g. heparin), or that are bound to plasma proteins (e.g. penicillin). Secretion of hydrogen ions is also very important for maintaining acid-base balance. The cells of the PCT and DCT produce a constant supply of hydrogen ions and bicarbonate (HCO$_3^-$) as a result of the normal cellular metabolism of oxygen and glucose.

$$O_2 + C_6H_{12}O_6 + \rightarrow ATP + CO_2 + H_2O$$

In the previous chapter, we saw that once carbon dioxide diffuses into an erythrocyte it quickly reacts with water (in the presence of the enzyme carbonic anhydrase) to form carbonic acid (H$_2$CO$_3$). This reaction also occurs in the cells of the PCT and, since carbonic acid is unstable, it dissociates into hydrogen ions (H$^+$) and bicarbonate (HCO$_3^-$).

$$CO_2 + H_2O \leftrightharpoons H_2CO_3 \leftrightharpoons H^+ + HCO_3^-$$

When carbon dioxide levels in the blood rise (and plasma pH falls), hydrogen ions are actively secreted into the nephron (in exchange for sodium ions) and bicarbonate diffuses into the peritubular capillaries (Figure 10.5). The secreted hydrogen ions combine with filtered bicarbonate in the tubular lumen to form carbonic acid (carbonic anhydrase is also present on the luminal surface of the cells) and,

predictably, dissociates into carbon dioxide and water.

$$H^+ + HCO_3^- \leftrightharpoons H_2CO_3 \leftrightharpoons CO_2 + H_2O$$

Carbon dioxide then diffuses from the nephron into the tubule cells where it triggers further hydrogen ion secretion. The upshot of all of this is that it is the presence/absence of both (acidic) hydrogen ions and (alkali) bicarbonate in the urine that determines acid-base balance of the plasma and the acidity of the urine. That is to say, if the amount of filtered bicarbonate is greater than the amount of secreted hydrogen ions, then bicarbonate will be lost in the urine (and urine will be more alkaline). If, on the other hand, the amount of secreted hydrogen ions is greater than the amount of filtered bicarbonate, then hydrogen ions will be lost in the urine (and it will be acidic to a greater or lesser degree). Fortunately for our urinary tract, this process is self-limiting and hydrogen ion secretion ceases when urine pH reaches about 4.5 (slightly less acidic than tomato juice – pH 4).

URINE

It is only once all three phases or urine production have been completed (filtration, reabsorption and secretion) that glomerular

TABLE 10.2 Typical composition of urine

Typical composition of urine	%
Water	96%
Urea	2%
Uric acid	
Creatinine	
Sodium	
Potassium	2%
Chlorides	
Phosphates	
Sulphates, etc	

filtrate can called or considered true urine. In the following section we will see how urine is concentrated in the distal convoluted tubule (DCT) and collecting duct but under 'normal' circumstances urine is about 96% water and contains variable quantities of waste products and ions (Table 10.2). This is why, in health, it is perfectly safe to drink your own urine. Not that I am advocating this practice but, if trapped in a boat at sea as theorised in Chapter 1, it is safer than drinking sea water which contains a much higher concentration of dissolved salt. Normal urine output is considered to be at least 0.5 ml/per kg/per hour (e.g. a 70 kg adult should produce at least 35 ml of urine per hour). Typically it is much higher.

FLUID BALANCE

Water is lost or excreted from the body in a number of ways: as expired air, sweat, faeces and urine. The amount of water lost each day in expired air (water vapour) and faeces remains fairly constant in health. The quantity of sweat produced (and evaporated from our skin) is dependent on temperature and environmental conditions but, in normal circumstances, it is also fairly consistent. The balance between water input and water output is determined, therefore, by the kidneys through the action of a number of hormones. We saw in Chapter 8, that long-term control of blood pressure is coordinated by the kidneys through the management of blood volume. When arterial blood volume begins to decline, the walls of the afferent arterioles are under less pressure and are therefore less stretched. This stimulates the cells of the juxtamedullary nephrons to secrete a hormone called renin which converts the chemical angiotensinogen (produced in the liver) into angiotensin I. Angiotensin I is then converted into angiotensin II by an enzyme called angiotensin-converting enzyme (ACE) secreted by endothelial cells in the lung and kidney (see Chapter 8, Figure 8.4). In simple terms, angiotensin II helps to increase blood pressure and circulatory volume in a number of ways. Firstly, it triggers vasoconstriction of the peripheral arterioles which increases vascular resistance

and systemic blood pressure as a whole. Secondly, angiotensin II also stimulates the secretion of antidiuretic hormone (ADH) which facilitates further reabsorption of water in the collecting ducts (see below). Finally, it stimulates the adrenal cortex to secrete a steroid hormone called aldosterone.

ALDOSTERONE AND ATRIAL NATRIURETIC HORMONE

Aldosterone encourages cells in the DCT to actively reabsorb more sodium and chlorine ions from the filtrate. This also facilitates the osmotic transport of water from a relatively hypotonic concentration (high percentage of water) in the distal tubules, to a relatively hypertonic concentration (lower percentage of water) in the renal cells and capillary blood. The principle actions of aldosterone, therefore, are to increase sodium reabsorption in the distal tubules, decrease urine output and increase blood volume. This does not occur instantly, however, and aldosterone exerts its effects slowly over a period of hours to days. Collectively, this process is known as the renin-angiotensin-aldosterone system or RAAS for short. Atrial natriuretic hormone (ANH), on the other hand, performs the exact opposite function of the RAAS. In Chapter 8, we noted that it is secreted by myocardiocytes (heart muscle cells) in response to atrial distention following an increase in blood volume and/or blood pressure. In order to reduce blood pressure and circulatory volume, atrial natriuretic hormone relaxes vascular smooth muscle (vasodilation) and suppresses the secretion of renin, aldosterone and antidiuretic hormone (ADH). This inhibits the reabsorption of sodium ions in the distal tubules which increases the quantity of sodium excreted in the urine (natriuresis) and the volume of urine produced (diuresis). Atrial natriuretic hormone also dilates afferent arterioles and constricts efferent arterioles which increases glomerular filtration rate and results in further natriuresis and diuresis. Finally, it also increases blood flow through the vasa recta ('straight' peritubular capillaries situated next to the loop of Henle of the juxtamedullary nephrons) which washes sodium and other solutes out of the medulla. This reduces the tonicity (pull) of the medullary interstitial fluid which, in turn, reduces reabsorption of water from the juxtaglomerular tubules. In short, atrial natriuretic hormone reduces blood pressure and circulatory volume by inhibiting most of the processes that promote vasoconstriction and sodium/water reabsorption.

ANTIDIURETIC HORMONE (ADH)

The final, and arguably most important, hormone that helps to maintain fluid balance is antidiuretic hormone (ADH) or vasopressin as it is also known. We noted earlier in the chapter, that the permeability to water of the

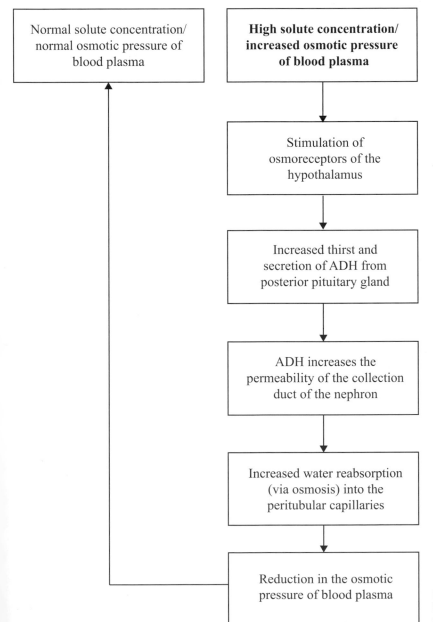

Figure 10.6 Antidiuretic hormone (ADH) and fluid balance.

PCT and descending limb of the loop of Henle cannot be adjusted. Consequently, water reabsorption occurs whenever the concentration of water within these structures is higher than that of the peritubular fluid. This passive process usually recovers about 85% of the total volume of filtrate produced each day and is known as obligatory water reabsorption since it cannot be prevented. The volume of water that is excreted each day as urine, therefore, depends on how much of the remaining 15% (10–20 l/d) is reabsorbed by the DCT and collecting duct. This is known as facultative water reabsorption since it occurs 'optionally' and is carefully regulated by ADH. When ADH levels are high, almost all of the filtrate is reabsorbed and only a very small amount of highly concentrated urine is produced. When ADH levels are low, on the other hand, very little filtrate is reabsorbed in the DCT and collecting duct, and large amounts of very dilute urine is produced. ADH is secreted by cells in the posterior pituitary gland (situated in the brain) in response to increased plasma osmolality (remember: the higher the drier). For example, if plasma omolarity begins to rise as a result of heavy sweating during strenuous exercise, sensory nerve cells in the hypothalamus called osmoreceptors detect the increase in osmotic pressure and trigger the sensation of thirst and the secretion of ADH from the posterior pituitary gland (Figure 10.6). ADH is transported in the blood to the kidneys, where it stimulates the insertion of additional water channel proteins called aquaporins (aqua + porin = water + opening) into the apical (facing) cell membrane of the collecting duct. This increases the permeability of these cells (they become more porous) and more water is osmotically transported back into the capillary circulation until plasma osmolality returns to normal and ADH secretion is inhibited (a negative feedback loop). In the absence of ADH, aquaporins are removed from the cell membrane by endocytosis and little or no water is reabsorbed.

ADH DEFICIENCY

A deficiency of pituitary ADH results in diabetes insipidus which is characterised by excessive diuresis and thirst. Treatment involves taking a manufactured version of ADH (Desmopressin) via tablet or nasal spray. Desmopressin can also be prescribed for bedwetting since it concentrates urine and helps to reduce the total volume of urine produced at night. Although this is not curative, it can provide short-term relief or contribute to other long-term management strategies. In short, ADH is essential for the concentration of urine when blood plasma levels are low and/or osmolality (solute concentration) is high. This explains why, should you be stuck in that boat I keep referring to, you cannot drink your urine indefinitely. Your body will continue to lose fluid from sweat and water vapour from your breath, and your urine will become progressively more concentrated as ADH compensates for this loss. Eventually urine production will stop altogether (the law of diminishing returns). On a completely unrelated note regarding the concentration of urine, the 17th-century German alchemist Hennig Brand experimented with urine in an attempt to produce gold! He boiled urine to reduce it to a thick paste before refining it into a waxy material. What he eventually produced was not gold (unsurprisingly) but a new substance that, much to his surprise, glowed pale green in the dark. He named this substance phosphorus from the Greek for 'light bearer'. It is possible to see the phosphorous in your own urine by examining it under ultraviolet light (black light) – something for the truly 'curious' only.

ALCOHOL

One of the most noticeable, and yet underappreciated, effects of alcohol on the body, is that it suppresses the secretion of ADH. Without ADH, there is little reabsorption of filtrate in the DCT and collecting duct, and the kidneys produce large quantities of dilute urine. This phenomenon explains why, after a few drinks at the pub, you must continually leave your seat to return to the increasingly familiar and usually overcrowded pub toilet. It also explains why, if you continue drinking alcohol, you will feel dehydrated and generally 'hung-over' the next morning. Alcohol also stimulates the conversion of glycogen into glucose (see Chapter 13) which may be lost in the urine as a result of diuresis. One 'unit' of alcohol is equivalent to 10 ml of pure alcohol (ethanol) and it is estimated that each unit consumed, forces the kidneys to generate an additional 120 ml of urine per hour. This fluid has got to come from somewhere, and excessive alcohol consumption inevitably results in cellular dehydration and electrolyte imbalance. This also results in the sensation of thirst since the osmoreceptors of the hypothalamus are extremely sensitive to increases in plasma osmolality. Unfortunately, drinking more alcohol simply results in further dehydration and continued thirst. Drinking water with alcohol provides a degree of compensation but you only retain 30–50% of this additional fluid. The only sure way to restore ADH secretion is to stop drinking alcohol altogether and allow plasma levels to decrease below the threshold value for ADH inhibition. Once this occurs the kidneys start to conserve water and urine becomes increasingly concentrated and less plentiful. As irritating as this mechanism is, sometimes referred to as 'breaking the seal', it prevents us from overloading our bodies with fluid (and alcohol) that could result in a number of dangerous and potentially fatal complications.

WATER INTOXICATION

Even drinking excessive quantities of tap water can be extremely harmful. For example, if you consume water faster than it can be excreted by the kidneys, it can decrease the sodium concentration (and osmolality) of the interstitial fluid and plasma (hyponatremia). This results in the osmotic movement of water from the interstitial fluid into the cells causing them to swell. This is known as water intoxication and can result in headaches, confusion, convulsions, coma and even death as cells in the brain swell and increase inter-cranial pressure. In 2007, an American woman died whilst taking part in a radio competition to drink the most water without going to the toilet. The radio station was eventually ordered to pay

her family $16 million in compensation since they had been warned that drinking large quantities of water was potentially dangerous. We saw in Chapter 1 that the average human being contains about 40 litres of water which accounts for 55–60% of total body weight. It is extremely important, therefore, that this fluid remains in the correct fluid compartments and that the kidneys continue to maintain normal fluid balance via the mechanisms discussed above.

FLUID REPLACEMENT

Fluid loss is dependent on internal and external variables but 'typically' about 1,500 ml is eliminated each day as urine, about 800 ml as water vapour and sweat (insensible loss) and 150–200 ml in normal faeces. Additional fluid loss due to excessive sweating, diarrhoea, vomiting (emesis), haemorrhage, burns, etc. may result in disruption of normal metabolic processes and a reduction in blood volume (hypovolaemia). In these (and other) instances, fluid replacement may be necessary to maintain blood pressure and to ensure cellular hydration. The simplest way to achieve this is by drinking water but, when this is not possible, an intravenous (IV) infusion may be necessary. Intravenous fluids are broadly divided into crystalloids and colloids. Crystalloids consist of small molecules that are able to diffuse across cell membranes (e.g. to provide cellular hydration and nutrition) as well as replace fluid from the intravascular compartment. Examples of crystalloid solutions include normal saline (0.9%), dextrose saline (5%) and Hartmann's solution (also known as compound sodium lactate or CSL). Colloids, on the other hand, consist of larger molecules that remain in the circulatory system for longer and help to sustain intravascular volume. That is to say, they are unable to cross the vascular membrane and help to maintain high colloid osmotic pressure in the plasma. Colloids can be blood-based products such as whole blood, packed cells (erythrocytes only) and clotting factors (platelets and fresh frozen plasma/FFP). They may also be synthetic plasma expanders such as Gelofusine which contains gelatine molecules and behaves much like blood filled with albumin. Although synthetic products are extremely useful for increasing intravascular volume when blood pressure is low, it is important to remember that they have no oxygen-carrying capacity or clotting factors. Laboratory results and investigation associated with fluid loss include increased serum osmolality, high urine specific gravity (see below), raised haematocrit (% of erythrocytes in blood) and increased plasma-urea concentration.

COLOUR, CLARITY AND ODOUR OF URINE

The colour, clarity and odour of urine can provide a great deal of information about a person's general state of health. Normal urine is typically transparent and ranges in colour from pale yellow to bright amber. Lack of colour is usually not a concern but may indicate excessive fluid consumption or diabetes insipidus (see above). Red or pinkish urine, on the other hand, suggests the presence of blood (haematuria). However, it is important to remember that certain foods such as beetroot and blackberries contain a red pigment which could be responsible for this change in colour. It is also important to discretely enquire whether menstrual blood could have coloured the sample. Cloudy urine often indicates urinary tract infection (UTI) and may contain white blood cells, bacteria, pus and large amounts of mucous. A foamy or frothy specimen is usually a sign of protein in the urine. If you have ever beaten eggs in a bowl and then washed it under a tap, you will have seen it froth and foam as protein from the eggs react with water. A slight odour is not uncommon in a normal urine specimen but strong or foul-smelling urine usually indicates that the sample is highly concentrated or infected. A sweet or fruity odour (acetone), on the other hand, is associated with ketone formation (see below) which may occur as a result of diabetes mellitus, starvation or dehydration. Some foods such as asparagus can also produce strong smelling urine. In this instance, what you can smell is the breakdown of a sulphur compound called methyl mercaptan or methanethiol. There is also a rare genetic condition called trimethylaminuria (fish odour syndrome) which causes urine, sweat and breath to smell strongly of fish.

URINALYSIS

All of the above can be observed simply by looking at and smelling the sample. More information, however, can be obtained by undertaking a reagent or dipstick test of the urine. Put simply, abnormal substances in the urine react with chemicals on the testing strips and cause colour changes that can be interpreted using a key. Reagent strips typically test for the following variables: bilirubin, urobilinogen, glucose, ketones, protein, pH, specific gravity, erythrocytes, leukocytes and nitrites. We saw in Chapter 5, that bilirubin is a waste product formed when erythrocytes are broken down in the liver and spleen, and is normally excreted from the body as a component of bile (via the gastrointestinal tract). If bilirubin is present in urine, therefore, it may indicate liver disease or damage since this process it not occurring normally. Urobilinogen results from the further breakdown of bilirubin in the gastrointestinal tract by commensal bacteria. If urobilinogen is detected in urine, it may also indicate liver disease/damage or possibly haemolytic (blood + splitting) anaemia. We noted earlier in the chapter that glucose should not be present in normal urine since it is entirely reabsorbed by the PCT in health. If glycosuria does occur, however, it usually indicates diabetes mellitus (see Chapter 13) but can occur during pregnancy or when taking certain medications (e.g. corticosteroids). More worrying, however, is the presence of ketones in the urine. These are acidic chemicals that are produced during the breakdown of fat to produce energy or fuel. This may occur as a result of prolonged vomiting, starvation (including some forms of dieting) and poorly controlled diabetes mellitus. We also noted earlier in the chapter, that protein molecules are too large to be filtered through the glomerulus and Bowman's capsule in health (Table 10.1). The presence of protein in the urine, therefore, may indicate damage to the glomerulus as a result of high blood pressure, renal inflammation or the formation of renal stones (calculi).

pH, SPECIFIC GRAVITY, ERYTHROCYTES AND LEUCOCYTES

The pH and specific gravity of urine are both variable. For example, although pH of urine is typically acidic (about 6), a vegetarian diet can result in a pH that is more alkali. This occurs because bicarbonate added to the blood from fruit and vegetables combines with hydrogen ions to form carbon dioxide and water. In short, this reduces the hydrogen ion concentration of plasma and increases the amount of bicarbonate filtered by the glomerulus and excreted in the urine (see above). Other reasons for alkaline urine include metabolic alkalosis and Fanconi's syndrome (a rare condition in which a number of compounds including bicarbonate are excreted in the urine rather than reabsorbed in the PCT). Highly acidic urine may also indicate acidosis, renal stone formation or a diet high in protein. Specific gravity (SG) simply refers to the overall concentration of solutes within the urine. The higher the value, the more concentrated the urine tends to be (the higher the drier). The presence of erythrocytes in urine (haematuria) usually indicates trauma to the urinary tract or urinary tract infection (UTI) but may also result from cancer (e.g. bladder or prostate) or as a side effect of anticoagulant medication (see Chapter 5). The presence of leukocytes indicates UTI (upper or lower) or renal inflammation. Finally, a positive nitrite test demonstrates that bacteria may be present in significant numbers (often escheria-coli/e-coli).

RENAL DISEASE

So far we have seen how the kidneys regulate the chemical composition of blood, maintain plasma osmolality and manage blood volume and pressure. In Chapter 5, we observed how the kidneys maintain a constant level of circulating erythrocytes through the secretion of erythropoietin (EPO) in response to hypoxaemia. In Chapter 4, we also noted that the absorption of dietary calcium from the gastrointestinal tract is dependent on the availability of a hormone called calcitriol. Calcitriol is the active form of vitamin D and is originally derived from calciferol (vitamin D_3) synthesised in the epidermis of the skin following exposure to ultraviolet light. Calciferol is converted into 25-hydroxy vitamin D by the liver before it is carried to the kidneys (bound to globulin) and converted into calcitriol by the cells of the PCT. Calcitriol facilitates the absorption of calcium (and phosphate) in the small intestine and increases reabsorption of calcium in the renal tubules. It also stimulates osteoclast activity which liberates calcium from the bone in order to increase plasma concentration (see Chapters 4 and 13). Finally, not content with all of these important regulatory functions, the kidneys are also able to synthesise glucose from amino acids and glycerol (gluconeogenesis) when levels decrease below normal. Bearing all of this in mind, it is easy to understand why kidney injury and renal disease are potentially so serious. For example, if the kidneys are unable to secrete erythropoietin or calcitriol it will result in renal anaemia and renal bone disease (osteomalacia). Moreover, if the kidneys are unable to excrete wastes and excess ions, it will result in toxic accumulation of urea, creatinine, potassium and other potentially harmful substances leading to nausea, vomiting, disorientation and other neuromuscular disorders. If the kidneys cannot produce or excrete urine in the normal way, there will also be fluid overload and possible oedema.

DIALYSIS

End stage renal failure occurs when about 90% of kidney function has been lost and the patient will require regular renal dialysis. Haemodialysis describes the process by which waste products and excess water are removed from the blood through a filter (dialyser) situated in the haemodialysis machine. Treatment usually takes place three times a week and lasts for 3–4 hours during which time the patient's entire blood volume (about 5 litres) circulates through the machine every 15 minutes or so. Peritoneal dialysis, on the other hand, takes place inside the patient's abdomen using their peritoneum as the dialysis membrane. A flexible plastic tube, known as a Tenckhoff catheter, is surgically inserted into the peritoneal cavity and allows dialysate to be inserted and drained. The dialysate remains in the abdomen for 4–6 hours (known as a 'dwell') before it is drained and replaced with fresh fluid. During this time, waste products diffuse across the peritoneum from the underlying blood vessels and are removed from the body when the dwell fluid is drained. Peritoneal dialysis is performed four times a day, every day. Although this sounds restrictive it is possible to empty and refill the dialysate fluid in a wide variety of locations and I have seen it done on a fishing boat!

CHAPTER 10: TEST YOURSELF

Q. What is the name for the thin muscular tubes that transport urine from the kidney to the bladder, and from the bladder out of the body?

A. Two ureters transport urine from the kidney to the bladder. One urethra transports urine from the bladder out of the body.

Q. Describe the gross (large) anatomy of the kidney from the outside in.

A. The kidney is enclosed in a protective layer of fat and fibrous tissue known as the renal capsule. The outer layer of the kidney is called the renal cortex. This surrounds the renal medulla which is divided into a number of cone-shaped renal pyramids. These drain urine into a number of cup-shaped structures known as calyces which, themselves, drain urine into the larger funnel-shaped renal pelvis. From here, urine drains into the ureters and bladder.

Q. What is meant by the term renal corpuscle and what does it do?

A. The renal corpuscle consists of the afferent arteriole, the efferent arteriole, the glomerulus and the Bowman's (or glomerular) capsule. The afferent arteriole transports blood towards the glomerulus and the afferent arteriole transports it away. When the blood is in the glomerulus, a pressure gradient pushes water and small molecules (e.g. glucose) through the semi-permeable walls of the glomerulus and Bowman's capsule (that surrounds it). In this way, water and solutes are filtered from the blood into the renal tubules (leaving larger molecules such as erythrocytes and proteins in the circulation).

Q. What are the sections of the renal tubule called?

A. Proximal convoluted tubule, loop of Henle, distal convoluted tubule and collecting duct.

Q. Anatomically, what is the difference between cortical and juxtamedullary nephrons?

A. Cortical nephrons are located almost entirely within the cortex (only a small section of the loop of Henle is contained within the medulla). Juxtamedullary nephrons, on the other hand, are located in the renal cortex (renal corpuscle, proximal and distal convoluted tubules) and medulla (loop of Henle).

Q. Both types of nephron produce urine by three precisely regulated processes: filtration, reabsorption, secretion. Briefly explain what is meant by reabsorption and secretion.

A. Reabsorption describes the movement of water and other substances, from the renal tubule back into the peritubular capillaries that surround it. Much of this process occurs immediately after filtration in the proximal convoluted tubule. Secretion moves substances out of the capillary blood and into the renal tubules where they mix with water and other waste materials in order to produce urine.

Q. What percentage of water is reabsorbed in the renal tubules in health?

A. About 99% of the 180 litres of water filtered from the blood is returned to the circulation via reabsorption.

Q. Why is secretion of hydrogen ions (H^+) important for health?

A. Secretion of H^+ is important for maintaining acid-base balance in the blood (pH 7.35–7.45).

Q. Normal urine output is considered to be at least 0.5 ml/per kg/per hour. What should the minimum urine output be for a 70 kg adult per hour?

A. $0.5 \times 70 = 35$ ml per hour.

Q. In addition to urination, how else do we lose water each day?

A. Expired air (water vapour), sweat (evaporation) and faeces.

Q. What is the name for the receptors (located in the hypothalamus) that detect when plasma osmolality is high (i.e. plasma volume is low)?

A. Osmoreceptors.

Q. Management of blood volume is controlled by the action of the renin – angiotensin – aldosterone system (RAAS) and antidiuretic hormone (ADH). Explain how ADH recovers water from the kidney during dehydration?

A. When dehydrated, osmoreceptors detect an increase in osmotic pressure and trigger the secretion of ADH from the posterior pituitary gland. ADH is transported in the blood to the kidneys, where it increases the permeability of the collecting ducts and facilitates the reabsorption of water into the capillary circulation.

Q. When undertaking urinalysis, what does the presence of leukocytes and nitrites indicate?

A. The presence of leukocytes indicates urinary tract infection and nitrites demonstrate that bacteria may also be present.

Q. What do ketones in the urine indicate?

A. Ketones are acidic chemicals that are produced during the breakdown of fat to manufacture energy. This may occur as a result of prolonged vomiting or starvation (including some forms of dieting) or, in the presence of glucose, as a result of diabetes mellitus.

Q. Why should glucose not be present in the urine of a healthy individual?

A. 100% of glucose is reabsorbed in the proximal convoluted tubule.

Q. Why should bilirubin not be present in urine?

A. Bilirubin is a waste product formed when erythrocytes are broken down in the liver (and spleen) and is normally excreted from the body as a component of bile. If it is present in urine, it may indicate liver disease or damage.

Contents

CHAPTER 11

DIGESTIVE SYSTEM

METABOLISM

The term metabolism refers to the cellular processes that result in the production and liberation of energy and the synthesis of substances necessary for life. For example, in Chapter 1, we observed that the human body is involved in a constant cycle of anabolism and catabolism. Anabolism is the phase of metabolism in which simple structures are transformed into complex molecules (e.g. amino acids into proteins). Catabolism, on the other hand, refers to the breakdown (destructive metabolism) of complex molecules into simple structures (e.g. protein into amino acids). Anabolism often requires chemical energy (ATP) to be expended, whilst catabolism results in its production or release. The energy required for anabolism is supplied by adenosine triphosphate (ATP). In Chapter 2, we saw that the 'energy' is actually stored in the covalent bonds between the phosphates with the greatest amount of energy in the bond between the second and third phosphate groups (remember: adenosine triphosphate). Put simply, adenosine triphosphate produces adenosine diphosphate + energy + phosphate (ATP → ADP + energy + P). Most of the energy from this balancing act is harnessed to drive cellular processes such as muscle contraction. The remainder is lost as heat and helps to maintain core temperature (Chapter 3). However, in order to ensure that this cyclical process continues in a healthy and uninterrupted fashion we must regularly ingest the necessary raw material or nutrients. These are subdivided into macronutrients which we need to consume in large amounts (carbohydrates, proteins and fats) and micronutrients which we consume in small quantities (minerals and vitamins). Water and fibre may also be considered nutrients and a balanced diet includes all of the above in an appropriate ratio.

CARBOHYDRATE

Carbohydrates are the most important metabolic fuel since they are broken down into monosaccharides (simple sugars) such as glucose and fructose. Around 35% of absorbed glucose is used immediately by cells whilst the rest is stored as glycogen in the liver until it is required (see Chapter 13). All carbohydrates are derived from plant sources except for lactose (milk sugar) and glycogen which is present in liver/meat. Carbohydrates are often described as either simple or complex. Simple carbohydrates are sugars whose chemical structure is composed of one or two sugars arranged in short chains (monosaccharides or disaccharides). Examples include glucose, fructose, sucrose, lactose and maltose which can be found in sugar beet, sugar cane, fruits, honey and milk. Complex carbohydrates, on the other hand, consist of a chemical structure made up of three or more sugars which are usually linked together to form a long chain (polysaccharides). Examples include starch, cellulose and dextrin which can be found in green vegetables, pasta, whole-grain bread, potatoes, corn, beans, lentils and peas. Since complex carbohydrates take longer to digest, they provide a more sustained source of energy than mono and disaccharides. However, not all polysaccharides can be digested, and cellulose, for example, passes through the human gastrointestinal tract (GIT) largely unchanged.

FIBRE AND PROTEIN

Cellulose is an example of dietary fibre and, although it is of little nutritional benefit, it provides a number of important functions. These include binding to intestinal fat (preventing it from being absorbed), providing a sensation of 'fullness', and adding bulk to faeces (poo) by retaining water (see below). Animals such as cows and sheep (known as ruminants) can acquire nutrients from cellulose (present in grass) by fermenting it in a specialised stomach and then regurgitating the partially digested material (cud) into their mouth for further chewing. This process of re-chewing the cud contributes to the further breakdown of cellulose and plant material and is known as rumination (hence ruminants). Proteins are made up of chains of amino acids which are necessary for the construction of muscles, tendons and bones, as well as enzymes, hormones, and plasma proteins including immunoglobulins (antibodies). Human proteins are constructed from a combination of 20 different amino acids. Nine of these are known as 'essential amino acids' and must be obtained from our diet since they cannot be synthesised by the body. Complete proteins (found in meat, fish, eggs, milk and soya) provide all of the essential amino acids. Incomplete proteins (found in pulses, grains and legumes) contain some of them.

FATS AND CHOLESTEROL

Dietary fats (lipids) are typically divided into three groups: saturated fat, unsaturated fat and cholesterol. Saturated fats are found mostly in animal products and have long been associated with an increased risk of cardiovascular disease. Examples include fatty and processed meats, cream, cheese, butter, lard

and (non-animal) coconut, chocolate and palm oil. Unsaturated or vegetable fats can be found in avocado, seeds, some vegetables, vegetable oil, olive oil and some fish oils. As a rule of thumb: saturated fats are solid at room temperature and unsaturated fats are liquid. Unfortunately, because unsaturated fats are difficult to transport in liquid form (and have a tendency to become rancid) some food manufacturers convert them into saturated fats by adding hydrogen. These are known as hydrogenated or trans-fats and have been implicated in the development of type 2 diabetes mellitus (see Chapter 13). Finally, cholesterol is synthesised by the liver and obtained in the diet from dairy products, egg yolk and fatty meat. Cholesterol combines with proteins in the blood to form lipoproteins known as low-density lipoprotein (LDL) and high-density lipoprotein (HDL). LDL transports cholesterol from the liver to the cells (which is good). However, if there is more cholesterol than the cells require it can accumulate in the artery walls. This is clearly undesirable and accounts for LDL's reputation as 'bad cholesterol'. HDL, on the other hand, transports cholesterol away from the cells and back to the liver (where it is added to the bile or converted into bile salts). For this reason, HDL is often referred to as 'good cholesterol' and higher levels are encouraged. Our relationship with dietary fat is complicated, therefore, and it is important to remember that, in the correct quantity, fat is a necessary part of a balanced diet. It is an essential component for the production of cell membranes, steroid hormones, prostaglandins and the myelin sheaths of axons (see Chapter 12). It is also a source of chemical energy and provides insulation and protection for our body as a whole.

VITAMINS AND MINERALS

Vitamins are chemical compounds that are required in small quantities for normal metabolism and health. Typically, they cannot be synthesised in sufficient quantities by the body and must be obtained from the diet. Vitamins are widely distributed in food and are divided into two main groups: fat-soluble vitamins

TABLE 11.1 Minerals

Mineral	Function
Sodium (Na)	Essential for muscular contraction, transmission of nerve impulses and the maintenance of electrolyte balance.
Potassium (K)	Essential for muscular contraction, transmission of nerve impulses and the maintenance of electrolyte balance.
Calcium (Ca)	Essential structural component of bone and necessary for muscle contraction and the coagulation of blood.
Phosphate (PO_4)	Essential for energy storage inside the cells as ATP. Essential structural component of bone and teeth.
Iron (Fe)	Essential for the formation of haemoglobin and erythropoiesis. Necessary for the synthesis of some enzymes.
Iodine (I)	Essential for the formation of thyroid hormones (thyroxin and triiodothyronine).

(A, D, E and K) and water-soluble vitamins (B complex and C). Minerals are also needed in trace amounts to ensure normal functioning of many cellular processes. They include sodium, potassium, calcium, phosphate, iodine and iron. We have observed in previous chapters, how many of these substances contribute to cellular health/homeostasis and Table 11.1 provides a brief summary.

PICA

Some people suffer from a condition called Pica where they compulsively eat items that have no nutritional value. It occurs most often in children and pregnant women and is usually transitory. Those affected generally eat relatively harmless substances such as ice, sand or soap (to name but a few) but some consume potentially dangerous items such as metal or flakes of dried paint which may contain lead. It is also interesting to note the trend amongst some people (particularly in the US) for consuming raw nutrients instead of food. In 2013 Robert Rhinehart, an engineering graduate from Atlanta, concocted a mixture of chemicals that would theoretically provide all of the essential nutrients he required to maintain health. By his own account, the early versions needed a bit a fine tuning and

initially he suffered from potassium poisoning (resulting in cardiac palpitations) amongst other problems. However, in May 2014 his product went on sale commercially (in the US) and he claims that 90% of his meals are now chemical. This is extreme to say the least but it is possible to use chemicals to successfully recreate flavours. For example, the chemical 2-heptanone, tastes exactly like Gorgonzola cheese, and 2-methyl-3-furanthiol, provides the flavour of chicken. Although the thought of laboratory-created food is distasteful to many (no pun intended) it is becoming increasingly possible.

HUNGER AND SATIETY

The hypothalamus is responsible for a variety of homeostatic functions including thermoregulation (see Chapter 3), fluid balance (see Chapter 10) and hunger and satiety (feeling full after eating). The lateral hypothalamus is responsible for hunger whilst the ventromedial hypothalamus controls satiety. When the stomach is empty, the gastric mucosa (lining of the stomach) secretes a hormone called ghrelin that stimulates receptors in the lateral hypothalamus and inhibits receptors in the ventromedial hypothalamus in order to produce the sensation of hunger. Ghrelin is also synthesised in lesser amounts by the small intestine, pancreas and hypothalamus itself, and is inhibited when the stomach is stretched. In some instances, however, this does not occur and ghrelin levels remain permanently elevated. For example, plasma ghrelin levels remain elevated in those suffering from the rare genetic disorder Prader-Willi syndrome (PWS) which causes a variety of symptoms including a constant feeling of hunger and a compulsion to eat. Ghrelin has also been shown to stimulate areas of the brain associated with reward and addiction (see Chapter 12). The 18th-century French soldier and 'showman' known as Tarrare is reported to have had an insatiable appetite (history doesn't record why). It is documented that he could eat huge quantities of meat, apples, stones, rubbish and live animals (including a whole cat and an eel). The French army even employed him to transport secret documents through enemy lines by swallowing them. Despite this, however, he was apparently slim and of average height. When he eventually died (of tuberculosis) an autopsy found that his oesophagus was abnormally wide and that his heavily ulcerated stomach occupied much of his abdominal cavity.

LEPTIN AND BODY MASS INDEX

The hormone leptin performs the opposite function to ghrelin and is produced by fat cells (adipocytes) in response to the total amount of body fat (adipose tissue) we store. Leptin acts upon receptors in the ventromedial hypothalamus which triggers the sensation of satiety. It also helps to regulate energy expenditure over a long period time and when leptin levels are high, the body stops storing additional fat and starts 'burning' it. However, in much the same way as persistently high blood glucose levels can lead to insulin resistance and type 2 diabetes mellitus (see Chapter 13), elevated leptin levels (as a result of a high percentage body fat) can lead to leptin-resistance. Consequently, although those who are severely obese generally exhibit high circulating concentrations of leptin, many do not experience a corresponding reduction in appetite because of leptin-resistance and desensitisation of the ventromedial hypothalamus. For adults, overweight and obesity ranges are often determined using weight (in kilograms) and height (in metres) to calculate what is known as body mass index or BMI. Although BMI does not measure body fat directly, for most people it provides a fairly accurate correlation to direct measures of body fat such as hydrostatic (underwater) weighing and dual energy xray absorptiometry (DEXA). It is important to note, however, that some individuals with high muscle mass may also have a high BMI. BMI is calculated by dividing the person's weight by their height squared (i.e. weight ÷ height ÷ height) in order to produce a numerical value (see Table 11.2). For example:

$$75 \text{ kg} \div 1.8 \text{ m} \div 1.8 \text{ m} = 23.1$$

TABLE 11.2 Body Mass Index (BMI) values

Category	BMI	BMI (Asian adults)
Underweight	< 18.5	< 18.5
Normal (healthy weight)	18.5 to 25	18.5 to 22.9
Overweight	25 to 30	23 to 27.5
Obese class I (moderately obese)	30 to 35	> 27.5
Obese class II (severely obese)	35 to 40	—
Obese class III (very severely obese)	> 40	—

THE PERITONEUM

The organs and structures of the digestive system can be divided into two groups: those of the gastrointestinal tract (GIT) and the accessory digestive organs such as the salivary glands, pancreas and liver (Figure 11.1). The GIT is essentially an uninterrupted tube that extends from the mouth to the anus. It consists of four separate layers: peritoneum,

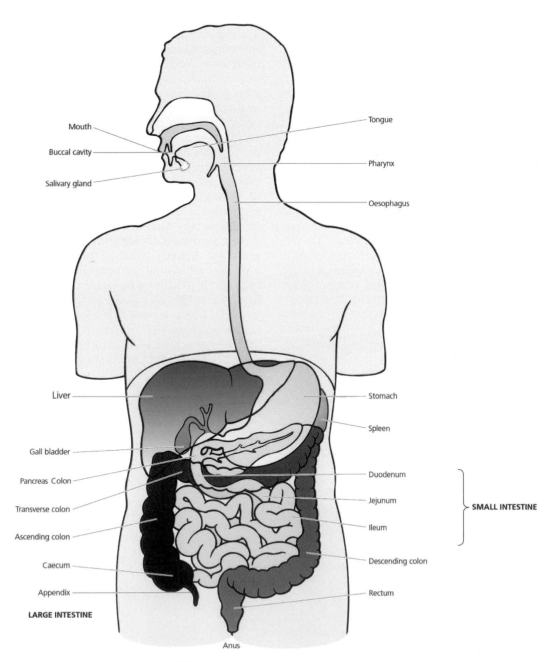

Figure 11.1 Gastrointestinal tract (GIT) and accessory digestive organs.

muscle, submucosa and mucosa (Figure 11.2). The outermost layer, the peritoneum, is a serous membrane (serosa) that lines the abdominal cavity and covers most of the abdominal organs. Some organs, such as the kidneys and pancreas, are only covered on their front (anterior) surface by the peritoneum and are said to be retroperitoneal (i.e. behind the peritoneum). Just like the serous membranes that cover the heart (pericardium) and lungs (pleura), the peritoneum is divided into an outer (parietal) and inner (visceral) layer. The parietal peritoneum is attached to the walls of the abdominal cavity whilst the thinner visceral peritoneum covers and surrounds most of the abdominal organs. The space between the two membranes is called the peritoneal cavity and contains serous fluid which allows the parietal and visceral layers to slide over one another in a frictionless fashion (like the heart and lungs). This is important since digested and partially digested material is regularly propelled through the GIT by rhythmic muscular contractions (peristalsis). The peritoneum also contains a series of large folds called the mesentery and omenta that hold the organs in place and provide a channel for blood and lymphatic vessels. The mesentery extends in a continuous fashion from the small to the large intestine and although

its function is still unclear at this time, it was designated an organ in 2016.[1]

GASTRIC SMOOTH MUSCLE AND MUCOSA

The next layer of the GIT (with the exception of the stomach) consists of two sheets of smooth muscle (muscularis): an inner circular layer and an outer longitudinal layer (Figure 11.2). This arrangement allows the muscles to churn and fragment partially digested material in order to ensure that it is mixed and blended with intestinal secretions (a process known as segmentation). It also allows peristaltic contractions to propel material through the GIT. Sandwiched between the two layers of muscle is a network of parasympathetic, sympathetic and sensory nerves called the myenteric or Auerbach's plexus. In simple terms, parasympathetic stimulation increases muscular activity within the GIT (resting and digesting) and sympathetic stimulation inhibits it (flight-or-fight). The third layer of tissue in the GIT is the submucosa (sub = 'under'). This is a layer of dense connective tissue containing nerve fibres and a rich supply of blood and lymphatic vessels. In some parts

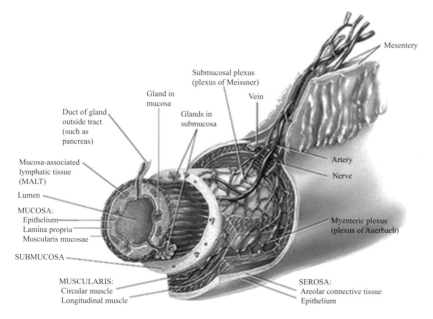

Figure 11.2 Layers of the gastrointestinal tract.

of the small intestine it also contains Peyer's patches (see Chapter 6) and exocrine glands that secrete enzymes and buffers into the lumen of the GIT. The final and innermost layer of the GIT is the mucosa or mucous membrane. This is subdivided into three further layers: the muscularis mucosa, the lamina propria and the epithelium (Figure 11.2). The muscularis mucosa is a thin layer of smooth muscle that provides involutions (inward projections) known as villi (see below). The lamina propria supports the blood vessels that nourish the epithelial cells and contains varying amounts of mucosa-associated lymphoid tissue (MALT: see Chapter 6). The innermost layer of the GIT is made up of columnar epithelium and has three main functions: protection, secretion and absorption of nutrients. This will be discussed in more detail below.

THE MOUTH AND SALIVARY GLANDS

The mouth or oral cavity is the point for normal ingestion of food and the first stage of mechanical and chemical breakdown. Chewing (mastication) takes place using the cheek muscles, teeth and tongue. The tongue is also the principal organ of taste but some taste buds (papillae) can be found on the roof of the mouth (palate) and the back of the throat (pharynx). This explains why children sometimes complain about 'tasting' nose drops as they run down the back of the nasal cavity into the pharynx. As the food is tasted in the mouth, it is mixed with saliva and rolled into a ball (bolus) prior to being swallowed. Saliva is produced and secreted by three pairs of salivary glands: sublingual (under the tongue), submandibular (under the mandible/jaw) and parotid glands. Although the parotid glands are by far the largest of the three pairs, the submandibular glands produce the most saliva (about 70% of the total). Saliva is essential to lubricate the mouth, assist with swallowing, protect the teeth against bacteria and to aid chemical digestion of food. It is essentially water (97–99%) mixed with varying amounts of mucus, mineral salts, lysozyme, immunoglobulin A (IgA) and the digestive enzyme

salivary (or alpha) amylase. We observed in Chapter 1 that salivary amylase breaks down (catabolises) complex carbohydrates (polysaccharides) present in rice, bread and potatoes into disaccharides such as maltose. Although salivary amylase only plays a minor role in the digestion of dietary carbohydrate overall, it is significant that this process commences as soon as carbohydrate enters the mouth since it (eventually) results in the production of glucose essential for the production of cellular energy (glucose + O_2 → ATP + CO_2 + H_2O). Salivation is regulated by the parasympathetic nervous system in response to the presence of food in the mouth or even the thought of food in the mouth. You may have heard of the experiments carried out by the Russian physiologist Ivan Pavlov on his hungry dogs. In summary, Pavlov presented a dog with a bowl of food and measured its drool. However, he quickly realised that any object or event that the dog associated with food (such as the lab assistant or, eventually, ringing a bell) triggered the same salivation response. What he demonstrated was that the (parasympathetic) salivation response can be manipulated or conditioned in response to the expectation of food. We all experience this to some degree and it is not uncommon for our 'mouth to water' in anticipation of a meal, particularly if we are hungry. However, it is not considered socially acceptable to actually drool on the floor. Sympathetic stimulation of the salivary glands, on the other hand, inhibits salivation and results in a dry mouth and difficulty swallowing. This is why your mouth becomes dry and you find it difficult to speak immediately before you have to give a presentation in front of your class or group of colleagues (flight-or-fight response). Finally, the viral infection mumps can cause the parotid salivary glands to become swollen and inflamed, resulting in the classic 'hamster-face' appearance.

SWALLOWING

Swallowing (deglutition) is partly a voluntary and partly an involuntary process. The tongue manipulates the food in the mouth and mixes it with saliva whilst the teeth tear and grind it into smaller pieces. These pieces are then compressed into a bolus and voluntarily moved towards the back of oral cavity by the tongue. The uvula (teardrop-shaped process 'dangling' from the middle of the soft palate) helps to prevent the bolus from entering the pharynx prematurely. However, most of us have experienced the crushing disappointment of sucking a sweet only for it to be unexpectedly swallowed as it moves too close to the back of the mouth. Once food enters the pharynx, swallowing occurs involuntarily as receptors in the uvula and palatal arch are stimulated. Palatal muscles elevate the uvula and soft palate to block the entrance to the nasopharynx during swallowing. At the same time, longitudinal muscle fibres in the walls of the pharynx lift the larynx and fold the epiglottis over the glottis to ensure that the bolus passes into the oesophagus and not the lower respiratory tract. Once in the oesophagus, the bolus is forced towards the stomach by peristaltic waves of muscular contraction. This process is assisted by gravity unless you happen to be eating upside-down or are on board the International Space Station. Solids typically take between four and eight seconds to pass from the oropharynx into the stomach whilst fluids take between one and two seconds. However, if the oesophagus or bolus is poorly lubricated it may be necessary to initiate secondary peristaltic waves to 'force' the food into the stomach. You may have experienced this whilst trying to swallow something unpleasant (e.g. medicine). Immediately before the swallowed material arrives at the stomach, the cardiac sphincter relaxes in order to allow it to enter and then closes again to prevent backflow (regurgitation) of acidic stomach contents into the oesophagus (Figure 11.3). A sphincter is simply a ring of muscle that surrounds and allows access to an opening or tube (in this case, the opening to the stomach, which happens to be located near to the heart – hence 'cardiac').

STOMACH

The stomach comprises the same four layers as the rest of the GIT (serosa, muscularis, submucosa and mucosa) with a number of important differences. For example, the epithelial cells of the stomach lining (mucosa) extend downwards into the lamina propria to form gastric pits, which contain specialised secretary cells called gastric glands (Figure 11.4). The stomach also has an additional layer of inner oblique muscle that allows it to churn and mix stomach contents with gastric secretions more effectively. When the stomach is empty, the muscularis contracts in order to fold the mucosa and submucosa into ridges called gastric rugae (Latin for 'wrinkles'). In this state, the adult stomach varies between 15 and 25 cm in length and is often compared to a large sausage. As food enters the stomach, however, the rugae flatten in order to allow it (and the muscles surrounding it) to stretch and expand. At full stretch, the stomach can accommodate as much as four litres of food (1–2 litres is more 'normal') and can occupy a considerable amount of space within the abdominal cavity (not as much as Tarrare, however). Since it is not possible to digest all of this food at once, the stomach acts as a holding area and releases partially digested material into the duodenum at a slow and measured rate. The first part of the stomach is called the cardia (because of its proximity to the heart) and acts as an entry point for food from the cardiac sphincter (Figure 11.3). It also contains a large number of mucus-producing glands (see below). Next to the cardia is the dome-shaped fundus where food is mixed with dilute gastric secretions and held until it is released into the next part of the stomach. The body of the stomach is situated below the fundus and acts as the principle mixing area for food and gastric secretions before it enters the final part of the stomach known as the pylorus (from the Greek word for 'gatekeeper'). The pylorus is often subdivided into the pyloric antrum ('gatekeepers cave') and pyloric canal which funnels partially digested, semi-liquid material called chyme towards the stomach exit (pyloric sphincter) and first part of the small intestine (duodenum). Chyme is highly acidic and exactly the sort of thing that you don't want to suddenly appear in your mouth following a sick-burp. A considerable amount of chemical digestion takes place in the pyloric antrum since food is often held here for a long period of time before being released into the next part of the GIT. Once food enters the stomach, peristaltic 'mixing waves' sweep over

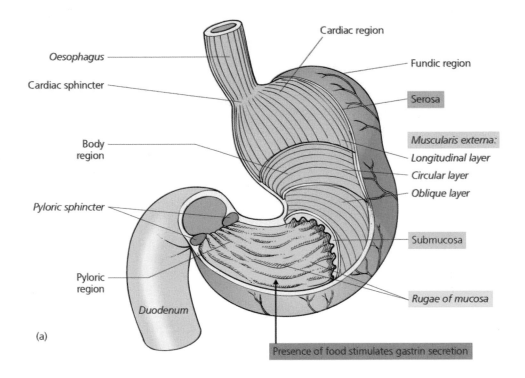

(a)

Oesophagus

Cardiac sphincter

Body region

Pyloric sphincter

Pyloric region

Duodenum

Cardiac region

Fundic region

Serosa

Muscularis externa:
Longitudinal layer
Circular layer
Oblique layer

Submucosa

Rugae of mucosa

Presence of food stimulates gastrin secretion

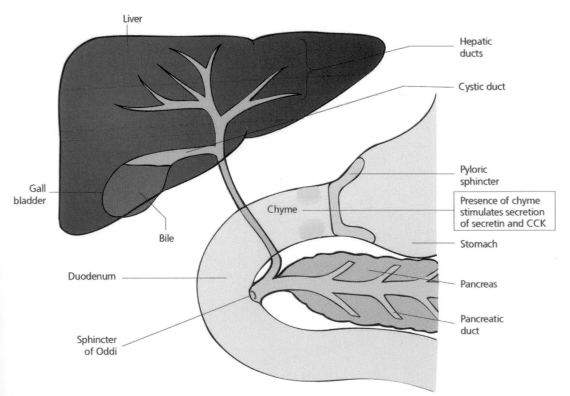

Liver

Gall bladder

Bile

Duodenum

Sphincter of Oddi

Hepatic ducts

Cystic duct

Pyloric sphincter

Presence of chyme stimulates secretion of secretin and CCK

Chyme

Stomach

Pancreas

Pancreatic duct

Figure 11.3 (a) Stomach. (b) Liver, pancreas and duodenum.

the body (of the stomach) and pylorus every 15–20 seconds. These intensify as they reach the pylorus and several millilitres of chyme is forced through the pyloric sphincter with each contraction. However, most of the chyme is pushed back into the body of the stomach where mixing and churning continue to take place. This process is regulated by both the autonomic nervous system (via Auerbach's plexus) and a hormone called gastrin.

GASTRIC SECRETIONS

Secretion of hormones, enzymes and buffers (collectively known as gastric juice) takes place in three phases: cephalic, gastric and intestinal. The cephalic phase refers to the production of saliva and other secretions before food reaches the stomach and occurs in response to parasympathetic stimulation discussed above. The gastric phase is initiated by the presence of food in the stomach and results in the secretion of the hormone gastrin from cells in the pyloric antrum and duodenum. We noted in the previous section, that the surface mucosa of the stomach contains numerous downward extensions called gastric pits (Figure 11.4). These are lined with columns of secretary cells called gastric glands and include G cells, parietal cells and chief cells. Gastrin is secreted by G cells in response to stretching (distension) of the pyloric antrum and the presence of undigested protein. It is inhibited by the increasing acidity of gastric secretions (typically a pH of less than 2). Gastrin promotes the contraction of gastric smooth muscle, the production of intrinsic factor by parietal cells and the secretion of pepsinogen by chief cells. Intrinsic factor is a glycoprotein (carbohydrate combined with a protein) that binds with vitamin B_{12} and allows it to be absorbed in the small intestine. Vitamin B_{12} (also known as cobalamin) is a water-soluble vitamin found in liver, meat, shell fish, eggs and dairy products. It is essential for erythropoiesis (red blood cell production) and the formation of DNA and myelin (see Chapter 12). A deficiency of intrinsic factor can be extremely serious and result in pernicious anaemia and damage to the central nervous system.

HYDROCHLORIC ACID AND PEPSIN

Gastrin also stimulates parietal cells to secrete hydrochloric acid (HCl) which helps to destroy the many microorganisms we ingest with food and unfold (denature) proteins so that they can be broken down by proteolytic (protein splitting) enzymes such as pepsin. Secretion of HCl maintains the pH of gastric juice between about 3.5 and 1.5. However,

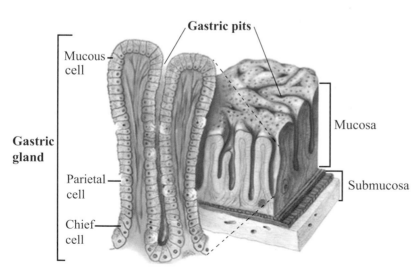

Figure 11.4 Gastric pits and glands.

in order to protect the parietal cells from the adverse effects of such strong acid, hydrogen ions (H+) and chloride ions (Cl-) are secreted separately into the stomach. Chief cells secrete two digestive enzymes into the stomach: gastric lipase and pepsinogen. Gastric lipase plays a limited role in the digestion of fats (lipids) and helps to split triglycerides into fatty acids and monoglycerides. Pepsinogen doesn't digest anything until it comes into contact with HCl, at which point it is transformed into its active form pepsin. Pepsin is an extremely aggressive protein-digesting enzyme that splits the bonds between amino acids, that make up proteins, in order to produce short chain peptides. The transformation of pepsinogen into pepsin is another example of positive feedback discussed in Chapter 3. That is to say, pepsinogen remains an inactive enzyme precursor (zymogen) until it nears the surface of the stomach (chief cells are situated deep within the gastric pits) and is converted into pepsin by HCl (and activated pepsin) in order to break down protein. This process continues until protein digestion has been accomplished. At this point, pH increases (i.e. acidity decreases) and the conversion of pepsinogin into pepsin stops. This is important, since it prevents auto (self) digestion of the protein present in gastric glands. The stomach is also protected from the potentially damaging effects of HCl and pepsin by a 1–3 mm layer of alkaline mucus secreted by mucus-producing cells situated on the surface of the stomach and in the neck of the gastric pits. This is why swallowing a bit (or a lot) of mucus is not necessarily a problem since it simply mixes with the mucus that is already present within the stomach. It also explains why, having vomited the acidic contents of your stomach into a bowl or other convenient receptacle, it is not unusual to find yourself retching mucus. Finally, it is estimated that the gastric glands produce, on average, an impressive 1.5 litres of gastric juice each day.

INTESTINAL DIGESTION

The duodenum is the first and shortest section of the small intestine. It extends in a C-shaped

arc around the head of the pancreas from the pyloric sphincter to the jejunum (Figures 11.1, 11.3). When chyme is delivered into the duodenum, it stimulates stretch receptors and chemical receptors (chemoreceptors) to inhibit gastrin production by the stomach and decrease gastric motility. It also stimulates the contraction of the pyloric sphincter which prevents the delivery of further chyme into the duodenum. This measured release of small amounts of acidic chyme through the pyloric sphincter helps to protect the delicate lining of the duodenum and ensures that intestinal digestion takes place at an appropriate rate. Chyme is also relatively hypertonic (i.e. it exerts osmotic 'pull' on water) and if it were released too quickly, it would attract large amounts of water resulting in poor digestion and absorption and, ultimately, diarrhoea. The fatty acids, peptides and glucose in chyme (in addition to its acidity) also trigger specialised (enterogastric) cells in the duodenum to secrete two hormones into the blood: secretin and cholecystokinin (CCK). Secretin stimulates cells in the liver and the pancreas' to secrete alkaline bicarbonate into the ducts that drain into the duodenum (Figure 11.3). This helps to neutralise the potentially damaging effects of acidic chyme by raising pH. Secretin also inhibits gastric motility and the production of gastric secretions. CCK derives its name from the Greek for bile + sac + move (chole + cysto + kinin) and stimulates the contraction of the gall bladder and the ejection of stored bile (produced in the liver). It also increases production of a number of digestive enzymes and secretions by the pancreas and relaxes the hepatopancreatic sphincter (also known as the sphincter of Oddi). This allows both pancreatic juice and bile from the liver/gall bladder, to be injected into the duodenum. Finally, CCK inhibits gastric activity in a similar fashion to secretin and may also inhibit the sensation of hunger.

PANCREAS

The pancreas is a retroperitoneal organ that is about 12–15 cm long and looks a little bit like a squashed banana in shape. It is subdivided into the head, body and tail and secretes digestive enzymes into the duodenum via the pancreatic duct (Figure 11.3). The pancreatic duct unites with the common bile duct to form a shared pathway called the hepatopancreatic ampulla (also known as the ampulla of Vater) which terminates at the hepatopancreatic sphincter mentioned above. The pancreas itself performs two important functions: the production and secretion of digestive juices into the pancreatic duct and duodenum (exocrine) and the production and secretion of hormones into the blood (endocrine). The hormone-producing endocrine tissue typically accounts for about 1% of the total mass of the pancreas and is organised into clusters of cells known as pancreatic islets. The hormones secreted by these cells help to regulate blood glucose (amongst other things) and are discussed in more detail in Chapter 13. The vast majority of pancreatic cells (99%), therefore, are exocrine acinar cells arranged in small clusters called acini. The Latin word *acinus* means berry and it is helpful to imagine or visualise a cluster of acinar cells as the different lobes of a raspberry or blackberry. These cells secrete a mixture of water, bicarbonate and digestive enzymes known collectively as pancreatic juice. The water and bicarbonate, as mentioned above, help to neutralise the acidic chyme from the stomach and create a more favourable environment for the pancreatic enzymes which work best at about pH 8 (slightly alkaline).

PANCREATIC ENZYMES

Pancreatic enzymes include pancreatic amylase that, like salivary amylase secreted in the mouth, helps to digest carbohydrate. The pancreas also produces protein-digesting enzymes called trypsin and chymotrypsin. Like pepsin, these are secreted as inactive enzyme precursors (trypsinogen and chymotrypsinogen) in order to protect the pancreas from auto-digestion. When trypsinogen passes through the hepatopancreatic sphincter, it comes into contact with an enzyme called enterokinase (also known as enteropepsidase) produced by cells in the duodenum. Enterokinase breaks

off (cleaves) part of the trypsinogen molecule to create trypsin which, in turn, converts inactive chymotrypsinogen into active chymotrypsin. Premature activation of these enzymes in the acinar cells can lead to pancreatic inflammation (pancreatitis). Interestingly (in my opinion at least) enterokinase was discovered by the same Ivan Pavlov who identified the conditioned reflex in dogs (see above). The final pancreatic enzyme (discussed here) is pancreatic lipase which, as its name suggests, helps to break down dietary lipids (fats, oils and triglycerides). We saw in Chapter 2 that lipids don't mix well with water (they are hydrophobic) and in the GIT they often clump together as large globules. These are difficult to digest and lipase is assisted in this process by bile secreted from the liver and gall bladder (Figure 11.3). Bile contains bile salts which, like the washing-up liquid discussed in Chapter 2, have hydrophilic and hydrophobic ends which envelop the fat and split large globules into numerous small molecules called micelles. These can be broken down (hydrolysed) by lipase into fatty acids and glycerol which are eventually absorbed through the mucosa of the small intestine. In addition to pancreatic enzymes, the epithelial cells of the small intestine (brush border) also secrete a number of enzymes which digest disaccharides into monosaccharides. For example, lactase converts lactose into galactose and glucose. Lactose intolerance is the inability to digest lactose because of lactase (enzyme) deficiency.

JEJUNUM AND ILEUM

The small intestine measures 6–7 m in length and is divided into three sections: the duodenum (discussed above), the jejunum and the ileum (Figure 11.1). The jejunum and ileum are suspended by the mesentery in sausage-like coils, and supplied with blood by the superior mesenteric artery. Digestion is (more or less) completed in the duodenum, where carbohydrates are broken down into monosaccharides (glucose, fructose and galactose); proteins into amino acids and peptides; and lipids into glycerol and fatty acids. Peristaltic

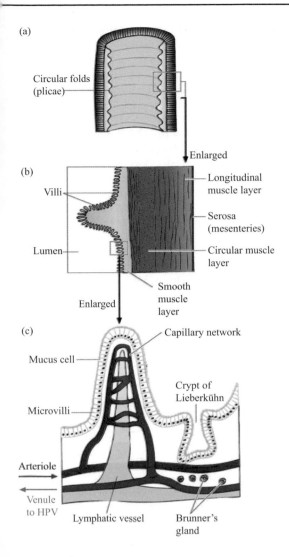

(a)

Circular folds (plicae)

Enlarged

(b)

Villi

Longitudinal muscle layer

Serosa (mesenteries)

Lumen

Circular muscle layer

Smooth muscle layer

Enlarged

(c)

Capillary network

Mucus cell

Crypt of Lieberkühn

Microvilli

Arteriole

Venule to HPV

Lymphatic vessel

Brunner's gland

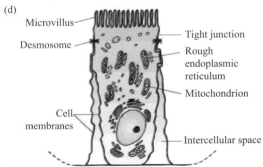

(d)

Microvillus

Desmosome

Tight junction

Rough endoplasmic reticulum

Mitochondrion

Cell membranes

Intercellular space

Figure 11.5 (a) Section of the duodenum. (b) Section through one circular fold. (c) Section through one villus (HPV = hepatic portal vein). (d) Intestinal cell.

contractions propel these simplified products of digestion through the duodenum, towards the jejunum and ileum, where they are gradually absorbed into the blood stream and lymph. However, in order for enough nutrients to be absorbed across the mucous membrane of this relatively short length of GIT, the intestinal fluid must come into contact with a large number of intestinal cells. Earlier in the chapter we noted that, in some parts of the GIT, the mucosa contains a thin layer of smooth muscle that provides inward projections known as villi (Figure 11.5). These finger-like involutions greatly increase the surface area available for absorption and it is estimated that in each mm^2 there are between 10 and 40 villi. Each villus measures 0.5–1.5 mm in length and contains one arteriole, one venule and a centrally located lymphatic capillary called a lacteal. The villi sway constantly to stir up the nutrients from the intestinal liquid and to increase the flow of blood and lymph. The simple columnar epithelial cells (enterocytes) that make up the villi are covered with additional microscopic projections called microvilli which form a brush border and further increase surface area. The brush border is also embedded with enzymes that complete the final stages of carbohydrate and protein digestion in the small intestine.

ABSORPTION

Monosaccharides are absorbed through the epithelial membrane into the bloodstream via a mixture of facilitated diffusion and active transport. Most proteins are absorbed into the bloodstream as amino acids via active transport (see Chapter 2). Finally, glycerol and fatty acids are absorbed via diffusion into the lacteals where they are mixed with lymph to form a milky substance called chyle. This is eventually transferred (via the lymph vessels) to the venous circulation where it is converted into lipoproteins, used for fuel or stored. However, most products of digestion (including vitamins and minerals) are transported via the superior mesenteric vein to the hepatic portal vein and the liver (see below). It is estimated that the villi of the jejunum and ileum absorb about 7.5 litres of fluid per day. Those who suffer from coeliac disease, however, are unable to absorb nutrients in the normal way because their villi become inflamed and sometimes permanently damaged. This occurs when the immune system mistakes substances found in gluten as a threat and launches a defensive response which attacks both gluten and the delicate lining of the small intestine.

LIVER

The liver is the second largest organ of the body (after the skin) and weighs about 1.5 kg. It is situated in the right upper quadrant of the abdominal cavity directly below the diaphragm. It consists of four lobes (of unequal size) which are themselves composed of 50,000–100,000 microscopic subunits called lobules (Figure 11.6). Lobules have a unique hexagonal shape and are formed from cells called hepatocytes (hepato + cyte = liver + cell). However, before we look at these structures in detail, it is important to understand the blood supply to and from the liver. We noted in the section above that nutrient-rich blood from the superior mesenteric vein drains into the hepatic portal vein and makes its way to the liver. This is interesting for two reasons. Firstly, it is unusual (but not unique) for a vein to supply blood to an organ (e.g. the heart). Secondly, the hepatic portal vein supplies about 80% of all the blood to the liver. The remaining 20% is provided by the

hepatic artery. Blood leaves the liver via the left, right and central hepatic veins (not to be confused with the hepatic portal vein) which drain into the inferior vena cava below the right atrium. Within the liver, the oxygenated arterial blood mixes with the deoxygenated venous blood in special vessels called sinusoids situated within the lobules. Sinusoids are essentially blood vessels with incomplete walls situated between two columns of hepatocytes. The oxygenated blood provides metabolic fuel for the hepatocytes whilst the deoxygenated blood contains the nutrients absorbed from the small intestine. Oxygen, carbon dioxide, nutrients, proteins and wastes are all exchanged through the thin walls of the sinusoids before the blood drains into a central venule which joins with veins from other lobules (Figure 11.6). Sinusoids also contain Kupffer cells (fixed macrophages) that destroy worn-out red blood cells, bacteria and other potentially harmful substances (Chapter 6).

FUNCTIONS OF THE LIVER

The liver has a wide variety of functions including the synthesis, breakdown (catabolism) and storage of macro and micro nutrients. For example, it stores fat-soluble vitamins (A, D, E and K), some water-soluble vitamins (B_{12}, C and folic acid), minerals (copper, iron and zinc) and glucose (as glycogen). It also transforms harmful substances (e.g. ammonia) into less harmful compounds (e.g. urea) and detoxifies

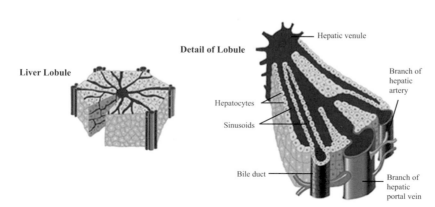

Liver Lobule

Detail of Lobule

Hepatic venule

Hepatocytes

Sinusoids

Bile duct

Branch of hepatic artery

Branch of hepatic portal vein

Figure 11.6 Hepatic lobule and sinusoid.

steroid hormones, drugs and alcohol. Other important functions include the production and secretion of bile, the manufacture of plasma proteins and clotting factors, and the generation of heat as a result of ongoing metabolic activity. With the exception of the brain, no other organ demonstrates such a variety of functional ability. This is particularly apparent when liver failure occurs and, although liver cells are able to renew themselves to some extent, damaged cells are often replaced with fibrous tissue (cirrhosis). Without going into too much detail, it is possible to quickly predict some of the consequences of end stage liver failure: inability to secrete bile results in jaundice and fatty diarrhoea (steatorrhoea), inability to produce plasma proteins results in albumin deficiency and fluid shift, inability to manufacture clotting factors results in haemorrhage, and inability to transform ammonia into urea results in toxicity and potentially lethal cerebral oedema. In short – please look after your liver.

LARGE INTESTINE

The large intestine or colon measures about 1.5 metres in length and is divided into four main parts: the ascending colon, the transverse colon, the descending colon and the sigmoid colon (Figure 11.1). Although it is shorter in length than the small intestine, the diameter of its lumen is much greater (about 6 cm). Other differences with the small intestine include the absence of villi, the abundance of mucus-secreting cells and the presence of three longitudinal bands of smooth muscle on the outer surface of the colon known as teniae coli. These thin ribbons of muscle contract lengthwise to produce pocket-like pouches known as haustra (Latin for 'bucket') which provide the colon with its segmented appearance. Haustral contractions occur every 25 minutes or so and propel the contents of the large intestine from haustrum to haustrum (or bucket to bucket). The principle function of the large intestine is the absorption of water from the material passing through it and the compaction of the remaining intestinal contents into semi-solid faeces.

Chyme arriving from the small intestine (ileum) passes through the ileocaecal valve into the pouch-like caecum (Latin for 'blind' as in blind-end). The caecum is attached to the vermiform (wormlike) appendix (discussed in Chapter 6) and commences the process of water absorption and compaction. As haustral contractions propel the chyme through the ascending, transverse and descending colon, more water is absorbed and the material becomes increasingly solid as it approaches the sigmoid colon and rectum. We noted in Chapter 6 that the colon also houses a variety of commensal bacteria which live symbiotically with their human host. The bacteria derive nourishment from cellulose found in plant cell walls, which the human digestive system (unlike that of cows and other ruminants) is incapable of breaking down. In return, the bacteria synthesise some B complex vitamins and vitamin K (necessary for the production of clotting factors). I once remarked to my children that it was possible 'to make vitamins up your bum' which simply resulted in much head-shaking and complaining about all the lies that I tell them.

COMMENSAL BACTERIA AND GAS

The other 'product' derived from the fermentation of cellulose by commensal bacteria in the large intestine is flatus or gas. Some of this gas (e.g. hydrogen sulphide and dimethyl sulphide) is quite odorous and it is estimated that, on average, a normal person 'expels' 500–1,000 ml of flatus each day. In health, the odour and volume is determined largely by dietary considerations such as the quantity of carbohydrate consumed (e.g. beans and broccoli). In Chapter 6, we saw that commensal bacteria compete with opportunistic and potentially pathogenic bacteria for essential nutrients, and also secrete inhibitory chemicals to eliminate them. We also noted that broad-spectrum antibiotics can damage and disrupt intestinal commensal activity and allow potentially pathogenic bacteria, such as Clostridium difficile, to multiply. A relatively new treatment for Clostridium difficile that is not responding to traditional therapy is called faecal transplantation (or stool transplant). It involves three stages: identifying a suitable poo donor, preparation of the donated 'material' and transplantation of the donated faeces into the recipient via an enema or, in a trial conducted 2012–2014, frozen in a capsule. Yes, this really does happen and has been demonstrated to be highly effective in many cases (although researchers warn that people should not be tempted to make 'home brews'). I also read that one team are developing a technique to introduce a bacteria found in baby poo into sausages in order to guard against disease in much the same way as probiotic yogurts are thought to. If you want to find out more about this exciting poo-sausage research, the article can be found in the wonderfully named journal *Meat Science* (Rubioa et al., 2014).

DEFECATION

It takes between 12 and 24 hours for material to pass completely through the colon. Once the majority of water and nutrients (including vitamins) have been absorbed from the chyme, the compacted semi-solid material is delivered to the rectum by powerful contractile waves appropriately known as mass movements. These occur in the transverse and descending colon about three or four times daily (typically during or after a meal). In order to prevent any physical damage to the colon during this process, mucus is secreted by the epithelial cells of the mucosa as the material passes over them. The mucus also helps to bind the undigested material into a consistent stool and normal 'healthy' faeces is made up of about 75% water and 25% solid matter (including undigested cellulose/fibre, dried digestive juices, protein, fat, cells shed by the intestine and bacteria). Of the 500 ml (or so) of chyme that enters the caecum each day, only about 150 ml becomes faeces. The finished product, so to speak, is excreted in response to a voluntary reflex triggered by stretching (distension) of the rectum as material enters it. Fortunately, defecation can be delayed by conscious controls (learned as a child) which allows voluntary constriction of the external anal sphincter at a time and place 'convenient' to us. Once you have passed the stool into an appropriate receptacle it is always worth having a look at it since much can be learned about our health from its appearance and consistency.

TOILET READING

The excellent Bristol Stool Chart was developed by Dr Ken Heaton at the University of Bristol and first published in 1997. It provides visual and descriptive indicators of the different types of stool likely to be produced (and encountered as a healthcare professional). It has become so popular that you can buy Bristol Stool Chart mugs, coasters, aprons, T-shirts, hoodies, etc. The descriptors range from type 1 ('separate hard lumps, like nuts, hard to pass') to type 7 ('watery, no solid pieces, entirely liquid'). However, my favourite descriptor is type 4: 'like a sausage or snake, smooth and soft'. Hard faeces (and constipation) tend to result from inadequate fluid intake (remember faeces = 75% water), insufficient dietary fibre, the effects of some medications (e.g. opiates such as morphine) and lack of exercise/physical activity. Diarrhoea, on the other hand, is usually the result of viral or bacterial infection (discussed in Chapter 6) or GIT disorders such as coeliac disease and ulcerative colitis. If you want to learn more about what your poo is telling you I thoroughly recommend the book of the same name by Josh Richman and Anish Seth.[2] This succinct but insightful work explores the physiology behind the déjà poo, the gift poo, floaters vs sinkers, as well as the advantages of the sit versus squat method of defecation. Essential reading for all serious students of the GIT in my opinion.

CHAPTER 11: TEST YOURSELF

Q. List the three macronutrients (principle food groups) and two micronutrients.
A. Macronutrients = carbohydrates, proteins and fats. Micronutrients = minerals and vitamins.

Q. Which part of the brain is responsible for hunger and satiety (feeling full after eating)?
A. The hypothalamus.

Q. Which hormone, secreted in the stomach and small intestine, stimulates the hypothalamus to produce the sensation of hunger?
A. Ghrelin.

Q. Which hormone, secreted by fat cells (adipocytes), stimulates the hypothalamus to produce the sensation of satiety?
A. Leptin.

Q. What does BMI stand for, how is it calculated and what is considered to be the healthy range?
A. Body Mass Index is calculated by dividing weight in kg by height in m^2 (i.e. weight ÷ height ÷ height = BMI). Normal range for an Asian adult is 18.5 to 22.9 and for a non-Asian adult, 18.5 to 25.

Q. What is the peritoneum?
A. The peritoneum is the outermost layer of the gastro intestinal tract (GIT). It is a serous membrane (serosa) that lines the abdominal cavity and covers most of the abdominal organs.

Q. List the three pairs of salivary glands and explain why saliva is important for digestion.
A. Sublingual, submandibular and parotid salivary glands secrete saliva to moisten and lubricate food prior to swallowing. Saliva also contains varying amounts of lysozyme, immunoglobulin A (IgA) and the digestive enzyme salivary amylase that breaks down carbohydrate.

Q. Explain what is meant by the term sphincter and name the two examples found in the stomach?
A. A sphincter is a ring of muscle that surrounds and allows access to an opening or tube. The cardiac sphincter is located at the entrance to the stomach and the pyloric sphincter at the exit of the stomach.

Q. Gastrin is secreted by G cells (in the stomach) in response to distension and the presence of undigested protein. What is the principle function of gastrin?
A. Gastrin promotes the production of intrinsic factor and hydrochloric acid by parietal cells, the secretion of pepsinogen by chief cells, and the contraction of gastric smooth muscle.

(Continued)

(Continued)

Q. What is the function of pepsinogen/pepsin in the stomach?

A. Pepsinogen is transformed into pepsin when it comes into contact with HCl. Pepsin is an extremely aggressive protein-digesting enzyme that splits the bonds between amino acids in order to produce short chain peptides.

Q. What is the function of mucus in the stomach?

A. Mucus protects the stomach from the potentially damaging effects of HCl and pepsin.

Q. What is the name of the partially digested liquid that exits the stomach into the first part of the small intestine?

A. Chyme.

Q. List the three parts of the small intestine in the correct order.

A. Duodenum, jejunum and ileum.

Q. Name the three pancreatic enzymes that break down protein, carbohydrate and fat.

A. Trypsin breaks down protein (into amino acids), Pancreatic amylase breaks down carbohydrate (into glucose) and Pancreatic lipase breaks down fat (into fatty acids and glycerol).

Q. How does bile (secreted by the liver/gall bladder) assist with the breakdown of fat?

A. Bile helps to split large globules of dietary fat into small molecules that are easier to break down.

Q. What is the name for the rhythmic muscular contractions that propel partially digested/digested material through the gastrointestinal tract?

A. Peristalsis.

Q. What is the name for the finger-like projections in the jejunum and ileum that increase surface area available for absorption of nutrients?

A. Villi.

Q. Which veins transport nutrients from the small intestine to the liver?

A. The mesenteric veins and the hepatic portal vein.

Q. List the different parts of the large intestine or colon in the correct order.

A. Ascending colon, transverse colon, descending colon, sigmoid colon, rectum and anus.

Q. What are the principle functions of the large intestine?

A. Absorption of water from the material passing through it, compaction of the remaining intestinal contents into semi-solid faeces and the breakdown of cellulose (by commensal bacteria).

Notes

1 Coffey, J.C. and O'Leary, D.P. (2016) The mesentery: structure, function, and role in disease. *The Lancet Gastroenterology & Hepatology*, 1(3): 238–247.

2 Richman, J. and Seth, A. (2013) *What's Your Poo Telling You?* London: Ebury Press.

Contents

CHAPTER 12

NERVOUS SYSTEM

CENTRAL NERVOUS SYSTEM

In Chapter 3, we observed how the body strives to maintain a stable internal environment (homeostasis) despite constant internal and external variation and disturbance. The nervous system is fundamental to this process and, together with the endocrine system (see Chapter 13), detects, responds to and regulates changes inside and outside the body. However, it is much more sophisticated than the simple 'sensor + integrator + effector' mechanisms that we have observed so far, and the nervous system is also responsible for sensory perception, voluntary movements, decision-making, personality, memory and emotion. The endocrine system also plays an important role in determining and regulating these qualities and activities but it is the nervous system that provides the primary means of communication via an integrated collection of nerve cells (neurons). However, before we look at neurons in more detail, it is important to understand how the nervous system is organised. Broadly speaking, it is divided into two parts: the central nervous system (CNS) and the peripheral nervous system (not to be confused with the parasympathetic nervous system – see below). The CNS consists of the brain and the spinal cord which are attached to one another at the base of the brainstem (remember that there is a hole in the underside of the cranium called the foramen magnum – see Chapter 4). We will look at the brain in

more detail later in the chapter and, for now, it is enough to say that it controls and coordinates conscious and unconscious thoughts and

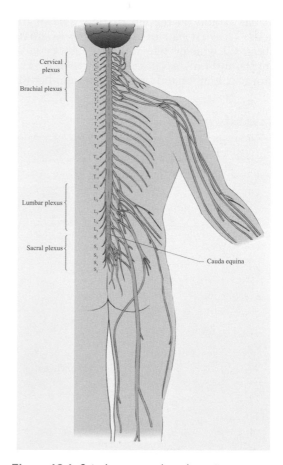

Figure 12.1 Spinal nerves and cauda equina.

actions. The spinal cord is essentially a cylinder of nervous tissue that conveys messages to and from the brain and the body as a whole. It measures 43–45 cm in length and extends from just above the first cervical vertebrae (C1) to the lower border of lumber vertebrae 1 (L1). Below this point, the spinal nerves fan-out as the cauda equina (Latin for 'horse tail') through the remaining lumber, sacral and coccygeal vertebrae (Figure 12.1).

PERIPHERAL NERVOUS SYSTEM

The peripheral nervous system refers to the nerves of the body that are not part of the brain and spinal cord (CNS). For example, 31 pairs of spinal nerves emerge from the spinal cord and relay information to/from a particular region on the left or right side of the body. The first pair of spinal nerves originate above C1 which is why there are eight cervical nerves and only seven cervical vertebrae. The thoracic, lumber and sacral nerves number the same as the corresponding vertebrae (e.g. 12, 5 and 5) and there is one pair of coccygeal nerves. In addition to the spinal nerves, there are also 12 cranial nerves that emerge directly from the brain and brainstem via a series of bony canals and small holes (foramina) in the skull. They are generally named according to their structure or function (Table 12.1) and a number of mnemonics have been devised to help students remember their order, function and whether or not they are motor nerves, sensory nerves or both.

The traditional mnemonic for remembering the cranial nerves is the somewhat surreal and (in my opinion) slightly sinister: On Old Olympus Towering Top A Finn And German Viewed A Horse.

You have to ask yourself: what are the Finn and German doing on Mount Olympus? Is the horse actually on the mountain (in which case how did it get up there) or is it at a distance (in which case why are the Finn and German so interested in it)? Luckily, there are more memorable aide-mémoires for cranial nerve order and function but it is probably inadvisable to print them here since they are

TABLE 12.1 Cranial nerves

Number	Nerve	Function
1	Olfactory	Smell
2	Optic	Vision
3	Oculomotor	Eye movements and pupils
4	Trochlear	Eye movements
5	Trigeminal	Facial sensation and chewing
6	Abducens	Eye movement
7	Facial	Facial expressions and taste
8	Auditory	Hearing and balance
9	Glossopharyngeal	Salivation and gag reflex
10	Vagus	Parasympathetic innervations and gag reflex
11	Accessory	Movement of head and shoulders
12	Hypoglossal	Movement of tongue, swallowing and speech

not at all politically correct. If you are interested, simply type 'medical mnemonics' into any search engine and your education can begin. I note that even the highly respectable Oxford Medical Education site has a section entitled: Less acceptable medical mnemonics (do not mention in exams).

MOTOR AND SENSORY NERVES

Nerves that travel away from the CNS are known as motor (or afferent) nerves, and control and coordinate movement. The muscles that are innervated by these nerves are known as myotomes. Nerves that travel towards the CNS are known as sensory (or efferent) nerves, and relay information toward the brain for interpretation or, in the case of reflexes, towards a corresponding motor nerve via the spinal cord (see below). Areas of sensory innervation in the skin are known as dermatomes (Figure 12.2). Both myotomes and dermatomes are of great importance when assessing spinal injury since immobility, or lack of sensation, may be the result of trauma to the corresponding area of the spinal cord or cauda equina. For example, the nerve entering the spinal cord just below thoracic vertebra 4 (T4) receives sensory information from the band of skin surrounding the torso that includes the nipples. If the spinal cord has been severed or severely damaged at this point, the patient will have no sensation or movement below this level since the means of communication to and from the CNS has been cut. Spinal cord injury that occurs as a result of traumatic injury to the neck is particularly dangerous since it can disrupt phrenic (diaphragm) nerve activity and result in death from diaphragmatic paralysis (see Chapter 9). The actor Christopher Reeve, who played Superman in the late 1970s and 1980s, had a horse riding accident in 1995 which resulted in the fracture of cervical vertebrae 1 and 2. As a result, he lost the use of all four limbs (tetraplegia) and required assistance breathing for the rest of his life (he eventually died aged 52 in 2004, having spent many years campaigning for greater research into spinal injury and

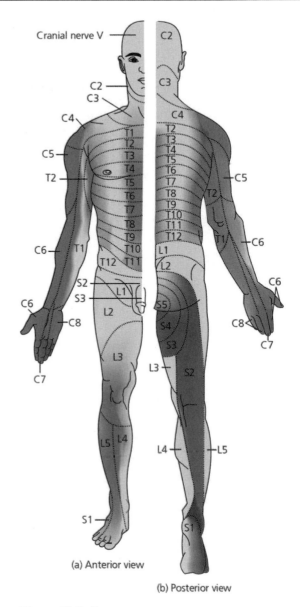

(a) Anterior view

(b) Posterior view

Figure 12.2 Dermatome map.

stem cell therapies). Sensory nerves include somatic (or cutaneous) receptors found in the skin (see Chapter 3), proprioceptors found in the muscle and joints (see Chapter 4), specialised structures such as baroreceptors (see Chapter 8) and peripheral chemoreceptors (see Chapter 9) found in the carotid and aortic bodies, and nerves associated with the five special senses: sound, sight, smell, taste and touch. Motor nerves of the peripheral nervous system can be divided into voluntary and involuntary divisions and, as we observed in Chapter 2, skeletal muscle is voluntary whilst smooth and cardiac muscle is involuntary. We have also observed on numerous occasions that involuntary muscular contraction and relaxation is determined by the autonomic nervous system which is subdivided into sympathetic (flight-or-fight) and parasympathetic (resting and digesting) pathways. For example, the vagus nerve (cranial nerve 10) extends from the brainstem to the abdomen and is responsible for parasympathetic control of the heart and digestive tract.

NEURONS

In Chapter 2, we observed that nervous tissue comprises two types of cell: neurons and supporting cells (e.g. glial cells or neuroglia). Neurons are often described as excitable since they have the ability to generate, transmit and receive electrical messages called action potentials. Although they share many of the same features and characteristics as other cells, they also possess a number of specialised structures that allow them to carry out this function. For example, most neurons consist of three main parts: a cell body, dendrites, and an axon (Figure 12.3). The cell body contains the usual organelles we would expect to find in a 'normal' cell including a nucleus, cytoplasm, mitochondria, ribosomes, golgi apparatus and endoplasmic reticulum (see Chapter 2). Although neurons possess a nucleus, once they reach functional maturity, they lose the

ability to undergo mitosis and replicate. This is not necessarily a problem, and providing they receive an adequate supply of oxygen and glucose, they should last a lifetime (80 years+). However, on the downside, neurons have an incredibly high metabolic rate and account for about 20% of the body's total oxygen consumption. If this supply is interrupted for more than a few minutes (e.g. during a stroke) cell death occurs, resulting in temporary or permanent loss of function (see below). Attached to the cell body are numerous dendrites (Greek for 'little tree' or 'branch') which provide an enormous surface area for the reception of signals from other neurons and tissue. For example, one neuron in the human brain can receive input from as many as 100,000 other neurons. Dendrites convey incoming messages called graded potentials towards the cell body that influence the creation of (outward) action potentials in a structure called the axon hillock. This cone-shaped elevation connects the cell body to a thin, cylindrical projection called an axon. Each neuron has only one axon which carries nerve impulses away from the cell body towards another neuron or tissue. Axons are usually longer than dendrites and (in the peripheral nervous system) can reach a length of about a metre.

MYELIN

The axon is surrounded by a specialised plasma membrane known as the axolemma and, in most cases, by a sheath of fatty material

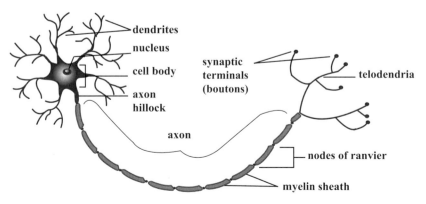

Figure 12.3 Neuron.

called myelin. Myelin sheaths are formed by Schwann cells in the peripheral nervous system and by oligodendrocytes in the central nervous system (see below). They consist of myelinated segments, separated by small gaps or interruptions called nodes of Ranvier (named after the French anatomist who discovered them in 1854). The fatty myelin helps to insulate the axon in a similar way to the rubber casing that insulates and protects electrical wire, and the nodes of Ranvier assist rapid transmission of nerve impulses along its length. Speed of conduction also depends upon the diameter of the axon and the larger the diameter, the faster the impulse. The fastest myelinated fibres can conduct action potentials (to skeletal muscle for example) at a rate of 120 metres per second. Even the slowest unmyelinated fibres conduct impulses at a respectable 0.5 metres per second. There is always more than one neuron involved in the transmission of a nerve impulse from its origin to its destination and they are organised into bundles much like fibre-optic cables. A cluster or group of neurons is called a nucleus when it occurs in the central nervous system and a ganglion in the peripheral nervous system. For example, each spinal nerve comprises a dorsal route ganglion (which innervates the posterior/dorsal aspect of the spinal cord and relays sensory information towards the CNS) and a ventral route ganglion (which innervates the anterior/ventral aspect of the spinal cord and relays motor information away from the CNS).

ACTION POTENTIALS

Electrical activity along the axon occurs because of the transient movement of sodium ions across the neuronal membrane. This sounds terribly complicated but is actually fairly straightforward. We know that sodium ions (Na^+) and potassium ions (K^+) have a positive charge. When a neuron is not transmitting an action potential, the inside of the cell is negatively charged relative to the outside. In this 'resting' state the neuron is said to be polarised. However, when it receives appropriate stimulation (e.g. from a dendrite) sodium channels in the neuronal membrane begin to

open and Na^+ from outside the cell rushes in. As the neuron becomes increasingly positively charged, it depolarises and an electrical charge (action potential) is created. To put it another way, the resting membrane potential of a neuron is about –70 millivolts (mV) or 70 mV LESS than outside the cell. The sudden influx of Na^+ across the neuronal membrane increases the positive charge and when it reaches about –55 mV an action potential is generated. Na^+ continues to enter the cell and the charge quickly reaches about +40 mV. At this point, Na^+ channels close (which prevents further Na^+ from entering the cell) and K^+ channels open, allowing (positively charged) K^+ to exit the cell. Depolarisation is rapidly reversed and repolarisation occurs (i.e. the potential difference changes from +40mV back to –70mV). The action potential travels along the axon as the membrane of the axon depolarises and repolarises in this way. The myelin sheath insulates the axon and prevents 'leakage' of the current as it travels away from the cell body. The nodes of Ranvier contain Na^+ and K^+ channels which allow the action potential to travel more quickly along the axon by 'jumping' from one node to the next. Local anaesthetics (e.g. Lidocaine) work by blocking this inward movement of sodium ions and therefore prevent not only the transmission of pain signals towards the CNS but everything else as well. If you have ever had a tooth extracted at the dentist, you will have experienced the effects of local anaesthetic on the nerves of your mouth. There is no sensation of any kind to the injected area (once the anaesthetic begins to work) but there is much dribbling as you fail to exert motor control.

SYNAPSES AND NEUROTRANSMITTERS

The axon eventually culminates in a series of fine extensions known as telodendria (end + 'tree/branch') at the end of which are a series of club-shaped processes called synaptic terminals or terminal boutons. These make contact with other neurons or tissue via a tiny junction or gap called a synapse. Synaptic terminals contain many small membranous sacs known as synaptic vesicles that store chemical messengers called neurotransmitters (nerve + transmitter). When an action potential (created by the wave of depolarisation along the axon) reaches the synaptic terminal, it triggers the migration of vesicles toward the presynaptic membrane. The vesicle membrane fuses with the presynaptic membrane and releases a neurotransmitter into the synapse. Neurotransmitters (think of them as chemical messengers) diffuse across the gap and bind with receptor sites on the opposing side (e.g. the surface of a dendrite). Examples of neurotransmitters include acetylcholine (Ach) and dopamine which help to regulate movement/motor control, motivation, arousal and reward (amongst other things). For example, the symptoms of Parkinson's disease occur when about 70% of dopamine-producing neurons, from an area of the brain called the substantia nigra, have been destroyed and include tremor, slowness of movement and muscular rigidity. Unfortunately, it is not possible to replace dopamine via a tablet or injection since it cannot cross the blood-brain barrier (see below). Consequently, the drug levodopa (L-dopa) is often used in combination with other therapies to treat Parkinson's symptoms since it is converted into dopamine by the body. However, only a small proportion manages to cross the blood-brain barrier and it has a number of side effects including nausea and involuntary muscle movements (dyskinesia). The book/film *Awakenings* outlines how neurologist Oliver Sacks (1933–2015) used L-dopa to revive (or 'awaken') a group of patients in the late 1960s who persisted in a catatonic (unresponsive) state following contraction of encephalitis lethargica ('sleepy sickness').

GLIAL CELLS

We observed in Chapter 2, that non-excitable glial (Greek for 'glue') cells nourish, protect and support excitable neurons. They are much more numerous than neurons and it is estimated that the brain consists of about 100 billion neurons and 30 trillion glial cells! Unlike neurons, glial cells are capable of dividing mitotically after maturation and do not possess axons or dendrites. The CNS contains several

types of glial cell including astrocytes, oligodendrocytes, microglia and ependymal cells. The most abundant are astrocytes which have numerous projections that radiate outwards from a central body like a star (the Greek word *ástron* means 'star'). These projections provide support for neurons and capillaries which they anchor in place. Astrocytes also regulate the chemical environment around the neurons and absorb and digest neurotransmitters and excess ions (including K^+) that could interfere with normal cell functioning. Finally, astrocytes are able to store glycogen which can be converted into glucose during periods of high metabolic activity and form scar tissue following CNS injury/damage. The next type of glial cell, oligodendrocytes, also provide a degree of structural support for neurons but their primary role is the production of myelin which wraps around and coats the axon. The word oligodendrocyte means 'cell of few branches' and individual oligodendrocytes cooperate with one another to myelinate segments of several/multiple axons (unlike Schwann cells which myelinate just one).

MICROGLIA, EPENDYMAL CELLS, SATELLITE CELLS AND SCHWANN CELLS

The next type of glial cell found in the CNS are microglia. As their name suggests, they are the smallest of the glial cells and function primarily as phagocytic immune cells. They are highly mobile and move through the nervous tissue removing cellular debris, waste products and other material including microorganisms. The final type of support cell found in the CNS are specialised epithelial cells called ependymal cells. Like epithelial cells found elsewhere in the body, many of these are ciliated (i.e. they possess tiny hair-like projections). Ependymal cells line the ventricles (cavities) of the brain and the central canal of the spinal cord, and contribute to the secretion of cerebrospinal fluid (see below). The beating of their cilia also helps to direct the flow of cerebrospinal fluid around the CNS and filter out debris and foreign particles. Since the peripheral nervous system is mainly composed of axons, there are only two types of support cell: satellite cells and Schwann cells. The first are similar in function to astrocytes and surround and support neuronal cell bodies found in clusters called ganglia. They also help to control and maintain the chemical environment around the neurons they support. Schwann cells are the principle glial cells of the peripheral nervous system and, as we already know, are functionally similar to oligodendrocytes. They manufacture myelin, maintain the axon and contribute to the removal of cellular debris.

NEURON DAMAGE

A number of different diseases cause damage to the myelin sheaths of neurons leading to temporary and/or permanent loss of sensation and function. For example, Guillain–Barré syndrome occurs when the body's immune system destroys the myelin sheaths that surround the axons of peripheral nerves resulting in ascending (symmetrical) weakness and possible paralysis of the diaphragm. Multiple sclerosis (MS) is another autoimmune disease that results in progressive demyelination of neurons and the destruction of myelin producing oligodendrocytes. The damaged myelin is eventually replaced by scar tissue or plaques (multiple + sclerosis = many + thickening) which inhibits and obstructs normal conduction along the affected axon/s. Symptoms are variable depending on the location and the extent of the damage but often include partial loss of vision and problems with speech, balance and motor coordination (including bowel and bladder control). Another disease that you have may have heard of as a result of the 'ice bucket challenge' initiative of 2014 is amyotrophic lateral sclerosis or motor neuron disease (MND). MND affects upper and lower motor neurons and leads to progressive weakness and wasting (atrophy) of skeletal muscles. It is a degenerative condition and, in the advanced stages of the disease, the individual may become totally unable to move. There is no cure for MND and most die from respiratory failure within 3–5 years of the onset of symptoms. There are of course exceptions and the physicist Steven Hawking was first diagnosed aged 21 in 1963.

PAIN TRANSMISSION

Before we look at the different parts of the brain and what they actually do, it is worth quickly examining the transmission of pain from the peripheral nervous system to the CNS. Pain is a complex phenomenon and difficult to define since it is such a subjective experience. The reason for this is that it is not only influenced by physiological processes but also by psychological and emotional factors. For example, the intensity of pain can be influenced by the context in which it occurs and there are numerous accounts of athletes and soldiers demonstrating disproportionately stoic responses to serious injury. For example, the Manchester City goalkeeper, Bert Trautmann, famously continued to play for a further 17 minutes after breaking several cervical vertebrae during the 1956 FA Cup final. Lord Uxbridge is said to have remarked (with evident surprise) to Lord Wellington at the Battle of Waterloo, 'By God, sir, I've lost my leg!' shortly after it was left in tatters by cannon shot. Such composure in the face of adversity makes you proud to be British – or German in the case of Trautmann. The US anaesthetist Henry Beecher was one of the first to measure this phenomenon and he recorded that only about a quarter of the soldiers he treated for serious injuries during the Second World War requested morphine, compared to 80% of civilians with similar injuries. He also wrote widely about the placebo effect after he witnessed an injured soldier settle and relax following an injection of normal saline he had been told was a large dose of morphine (the field hospital had run out).

ACUTE AND CHRONIC PAIN

Broadly speaking, pain can be divided into two categories: acute and chronic. Acute pain typically persists for a relatively short period of time, is focal to the site of injury and acts as a protective mechanism. That is to say, it signals to the brain that there is an actual or potential problem that requires some kind of protective response. Chronic pain, on the other hand, may have no identifiable cause and serves no biological function. In this sense, it exhibits the characteristics of a disease state rather than a self-limiting symptom. At one time or another, we have all thought 'wouldn't it be nice to have no pain at all'. However, without acute pain at least, we would be at constant risk of tissue damage and serious injury. Those who suffer from the rare genetic condition congenital analgesia experience precisely this problem and often fail to perceive and respond to injury. One particularly gruesome anecdote told by a sufferer relates to his failure to notice he was chewing his tongue whilst eating breakfast. The polar opposite of this condition is phantom limb pain, where sufferers experience pain or other sensations (e.g. itching, tingling and/or cramp) in a part of the body that has been amputated or surgically removed. We will explore why this might occur later in the chapter.

NOCICEPTION

In Chapter 3, we observed that pain perception (nociception) is the process by which a painful stimulus is detected and relayed towards the CNS. The noxious stimulus is converted (transduced) into electrical energy that, when it reaches a threshold value, generates an action potential and allows for the conscious awareness of pain. Nociceptors have two different types of axon: alpha-delta (Aδ) fibres and C-fibres. Aδ fibres are myelinated and allow action potentials to travel at speeds of 5–30 metres per second. Pain associated with Aδ fibres is often referred to as 'fast pain' and tends to present as an initial, sharp pain which recedes relatively quickly. C-fibres, on the other hand, are non-myelinated and facilitate conduction at a much slower rate of 0.5–2 metres per second. This 'slow pain' is less intense, more prolonged, and often described as a dull ache. It is estimated that C-fibres account for about 70% of all nociceptive fibres. Sensory and nociceptive fibres relay action potentials towards the spinal cord through the dorsal route ganglion (Figure 12.4). This simply refers to the collection or cluster of neurons (ganglia) that interface with the posterior (dorsal) portion of a particular part of the spinal cord (e.g. T1). The dorsal route ganglion synapses with an area of grey matter called the dorsal horn and transmits sensory information towards the brain through an area of white matter known as

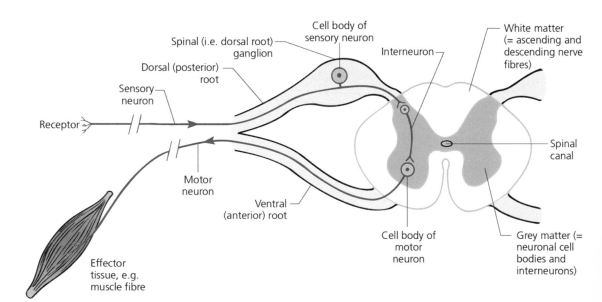

Figure 12.4 Dorsal and ventral root ganglion of the spinal cord.

the spinothalmic tract (STT). The grey matter contains neuron cell bodies, dendrites and axon terminals, whilst the white matter consists of bundles of myelinated axons and glial cells. The myelinated axons of the STT act like a motorway where 'traffic', nerve impulses relayed from lower segments of the spinal cord, drive up towards the brain. Signals travel through the brainstem and synapse on neurons in the thalamus (the brain's relay centre) before reaching the sensory cortex of the cerebrum (see below). It is thought that noxious information does not become pain until the brain interprets and adds meaning to it. This may account for the fact that different people often exhibit contrasting responses to similar levels of pain and trauma. Sensory neurons and pain receptors from the face and head access the CNS via the trigeminal nerve (Table 12.1).

REFLEXES

Reflexes are the simplest form of movement and are involuntary responses to external stimulation. They may be coordinated by the spinal cord or by the brainstem. Examples of spinal reflexes include simple withdrawal reflexes that occur in response to pain (see below) and the knee-jerk (or patella-tap) reflex used to assess L2, L3 and L4. Examples of brainstem reflexes include coughing and gagging, when the throat is irritated, and the constriction of the pupils in response to bright light (pupillary light reflex). When brainstem reflexes are absent or depressed it may indicate damage to the brain (reversible or otherwise) or it could be the result of drug overdose (e.g. tricyclic antidepressants or opiates) or severe hypothermia (remember the cheerful motto: not dead until warm and dead). In simple terms, a reflex consists of an arc whereby sensory information (e.g. pain) is detected by a peripheral nerve receptor (nociceptor) and relayed to the spinal cord or brainstem by a sensory neuron. The neuron makes synaptic contact with a motor nerve fibre (via an inter-neuron) and the message travels directly to a muscle where it stimulates a response (Figure 12.4). Because reflex movements do not require the

involvement of the higher centres of the brain, they are both rapid and involuntary. All of us can remember an example of a sudden and unintended limb movement in response to painful stimuli. For example, I remember walking to the beach with my eldest son when I unexpectedly jumped into the air. Four things went through my mind in quick succession before I landed: (i) Why have I jumped into the air? (reflex action); (ii) I think I may have stepped on a nail (correct); (iii) Remember to land on the other foot (iv); I hope my son didn't hear the expletive I am pretty sure I just shouted. Fortunately, he didn't since he was too surprised and embarrassed by the whole leaping into the air business.

SPECIAL SENSES

Before we examine the different regions of the brain, it is worth quickly considering the five special senses. As noted above, they consist of touch, taste, smell, sound and sight. In Chapter 3, we saw that nerve endings situated in the dermis of the skin (and elsewhere) transmit sensory nerve impulses relating to pressure, pain and temperature, towards the central nervous system. These signals are interpreted by the primary sensory cortex (situated in the parietal lobe of the cerebrum) discussed below. Our sense of taste (gustation) and smell (olfaction) are closely linked because both use chemical receptors (chemoreceptors) to generate sensory information/nerve signals. In Chapter 11, we noted that taste buds (papillae) are situated on the tongue and, to a lesser extent, on the roof of the mouth (palate) and in the pharynx. These tiny, peg-like projections give the tongue its slightly abrasive feel and respond to five taste sensations: salty, sour, bitter, sweet and umami (a word derived from the Japanese for 'delicious taste'). Salty taste is largely produced by sodium ions (Na^+) dissolved in solution/saliva and sour taste by hydrogen ions (H^+). Bitterness is the most sensitive of the tastes and is thought to warn of potentially toxic ingredients. However, many food and drinks also have a bitter quality including coffee, turmeric, rocket, etc. Sweet taste is produced by the presence of saccharides and a few other substances including aldehydes and ketones. Finally, umami is usually described as a 'savoury' or 'meaty' taste and cannot be replicated by combining the other four tastes. Umami is essentially the taste of glutamate found in fish, mushrooms, tomatoes, beans and many fermented foods including soy sauce, cheese and Marmite. Monosodium glutamate (MSG) is often added to food as a flavour enhancer. The mouth and tongue also contain mechanoreceptors, nociceptors and thermoreceptors which indicate when food and drink is hot or cold. All five taste sensations are enhanced and influenced by olfaction and if you lose your sense of smell, or simply hold your nose when eating, taste is impaired. It is estimated that about 80% of taste is actually smell, so to speak. The olfactory receptors cover the superior nasal concha on either side of the nasal septum (see Chapter 9, Figure 9.2) and detect airborne chemicals (odorants) that have been dissolved in mucus. Once a nerve impulse has been generated, it

is driven towards the limbic system via the olfactory bulb discussed in more detail below. The location of the olfactory receptors within the nose means that we often have to sniff to ensure odorants can be detected. Interestingly, the mucus that 'captures' and dissolves these chemicals is constantly renewed which means that strong or unpleasant odours are quickly reduced in intensity. This partly explains why people who work in smelly environments become desensitised to noxious odours and are still able to enjoy their lunch!

SOUND AND BALANCE

The ear can be divided into three anatomical regions: the external ear, middle ear and inner ear (Figure 12.5). The external ear consists of the auricle and the auditory canal. The auricle is simply a flap of elastic cartilage that funnels sound waves into the auditory canal. In

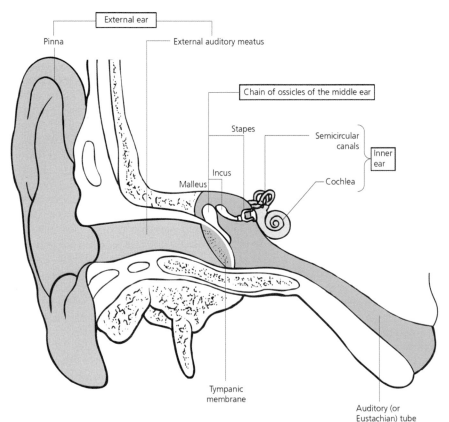

Figure 12.5 Outer, middle and inner ear.

Chapter 3, we observed that apocrine glands in the auditory canal secrete wax (cerumen) in order to protect the ear from water, bacteria and foreign bodies, etc. At the far end of the auditory canal, the eardrum or tympanic membrane represents the first part of the middle ear. In Chapter 4, we noted that three tiny ossicles (malleus, incus and stapes) collectively transmit sound waves from the tympanic membrane to the fluid-filled inner ear via the oval window. In Chapter 9, we also observed that the Eustachian tube opens into the middle ear in order to maintain constant air pressure and to provide drainage (into the nasopharynx) if necessary. The final part of the ear is the inner ear which contains the semicircular canals, vestibule and cochlea. These three structures are collectively known as the bony labyrinth and filled with fluid called perilymph. Perilymph, in turn, surrounds a series of ducts and sacs called the membranous labyrinth which contains fluid called endolymph. Motion receptors within the endolymph respond to movement of the fluid and allow us to orientate ourselves in response to rotation, gravity and acceleration. For example, receptors in the semicircular ducts (anterior, posterior and lateral) detect rotational movement in the three different planes, whilst receptors in the vestibule respond to gravity and acceleration. Receptors in the spiral-shaped cochlea, on the other hand, are stimulated by pressure waves generated by the vibration of the tympanic membrane, ossicles and oval window. These pressure waves create a corresponding wave-motion in the perilymph and endolymph that excites specialist hair cells in the cochlea. This results in the creation of nerve impulses that are transmitted towards the brain by the auditory nerve. Very loud noise can damage these delicate hair cells leading to temporary or permanent hearing loss. Hearing loss may also result from problems in the outer ear (e.g. earwax plug), middle ear (e.g. infection such as otitis media) and auditory regions of the brain (see below).

SIGHT

The fifth and final special sense is sight and it is estimated that about 70% of the body's sensory receptors are located in the eye. Although the adult eye measures about 2.5 cm in diameter (slightly smaller than a ping-pong ball), only a small percentage of the anterior surface is visible between the eye lids (palpebrae). The rest is enclosed within the bony orbits of the skull (see Chapter 4). Consequently, the most obvious or recognisable parts of the eye are the external structures: the sclera, iris and pupil (Figure 12.6). The sclera, or 'white of the eye', is a protective layer composed of dense connective tissue that covers approximately five-sixths of the eye's surface (the majority of which is enclosed within the orbit). The sclera 'surrounds' the coloured iris which, in turn, surrounds the 'black' pupil. The iris consists of two layers of pigmented smooth muscle that not only provide the eye's colour but also contract and dilate to make the pupil larger (mydriasis) and smaller (miosis) respectively. In Chapter 2 we noted that some drugs stimulate these reactions but, under normal circumstances, pupillary dilation is a sympathetic (nervous system) response to low levels of light (and fear, etc.) and pupillary constriction is a parasympathetic response to increased levels of light. The pupil is not a physical structure, therefore, but simply an opening or aperture that allows light to pass into the eye. Both the iris and the pupil are covered and protected by a transparent and highly sensitive membrane called the cornea (continuous with the sclera). In order to ensure transparency, the cornea does not have any blood vessels, and nutrients are absorbed from the fluid (aqueous humour) that circulates between the cornea and the iris in what is known as the anterior chamber. The aqueous humour helps to maintain the shape of the eye and also remove waste products generated by cell metabolism. One of the reasons eyes often appear cloudy or opaque in the hours following death is because the cells of the cornea no longer derive nourishment from the aqueous humour. The lens of the eye is situated directly behind the pupil and is controlled by ciliary muscles that stretch and relax it in order to bend (refract) and focus light onto the retina behind. This process is known as accommodation and allows us to view objects at varying distances (something that becomes increasingly difficult after the age of 40). The area between the lens and the retina is known as the posterior chamber and

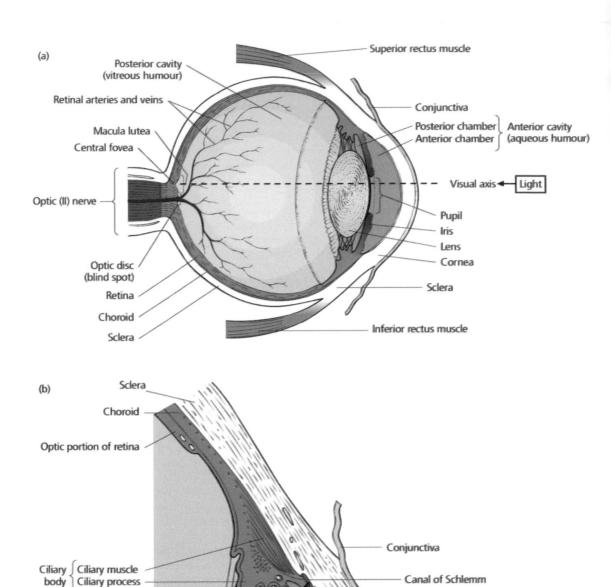

Figure 12.6 (a) Eye (including visual axis). (b) Iris, ciliary body and circulation of the aqueous humour.

is filled with a jelly-like substance called vitreous humour. This helps to maintain the spherical shape of the eye and secures the retina in place. The retina is the innermost layer of the eye and covers about three-quarters of the posterior surface. It contains two types of photosensitive receptor cells called rods and cones that convert light into nerve impulses. Each retina has about 120 million rods that allow us to see in low or dim light but are unable to discern colour. Cones, on the other hand, are much less numerous (about 6 million per retina) but are highly sensitive to colour and are stimulated by bright light. Cones are concentrated in a central yellow spot on the retina called the macula. At the centre of the macula, the fovea centralis contains the densest concentration of cones. In simple terms, rods and cones convert light into nerve impulses that are sent via the optic nerve (cranial nerve 2) to the visual cortex of the brain (see below). We noted earlier in the chapter that direction of gaze, position of the eyelids, lens shape and the size of the pupils are controlled by cranial nerves 3, 4, and 6 (Table 12.1).

BRAINSTEM

The brain comprises three main regions or areas: the brainstem, the cerebellum and the cerebrum (Figure 12.7). In the previous chapters, we have discussed some of the actions of the brainstem, particularly in relation to the cardiovascular and respiratory centres. However, it is useful to recap some of this information here and take a further look at the different areas in context. We noted at the beginning of this chapter that the brainstem is attached to the spinal cord just above the level of C1 through the foramen magnum. Consequently, it is the lowest and the most primitive part of the brain and provides a common pathway for motor and sensory nerve impulses travelling to and from the spinal cord. It also coordinates many of the body's autonomic responses necessary for homeostasis and life support in general. The brainstem is divided into three discrete parts (in ascending order): the medulla oblongata, the pons and the midbrain. The medulla is a continuation of the superior part of the spinal cord and measures about 3 cm in length. However, despite its small size, it houses the cardiovascular and respiratory centres, and coordinates a number of autonomic activities such as swallowing, coughing, sneezing, vomiting and hiccupping. Situated directly above the medulla is the widest section of the brainstem known as the pons (Latin for 'bridge'). The pons attaches the brainstem to the cerebellum behind and contains the apneustic and pneumotaxic centres that help regulate respiratory rate and depth (see Chapter 9).

MIDBRAIN AND RETICULAR FORMATION

The third and most superior section of the brainstem is the midbrain, situated above the pons and below the diencephalon or interbrain (see below). At the front of the midbrain, two cylindrical bundles of nerve fibres called cerebral peduncles (Latin for 'little feet') help to support the cerebrum and conduct nerve impulses from the higher centres of the brain. The midbrain also contains the substantia nigra (Latin for 'black substance') that contributes to the production of the hormone dopamine, which plays an important role in motor coordination, addiction and reward. The substantia nigra derives its name from the colour of the dopaminergic cells that

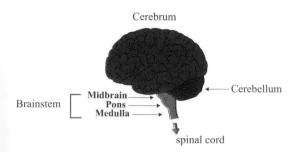

Figure 12.7 Cerebrum, cerebellum and brainstem.

(a)

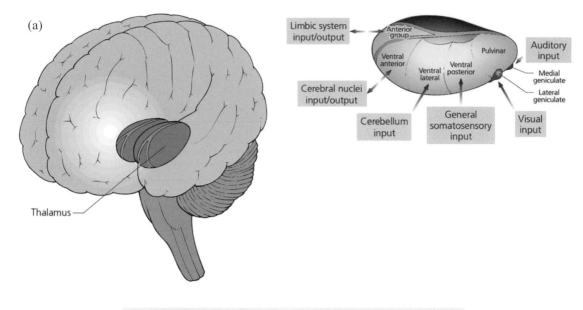

(b)

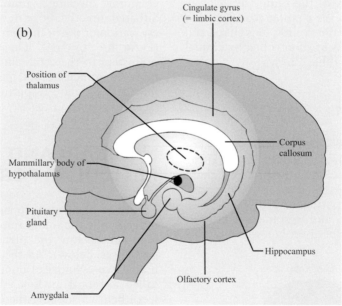

Figure 12.8 (a) Thalamus. (b) Diencephalon and major components of the limbic system.

contain high levels of neuromelanin – a dark pigment closely related to melanin (see Chapter 3). Finally, the midbrain houses a number of nuclei (clusters of neurons) that process visual and sound (auditory) information and control reflexes triggered by these stimuli (e.g. the startle reflex in response to loud, unexpected noise). The medulla oblongata, pons and midbrain all contain an intricate network of interconnected neurons called the reticular formation which extend from the spinal cord (through the brainstem) to the diencephalon above (Figures 12.7, 12.8). The reticular formation helps to regulate the sleep-wake cycle as well as a number of vital autonomic functions. It also acts rather like a filter for sensory input and helps the cerebrum to ignore information that is repetitive, familiar and/or unimportant. This explains why it is possible to sleep through noisy rain, traffic and other familiar, non-threatening sounds, but wake suddenly when something goes bump in the night.

CEREBELLUM

The cerebellum (Latin for 'little brain') is situated directly behind the brainstem and immediately below the occipital lobe of the cerebrum (Figure 12.7). It is secured to the brainstem by three pairs of cerebellar peduncles (inferior/middle/superior = medulla/pons/midbrain) and is often compared to a head of cauliflower in appearance. The main role of the cerebellum is to monitor and regulate coordinated movement in order to maintain balance and equilibrium. It receives information from proprioceptors situated in muscles and joints (see Chapter 4) and compares it to other signals received from the cerebrum. This allows the cerebellum to calculate and fine-tune the most efficient way to ensure muscle contraction achieves the desired result, whilst maintaining posture and balance. This information is quickly relayed (via the superior cerebellar peduncles) to the motor cortex of the cerebrum in order to coordinate muscular activity and movement. One of the reasons we stagger, and generally behave in an uncoordinated fashion, when drunk is because alcohol inhibits and impairs cerebellar proprioceptive sense. The cerebellum is also important for the timing of rhythmic movement during dancing which, in my experience at least, can also be significantly impaired by alcohol. Injury to the cerebellum does not cause paralysis but results in loss of muscle tone, uncoordinated movement (ataxia) and, on occasion, impaired thoughts about movement.

DIENCEPHALON

The diencephalon is a deep, central area of the brain situated between the midbrain and the cerebrum (Figure 12.8). It consists of a number of important structures including the thalamus, hypothalamus, pituitary and pineal glands. The largest of these structures is the egg-shaped thalamus (Greek for 'inner room') which makes up about 80% of the diencephalon. More accurately, the thalamus resembles two small eggs (connected by a central body known as the massa intermedia) and its inner (medial) walls help to enclose the third ventricle. The thalamus consists of a large number of different nuclei that relay ascending sensory information to specific areas of the cerebrum and limbic system and, like the reticular formation, help to filter unimportant or unnecessary input. It also plays an important role in memory, learning and conscious perception. For example, synaesthesia is a rare neurological condition in which sensory experiences become blended or combined (e.g. numbers or sounds may appear to have certain colours or tastes). One of the explanations for this phenomenon is that the thalamus relays sensory information to the wrong part of the brain where it is interpreted as if it were a different sensation.

HYPOTHALAMUS AND PITUITARY GLAND

The next part of the diencephalon is the hypothalamus which, as its name suggests, is situated below (and anterior to) the thalamus (Figure 12.8). Although it is a relatively small structure, it consists of 12 separate nuclei that direct and regulate a large number of important autonomic and homeostatic mechanisms. For example, it is essential for the regulation of temperature and the sleep-wake cycle (see Chapters 3 and 11), fluid balance and thirst (see Chapter 10), and satiety and hunger (see Chapter 11). It also helps to regulate the autonomic centres of the brainstem that control heart and respiratory rate (see Chapters 7, 8 and 9) and plays an important role in sexual arousal and strong emotion/emotional behaviour. Finally, the hypothalamus is essential for the operation and management of the endocrine system. This will be discussed in more detail in Chapter 13 but, in brief, it is connected to the pituitary gland by a narrow stalk of cells called the infundibulum (Latin for 'funnel'). The pituitary gland is often referred to as the heart of the endocrine system and secretes a number of important hormones in response to direct stimulation (nervous and hormonal) from the hypothalamus.

EPITHALAMUS AND PINEAL GLAND

The final part of the diencephalon is the epithalamus, which is situated above and behind the thalamus. It forms part of the choroid plexus of the third ventricle and connects the diencephalon to the limbic system (see below). The epithalamus also houses a small, cone-shaped gland known as the pineal gland (from the Latin for 'pine cone' or 'pine nut'). This secretes a hormone called melatonin which contributes to the regulation of the sleep-wake cycle. The 17-century French philosopher René Descartes (considered to be the father of modern philosophy) believed that the pineal gland was the principal seat of the soul and the place where all of our thoughts are formed. He based this assumption on the fact that it occupied a central position within the brain and is the only structure he could identify that was not paired or mirrored in some way. He also believed that the pineal gland was full of animal spirits that manifested themselves as a kind of fine wind (or flame) and were capable of inflating the ventricles. This goes to show that you can't be right about everything.

LIMBIC SYSTEM

The limbic system (from the Latin word for 'border') is situated on either side of the thalamus and directly below the cerebrum. It is often referred to as the 'emotional brain' since it plays an important role in the regulation of emotions including pain, pleasure, affection and anger. It is also responsible for the formation of memory and the body's response to odour. Like the diencephalon, the limbic system consists of a number of different, interrelated structures which include the hippocampus, fornix, amygdala, cingulate gyrus, mammillary bodies and olfactory bulbs (Figure 12.8). The hippocampus (Greek for 'sea horse') helps to transform new sensory information into long-term memories and assists with memory retrieval. It also plays an important role in spatial navigation and the 2014 Nobel Prize for physiology/medicine was awarded to three scientists who identified a series of cells in the hippocampus that allow us to judge distance and physical position (a kind of internal GPS system). Damage to the hippocampus can affect memory and those who suffer from Alzheimer's disease experience difficulty recalling recent events (short-term memory loss) and disorientation. In the film *Memento*, the protagonist (Leonard Shelby) suffers from anterograde amnesia (often caused by damage to the hippocampus or mammillary bodies) which renders him unable to acquire and retain new memories. The film involves his struggle to differentiate between fact and deception as he tries to uncover the identity of his wife's killer using only notes, pictures and tattoos. If that wasn't complicated enough, the film's chronological narrative takes place simultaneously backwards (in colour) and forwards (in black-and-white) with the intentional result that the viewer must pay as much attention to what is taking place as Leonard.

FORNIX AND AMYGDALA

The fornix (Latin for 'arch') is a c-shaped bundle of axons (white matter) that transmits information from the hippocampus to the hypothalamus and elsewhere. For example, the posterior fibres of the fornix continue through the hypothalamus to the mammillary bodies (see below) and thalamus. The amygdala or amygdaloid body is an almond-shaped cluster of neurons (nuclei) situated on either side of the thalamus at the lower end of the hippocampus. It is responsible for the formation and storage of memories associated with emotional events and helps us to interpret the emotions and emotional responses of others. The amygdala also plays an important role in the perception of fear and coordinates the flight-or-fight mechanism (in response to fear-provoking stimuli) as well as the way in which aggression and anger are expressed. It is thought that conditions such as autism, depression and post-traumatic stress may be linked to abnormal functioning of the amygdala as a result of damage, inadequate developmental or neurotransmitter imbalance.

CINGULPATE GYRUS AND MAMMILLARY BODIES

The next part of the limbic system is a large, arch-shaped structure known as the cingulate gyrus (Figure 12.8). It is situated directly above the corpus callosum and below the cerebrum, and helps to process and regulate acute pain and emotion. It is also thought to play an important role in learning to predict and avoid negative consequences. The mammillary bodies are two small nuclei situated directly below the thalamus that are connected to the hypothalamus and thalamus via the fornix. They are essential for the development of episodic or recollective memory. That is to say, long-term memory that involves the recollection of specific events and experiences and the emotions associated with them (e.g. your first day at school or your first kiss). Episodic memories are often autobiographical and can be triggered by sensory stimulation such as a particular smell or piece of music. Chronic alcohol consumption (resulting in vitamin B1 deficiency) can damage the mammillary bodies and lead to impaired memory and, in extreme cases, anterograde amnesia (see above).

OLFACTORY BULBS

The final part of the limbic system (to be discussed here) are the olfactory bulbs that transmit sensory information regarding odours to the amygdala, hippocampus, thalamus and cerebrum via the olfactory tract. The olfactory receptors are embedded in a specialised area of mucous membrane in the roof of the nasal cavity. The olfactory bulbs are situated directly above on either side of the cribiform plate of the ethmoid bone and are innervated

by the olfactory nerve (cranial nerve I). The association between smell and memory is particularly strong because of the connection between the olfactory bulb and other parts of the limbic system such as the amygdala and hippocampus. Some smells are closely associated with particular events, people, moods and emotions, and can prompt very different responses from people depending on their experiences. For example, the smell of chlorine might be associated by one person with the swimming pool (good experience) and by another with the hospital (bad experience). I know somebody who still feels nauseous every time they smell a particular soft drink because it was the last thing they drank before surgery some thirty years previously.

CORPUS CALLOSUM AND HEMISPHERIC LATERALISATION

The cerebrum is the largest part of the brain and is divided into two halves or hemispheres by a deep cleft known as the longitudinal fissure (Figure 12.9). The two hemispheres are connected to one another by a thick bundle of nerve fibres called the corpus callosum (Latin for 'calloused body'). The corpus callosum is situated below the cerebrum (and cingulate gyrus, Figure 12.8) and consists of about 200 million axons (whiter matter). It allows each hemisphere to control movement on the opposite (contralateral) side of the body. That is to say, the left side of the brain controls the right side of the body and the right side of the brain controls the left side of the body. This is thought to contribute to the concept of 'handedness' and those who are right-handed are said to be left-brain dominant and those who are left-handed are right-brain dominant. Each hemisphere also performs a number of unique and specialised functions, a trait known as hemispheric lateralisation. For example, in the mid-19th century, the French neurosurgeon Paul Broca identified an area of the left hemisphere that plays an important role in the production of spoken and written language (Broca's area, Figure 12.10).

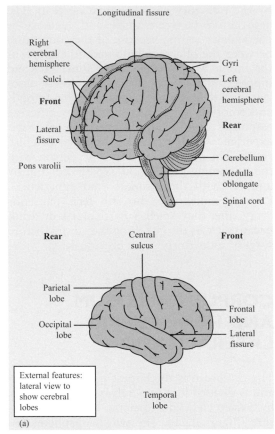

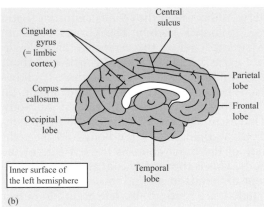

Figure 12.9 (a) Cerebral hemispheres and lobes. (b) Inner surface of the left hemisphere.

Not long after he had published his findings, a German neurologist called Karl Wernicke identified another area of the left hemisphere that is involved in language comprehension (Wernicke's area). It is estimated that as many

as 97% of the population (including those who are left-handed) exhibit left hemisphere language specialisation. The left hemisphere also seems to be important for numerical and scientific reasoning and is often characterised as the logical or rational brain. For example:

It deson't mttaer in waht oredr the ltteers in a word aepapr, the olny iprmoatnt tihng is taht the frist and lsat ltteers are in the rghit pcale. The rset can be a toatl mses and y8u cn sitll raed it without a pobelrm.

The right hemisphere is thought to be more creative and plays an important role in artistic, musical and emotional awareness, as well as facial recognition and spatial perception. That is not to say those who are right-handed (left-brain dominant) cannot be artistic or creative; or those who are left-handed (right-brain dominant) cannot excel at writing or rational thought. In reality, we use both sides of our brain to a greater or lesser extent.

SPLIT-BRAIN

US neuroscientists Roger Sperry and Michael Gazzaniga performed a number of experiments on individuals whose corpus callosum had been removed (split-brain patients). One of the experiments involved presenting one object to the left eye and a different object to the right eye. The split-brain patient was then asked to place their left hand under a screen and draw what they had observed with their left eye. When asked to explain the picture, however, they always described what they had seen with their right eye. This and other experiments helped to demonstrate that without the corpus callosum, the left and right hemispheres are unable to communicate with each other. Agenesis of the corpus callosum is a rare congenital disorder where the corpus callosum is partially or totally absent at birth. Typical characteristics associated with this condition may include visual and hearing impairment, poor motor coordination, difficulty with abstract reasoning, misinterpretation of non-verbal communication and poor perception of pain. The most notable person to have agenesis of the corpus callosum was Kim Peek (1951–2009) who became famous as the inspiration for the character Raymond Babbitt in the film Rain Man. Peek had an exceptional memory and was able to read two pages of a book simultaneously. He read one page with his left eye and the other with his right and it took him about ten seconds in total.

CEREBRUM

The ridged appearance of the cerebrum is created by a series of surface folds of varying depths. These are known as gyri (Latin for 'circle') and are separated from one another by fissures called sulci (Latin for 'trench'). These folds greatly increase the total surface area of the cerebrum and it is estimated that, unfolded, it would measure 1,500–2,000 cm². Each hemisphere of the cerebrum is further divided into four sections or lobes which share the same name as the cranial bones they sit beneath: frontal, parietal, occipital and temporal (Figure 12.9). The frontal lobe, as its name indicates, is situated at the front of the brain and is associated with reasoning, motor skills, higher cognitive functions and expressive language. It is divided into a number of substructures or regions including Broca's area (see above), prefrontal cortex, primary motor cortex and premotor cortex (Figure 12.10). The prefrontal cortex plays an important role in the management and regulation of key cognitive processes such as decision-making, planning, problem-solving and the inhibition of inappropriate social behaviour. These are collectively known as higher or executive functions and the prefrontal cortex coordinates information relayed from other parts of the brain in order to guide voluntary control of our actions. Those who sustain damage or injury to these pathways can undergo significant personality changes and behave in a manner that is unfamiliar to those who knew them before the accident. The most famous example of damage to this area is provided by the case of Phineas Gage. In 1848, Gage suffered extensive damage to his prefrontal cortex when an explosion drove a large iron bar through his skull whilst he was working on the railway. Despite the traumatic nature of his injury (according to a witness statement, the iron bar was found some 25 m away 'smeared with blood and brain'), Gage recovered with his memory, speech and motor skills intact. However, according to his physician, Dr John Harlow, he became:[1]

> fitful, irreverent, indulging at times in the grossest profanity (which was not previously his custom), manifesting but little deference for his fellows, impatient of restraint or advice when it conflicts with his desires . . . Previous to his injury . . . he possessed a well-balanced mind, and was looked upon by those who knew him as a shrewd, smart business man, very energetic and persistent in executing all his plans of operation. In this regard his mind was radically changed, so decidedly that his friends and acquaintances said he was 'no longer Gage'.

PRIMARY MOTOR CORTEX

The next region of the frontal lobe is the primary motor cortex situated directly in front of the central sulcus that separates the frontal lobe from the parietal lobe (Figure 12.10). It generates nerve impulses that activate skeletal muscle and control the execution of movement on the opposite (contralateral) side of the body. The primary motor cortex is mapped so that specific areas control the movement of particular body parts. For example, foot and leg movements map to the part of the primary motor cortex closest to the midline. Parts of the body capable of a high degree of movement, such as the hands and lips, are represented by large areas of the primary motor cortex. The premotor cortex consists of a narrow strip of tissue situated between the prefrontal and primary motor cortices. It helps to anticipate and plan voluntary movement and controls learned motor skills necessary to play a musical instrument or type. It also seems to play a role in the initiation and onset of laughter in response to others laughing.

association area. The former receives visual information from the retina of the eye via the optic nerves and a series of neurons that originate in the lateral geniculate nuclei of the thalamus (see above). The latter interprets this information in relation to past visual experiences and allows us to recognise and understand what we are 'seeing'. For example, when you see the characters y, e and s, your visual association area recognises that collectively they form the word 'yes'. The same is true when you recognise a familiar face or differentiate between a tennis ball and a cricket ball. Damage to this area can result in difficulty identifying objects, colours and words and, in some cases, trigger visual hallucinations or recurrent visual disturbances known as palinopsia (Greek for 'again' and 'seeing').

TEMPORAL LOBE

The final lobe of the cerebrum is the temporal lobe which is separated from the frontal and parietal lobes by the lateral sulcus (Sylvian fissure). It consists of the primary auditory cortex, the auditory association area and a number of limbic system structures including the hippocampus (Figure 12.10). The primary auditory cortex receives sound information in terms of pitch, rhythm and volume from the inner ear via the auditory nerve. The auditory association area interprets and translates these noises as speech, music or other familiar/unfamiliar sounds. Memories of sounds heard in the past are also stored in the temporal lobe, and we observed earlier in the chapter that the hippocampus is closely associated with the formation and retrieval of memories. The temporal lobe also seems to play an important role in face and object recognition and speech and language processes (Wernicke's area is situated where the temporal and parietal lobes meet). Damage to the temporal lobe can result in a condition called agnosia where individuals are unable to recognise common objects, sounds, shapes or smells. The type of agnosia is dependent on which part of temporal lobe (or elsewhere) has been affected. For example, auditory agnosia often occurs following damage to the superior temporal lobe whereas visual agnosia occurs as a result of damage to the middle-inferior temporal lobe or posterior occipital lobe.

STROKE

A stroke, or cerebral vascular attack (CVA) as it is also known, occurs when there is a disturbance in the blood supply to an area of the brain. We observed earlier in the chapter that neurons consume about 20% of the body's oxygen and if this supply is interrupted for more than a few minutes, cell death occurs, resulting in temporary or permanent loss of function. The most common cause of stroke is when a cerebral artery becomes blocked by a blood clot (thrombus). This is known as an ischaemic stroke or cerebral infarct, and is essentially the same mechanism that occurs during a heart attack (the term 'brain attack' is used in Canada and the US). The other major cause of stroke is when a blood vessel ruptures and spills blood into the cerebrum or the meninges (see below). This is known as a haemorrhagic stroke and, as well as disrupting the supply of oxygen and glucose to a particular area of the brain, the escaping blood also causes damage by compressing surrounding tissue and triggering inflammation (see Chapter 6). It is difficult to tell the difference between the two types of stroke without a brain scan (e.g. computed tomography) since typically both result in similar symptoms. These include dizziness, confusion, slurred speech, difficulty swallowing and weakness, numbness or paralysis to one side of the body. Symptoms are highly dependent, therefore, on the extent of the damage and the area/side of the brain affected. A stroke affecting the left side of the brain causes symptoms (e.g. weakness) to the right side of the body. Treatment for ischaemic stroke is very similar to that for heart attack and involves providing a thrombolytic (clot + splitting) drug that quickly breaks down and dissolves the thrombus obstructing the vessel. Clearly this treatment is not suitable for somebody experiencing a haemorrhagic stroke since it would exacerbate the bleeding and it is essential that a firm diagnosis is made before treatment is commenced.

MENINGES

The brain and spinal cord (CNS) are surrounded by three protective membranes collectively known as meninges. The outermost of these is called the dura mater from the Latin for 'tough mother'. It is a strongest and thickest of the three membranes and is divided into outer and inner layers (Figure 12.11). The outer layer is attached to the periosteum of the cranium (Chapter 4) whilst the inner layer has multiple folds that mirror the outline of the brain beneath. For the most part, the two layers are fused together to provide support and stabilisation for the brain. However, in some areas, they separate to accommodate a number of dural venous sinuses that drain cerebrospinal fluid (CSF) and venous blood from the brain, and return it to the internal jugular veins of the neck. The middle meninx (singular of meninges) is the arachnoid mater from the Greek for 'spider-like'. It is separated from the dura mater by the subdural cavity which is lubricated by a thin film of fluid. Finger-like projections called arachnoid villi project upwards from the arachnoid mater into the largest of the dural venous sinuses (the superior sagittal sinus) in order to absorb CSF mentioned above. Directly beneath the arachnoid mater is the subarachnoid space which is filled with CSF. The arachnoid mater derives its name ('spider-like mother') from the thousands of web-like extensions that span this space and anchor it to the third and innermost meninx, the pia mater.

PIA MATER AND CEREBROSPINAL FLUID

The pia mater ('tender mother') is an extremely thin and delicate membrane that sticks to the outer surface of the brain and extends into its various folds and involutions. The pia mater is also impermeable to fluid which allows it to retain cerebrospinal fluid (CSF) in the subarachnoid space above. CSF is similar in composition to blood plasma (i.e. it is mainly water) and circulates around the brain and spinal cord via the subarachnoid space. It is secreted at a rate of about 0.5 ml per minute by the choroid plexus, a network of blood vessels made up of modified ependymal cells that project into each of the

(a)

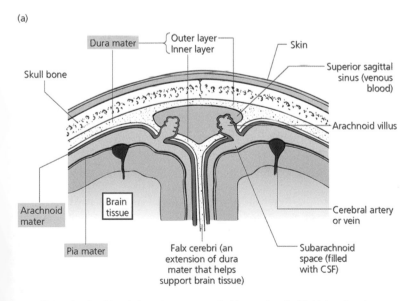

Note: Arachnoid and pia mater are connected by a network of bridging strands (called trabeculae) that help to maintain the patency of the subarachnoid space

Figure 12.11 Meninges.

four ventricles of the brain. Since secretion keeps pace with reabsorption (via the superior sagittal sinus), the average volume of CSF in the ventricles, subarachnoid space and everywhere else in the central nervous system remains about 150 ml. This is important since it maintains a constant and uniform inter-cranial pressure. It also provides buoyancy for the brain which prevents it from being crushed or compressed by its own weight. Finally, CSF cushions the brain and spinal cord from trauma, and provides nourishment for the tissue that it bathes. Hydrocephalus (from the Greek words for 'water' and 'head') occurs when there is an accumulation of CSF in the brain as a result of excessive production or poor reabsorption. In adults and older children, this causes an increase in inter-cranial pressure which, if unrelieved, can result in permanent brain damage. In babies and infants whose cranial sutures have not yet fused (see Chapter 4), the bones are able to expand to accommodate the excess fluid to some extent. Treatment normally involves inserting a tube called a shunt into one of ventricles to drain the CSF. The shunt contains a valve to ensure the fluid only travels in one direction (i.e. out of the brain and into the venous circulation).

CHAPTER 12: TEST YOURSELF

Q. The nervous system can be broadly divided into the central nervous system (CNS) and the peripheral nervous system. What is the difference between the two?

A. The CNS consists of the brain and the spinal cord (attached to one another at the base of the brainstem). The peripheral nervous system refers to the nerves of the body that are not part of the CNS, including 31 pairs of spinal nerves.

Q. How many pairs of cervical, thoracic, lumber, sacral and coccygeal nerves are there?

A. 8 cervical, 12 thoracic, 5 lumber, 5 sacral and 1 coccygeal.

Q. How many cranial nerves are there?

A. Twelve.

Q. What is the difference between motor (efferent) and sensory (afferent) nerves?

A. Motor nerves travel away from the CNS and coordinate movement. Sensory nerves travel towards the CNS and relay information toward the brain for interpretation or, in the case of reflexes, towards a corresponding motor nerve via the spinal cord.

Q. What is the function of the axon hillock and axon in a neuron?

A. The axon hillock is a small elevation situated between the cell body and the axon. It triggers the creation of a nerve impulse (action potential) that is driven along the length of the axon towards the synaptic terminals.

Q. Most axons are surrounded by a sheath of fatty material called myelin. What does myelin do?

A. Myelin insulates the axon and helps to increase the speed of nerve transmission along its length.

Q. What is the function of a synapse and a neurotransmitter?

A. A synapse is a small junction or gap between a synaptic terminal of one neuron and the dendrite of another neuron/receptor tissue. When a nerve impulse reaches the synaptic terminal, it triggers the secretion of a neurotransmitter (chemical messenger) into the synapse. The neurotransmitter diffuses across the gap and binds with a receptor on the opposing side.

Q. What is a reflex and why does it occur?
A. A reflex is a rapid, involuntary response to external stimulation. It consists of an arc whereby sensory information (e.g. pain) is detected by a sensory nerve receptor and relayed to the spinal cord. The neuron makes synaptic contact with a motor nerve fibre (via an inter-neuron) and the message travels directly to a muscle where it stimulates a response (e.g. withdrawal).

Q. What are the five special senses?
A. Touch, taste, smell, sound and sight.

Q. List the three principle regions of the ear.
A. External ear, middle ear and inner ear.

Q. The retina of the eye contains two types of photosensitive receptor cells: rods and cones. Explain how they differ in terms of function and location.
A. The retina contains numerous rods that allow us to see in dim light but are unable to discern colour. Cones are highly sensitive to colour and concentrated in the macula. They are much less numerous.

Q. What are the three main regions of the brain?
A. Brainstem, cerebellum and cerebrum.

Q. List the three parts of the brainstem in ascending order?
A. Medulla oblongata, pons and midbrain.

Q. Briefly describe the principle functions of the medulla (think back to Chapters 7, 8 and 9).
A. The medulla houses the cardiovascular and respiratory centres, and coordinates a number of autonomic activities including coughing, sneezing, vomiting and hiccupping.

Q. Briefly describe the main role of the cerebellum?
A. The cerebellum monitors and regulates coordinated movement in order to maintain balance and equilibrium.

Q. Briefly describe the principle functions of the thalamus (located in the diencephalon).
A. The thalamus relays sensory information to specific areas of the cerebrum and limbic system. It also helps to filter unnecessary information and plays an important role in memory and learning.

Q. What is the limbic system?
A. The limbic system consists of a number of interrelated structures situated on either side of the thalamus (below the cerebrum). It plays an important role in the regulation of emotions including pain, pleasure and anger. It is also responsible for the formation of memory.

Q. The cerebrum is the largest part of the brain and is divided into two halves (hemispheres) by the longitudinal fissure. What is the name of the structure that allows the hemispheres to communicate?
A. The corpus callosum.

Q. What are the four lobes of the cerebrum called?
A. Frontal lobe, parietal lobe, occipital lobe and temporal lobe.

(Continued)

(Continued)

Q. Where are the primary motor and primary sensory cortex located?

A. The primary motor cortex is located in the frontal lobe and the primary sensory cortex in the parietal lobe.

Q. Which parts of the brain receive and interpret visual information?

A. The occipital lobe receives and interprets visual information from the optic nerve. The thalamus also interprets this information in relation to past visual experiences and allows us to recognise and understand what we are 'seeing'.

Q. Which part of the brain receives and interprets auditory (sound) information?

A. The temporal lobe receives sound information in terms of pitch, rhythm and volume via the auditory nerve and interprets and translates these noises as speech, music or other familiar/unfamiliar sounds. The limbic system (hippocampus) is associated with the formation and retrieval of memories associated with sound.

Q. What are the names of the three meninges that surround the brain and spinal cord (from the outside in)?

A. Dura mater, arachnoid mater and pia mater.

Q. What is the function of cerebrospinal fluid (CSF)?

A CSF maintains a constant inter-cranial pressure and provides buoyancy for the brain. It also protects the brain and spinal cord from trauma and provides nourishment for the tissue that it bathes.

Note

1 Harlow, J.M. (1868) Recovery from the passage of an iron bar through the head. *Publications of the Massachusetts Medical Society*, 2: 327–347.

Contents

CHAPTER 13

ENDOCRINE SYSTEM

HORMONES

In the previous chapter, we observed that the nervous system uses electrical signals to maintain a stable internal environment, as well as interpret sensory stimulation, generate voluntary movement and undertake mental activities involved in memory, intelligence and moral sense. The endocrine system, on the other hand, employs chemical messengers called hormones (from the Greek for 'set in motion') to influence and regulate cellular activity throughout the body. Although hormones are a much slower method of communication than nerve impulses (which can travel at a rate of up to 120 metres per second) they are capable of influencing many cells simultaneously and can exert a much longer duration of action. We produce more than 80 different hormones which govern and control every aspect of the human body to a greater or lesser extent. Although we will only discuss a few of these chemical messengers in this chapter, we should not underestimate how important they are to everyday health and well-being and it is no coincidence that we have already referred to many of them in the preceding chapters. It is also important to stress that the nervous and endocrine systems do not operate in isolation from one another, they work collaboratively in order to control and regulate cellular activity and to maintain homeostasis.

PEPTIDES, AMINO ACID DERIVATIVES AND LIPID DERIVATIVES

There are three main groups of hormones based upon their chemical composition: peptides, amino acid derivatives and lipid derivatives. Peptide hormones are synthesised from chains of amino acids using a messenger RNA template (see Chapter 2). They are soluble in water and include all the hormones secreted by the hypothalamus and pancreas, and most of the hormones secreted by the pituitary gland. Amino acid derivatives are relatively small molecules derived from the amino acids tyrosine and tryptophan. There are two types of tyrosine-derived hormones: thyroid hormones and catecholamines (secreted by the medulla of the adrenal gland). Tryptophan, on the other hand, is a precursor to melatonin which we noted in Chapter 12 is produced by the pineal gland. Most amino acid derivatives are soluble in water but some, such as the thyroid hormones, are fat soluble only. Lipid derivative hormones are made from either cholesterol or fatty acids. Those made from cholesterol are known as steroids and include all the hormones secreted by the cortex of the adrenal gland, as well as those secreted by the male and female reproductive organs (gonads). Steroid hormones are fat soluble and are transported in the blood by carrier proteins (e.g. albumin and globulin). This means that they remain in the circulation much longer than peptide or amino acid derived hormones. For example, cortisol takes 60–90 minutes to reach half its original value (half-life) compared to adrenaline which takes about 2 minutes. Lipid derivative hormones made from fatty acids are known as eicosanoids and include leukotrienes and prostaglandins discussed in Chapter 6. They are also fat soluble but typically function close to their site of production and degrade relatively quickly.

RECEPTORS

Hormones are secreted into the blood by an endocrine gland or by specialised cells situated within an organ (e.g. pancreatic beta cells secrete the peptide hormone insulin). Endocrine glands differ from exocrine glands (such as sweat, salivary or mammary glands) in that they don't discharge their products into a duct or onto the surface of the skin. Consequently, they are often referred to as ductless glands and secrete hormones into the interstitial fluid surrounding the secretory cells where they diffuse directly into the capillary blood. Hormones are transported in the bloodstream (dissolved in plasma or attached to a protein carrier) to a part of the body known as the target. Hormones bind to receptors situated on, or within, the target cells in order to influence their activity (Figure 13.1). For example, the cells of the breast, uterus and vagina all possess receptors for the steroid hormone oestrogen.

WATER- AND FAT-SOLUBLE HORMONES

In Chapter 2, we observed that the cell membrane comprises a hydrophilic (water-loving) and hydrophobic (water-hating) phospholipid bi-layer that ensures water and ions remain in the correct concentrations inside and outside the cell. Water-soluble hormones are unable to penetrate this fatty barrier and must bind to receptors located on its surface. This triggers a chemical reaction which activates enzymes within the cell in order to increase/decrease cellular activity. In general terms, water-soluble hormones act quickly but have a short duration of action since they are broken down rapidly in the interstitial fluid. For example, the peptide hormone insulin (see below) acts within minutes to lower plasma glucose but has a half-life of 4–6 minutes. Fat-soluble or steroid hormones, on the other hand, are able to pass through the phospholipid membrane with ease and bind with receptors situated on the nuclear membrane. This produces a hormone receptor complex that migrates into the nucleus to bind with a section of DNA and triggers enzyme activity which influences biochemical processes within the cell (Figure 13.2). In contrast to water-soluble hormones, steroid hormones are often slow to start but tend to have a longer duration of action. Finally, the number of receptors found on the cell and nuclear membranes does not necessarily remain static. Some cells produce more receptors in response to high levels of a particular hormone – a process known as up-regulation. In other cases, exposure to elevated hormone levels can desensitise target cells

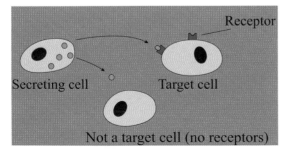

Figure 13.1 Target cells and cell membrane receptors.

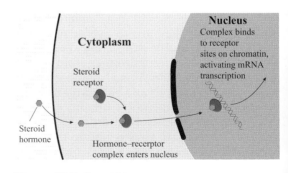

Figure 13.2 Steroid hormone receptors.

and lead to loss of receptors. This is known as down-regulation and seems to protect the cell from over-activity and stimulation in the presence of persistently high hormone levels.

HYPOTHALAMUS

In health, hormone levels in the blood are variable and self-regulating within their normal range. This is usually achieved through a negative feedback mechanism but some examples of positive feedback also exist. In Chapter 3, we observed that homeostasis is maintained by a number of control systems that detect and respond to changes in internal and external environment. In the case of the endocrine system, it is the hypothalamus and pituitary gland that control and regulate the activity of most of the other endocrine glands. The hypothalamus is connected to the pea-like pituitary gland by a narrow stalk of cells called the pituitary stalk or infundibulum (see also Chapter 12). The anterior lobe of the pituitary gland is also connected to the hypothalamus by a network of blood vessels called the hypophyseal portal system (the Latin name for pituitary gland is *hypophysis*). The hypothalamus produces and secretes a variety of regulatory hormones (peptides) which are delivered to the anterior pituitary gland via the hypophyseal portal system (Figure 13.3). These hormones control the activity of the endocrine cells of the anterior pituitary gland and are referred to as hypothalamic-releasing and hypothalamic-inhibiting hormones (see below). The posterior lobe of the pituitary gland, on the other hand, comprises nervous tissue and only secretes two (peptide) hormones: oxytocin and antidiuretic hormone (ADH). Finally, in the previous chapter, we also noted that the hypothalamus contains 12 separate nuclei that direct and regulate a large number of important endocrine and autonomic mechanisms. For example, when the sympathetic nervous division of the hypothalamus is stimulated, it immediately activates the neuroendocrine cells in the adrenal medulla which produce the hormones adrenaline and noradrenaline (see below).

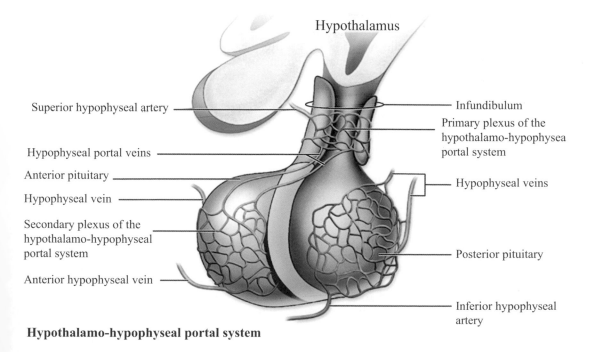

Hypothalamus

Superior hypophyseal artery

Infundibulum

Primary plexus of the hypothalamo-hypophysea portal system

Hypophyseal portal veins

Anterior pituitary

Hypophyseal veins

Hypophyseal vein

Secondary plexus of the hypothalamo-hypophyseal portal system

Anterior hypophyseal vein

Posterior pituitary

Inferior hypophyseal artery

Hypothalamo-hypophyseal portal system

Figure 13.3 Anterior pituitary gland and hypophyseal portal system.

OXYTOCIN AND ADH

In Chapter 3, we saw how the posterior pituitary gland secretes oxytocin to stimulate contraction of the uterus during labour, and the let-down reflex during breast feeding (both examples of positive feedback). Oxytocin also has a number of other interesting qualities including the ability to heighten sociability and reduce anxiety. Consequently, it is often referred to as the 'love' or 'cuddle' hormone since it is thought to encourage bonding between mother and child after the physiological stress of birth. Interestingly, it can be administered via a nasal spray to help to improve communication and sociability in children and teenagers with autism. It has also been tested as an aid to cooperation for couples discussing issues that may cause conflict or disagreement (by increasing empathy for the person with the opposing view). Finally, oxytocin also contributes to feelings of sexual arousal and is the hormone responsible for stimulating male and female orgasm (see Chapter 14). ADH (also known as vasopressin) is secreted when hypothalamic osmoreceptors detect an increase in the concentration of blood plasma often in response to dehydration (see Chapter 10). ADH is then transported in the blood to the kidneys where it stimulates the insertion of additional water channel proteins (aquaporins) into the cell membrane of the collecting ducts. This increases permeability, and more water is osmotically transported back into the capillary circulation until plasma osmolality returns to normal, and ADH secretion is inhibited (a negative feedback loop). ADH has a half-life of 5–20 minutes which allows for rapid adaptation to fluctuations in plasma osmolality. Although both oxytocin and ADH are secreted by the posterior pituitary gland, they are synthesised by cell bodies in the hypothalamus where they are packaged into secretory vesicles. They are then transported along axons situated in the infundibulum (hypothalamic-hypophyseal tract) to the posterior lobe of the pituitary gland for storage (Figure 13.3). These 'readymade' hormones can then be secreted into the bloodstream as and when required. This process is made possible because the posterior pituitary gland and hypothalamus consist of the same nervous tissue, and the former is essentially a down-extension of the latter.

ANTERIOR PITUITARY HORMONES

Unlike the posterior lobe of the pituitary gland, which is composed of the same nervous tissue as the hypothalamus, the anterior lobe consists entirely of glandular epithelium. We noted above that the hypothalamus communicates with the anterior pituitary gland through the secretion of releasing and inhibiting hormones into the hypophyseal portal system (Figure 13.3). The short distance travelled by these peptide hormones ensures that they are not diluted in the plasma before they reach the anterior pituitary gland and communication is rapid and efficient. The main releasing hormones secreted by the hypothalamus are growth hormone releasing hormone (GHRH), thyroid-releasing hormone (TRH), corticotropin-releasing hormone (CRH) and gonadotropin-releasing hormone (GnRH). The main inhibiting hormones are growth hormone inhibiting hormone (GHIH) and dopamine (also known as prolactin-inhibiting hormone or PIH). As their names suggest, these hormones either encourage or inhibit the release of a hormone from the anterior pituitary gland. For example, growth hormone inhibiting hormone not only inhibits the release of growth hormone it also inhibits the release of thyroid-stimulating hormone, cholecystokinin (CCK) and insulin (see below). Hormones secreted by the anterior pituitary gland are often referred to as tropic hormones (the Greek word *tropos* means 'turn' or 'change') since they turn on/off endocrine glands elsewhere in the body. There are seven anterior pituitary hormones in total: growth hormone, thyroid-stimulating hormone, adrenocorticotropic hormone, prolactin, melanocyte-stimulating hormone, follicle-stimulating hormone and luteinising hormone. Melanocyte-stimulating hormone, as it name suggests, stimulates the melanocytes of the skin and hair to produce the brown/black pigment melanin (see Chapter 3). We will discuss follicle-stimulating hormone (FSH) and luteinising hormone (LH) in Chapter 14 when we consider and explore (figuratively speaking) the male and female reproductive systems.

GROWTH HORMONE

The most abundant hormone produced by the anterior pituitary gland is growth hormone (GH) or somatotropin. GH encourages cells in the bone, cartilage, skeletal muscle and elsewhere to secrete small protein hormones called insulin-like growth factors (IGFs) that increase the rate at which amino acids enter cells and are used to synthesise proteins. This stimulates cell growth and tissue repair particularly during childhood and adolescence (see Chapter 4). GH also plays an important role in regulating protein, fat and carbohydrate metabolism. For example, it inhibits glucose metabolism by muscle and adipose tissue, and increases the synthesis of glucose from amino acids and glycerol by the liver (gluconeogenesis). This helps to counteract the effects of fasting (e.g. overnight) and GH is known as a glucose-sparing hormone since it spares glucose for use by the neurons when levels are low. The amount of GH secreted by the anterior pituitary gland varies over the course of the day and at different points during our lives. For example, GH levels are at their highest during adolescence and peak in late puberty. Secretion declines significantly as we get older which contributes to loss of muscle mass and skin thickness. On a day-to-day basis, secretion occurs in regular bursts or pulses but is most abundant at night particularly during deep sleep. Other factors also contribute to the secretion of GH including vigorous exercise, strong emotions and physical stress.

HYPER- AND HYPO-SECRETION OF GROWTH HORMONE

We noted above, that secretion of GH is regulated and controlled by two hypothalamic hormones: growth hormone releasing hormone (GHRH) and growth hormone

inhibiting hormone (GHIH). However, over- and under-production of GH can occur in children and adults often because of a benign tumour of the pituitary gland. Hyper-secretion of GH in adults results in a condition known as acromegaly (from the Greek words for 'extremities' and 'enlargement'). Symptoms typically develop slowly over a number of years and include thickening of the bones, due to ossification of the periosteum (particularly the lower jaw and brow), and soft tissue swelling resulting in enlarged hands, feet, tongue, etc. Linear bone growth does not occur since the epiphyseal growth plates have already ossified and closed. Hyper-secretion of GH during childhood or early adolescence, on the other hand, results in gigantism since the growth plates remain active and bone, muscle and connective tissue develop at an accelerated rate. The most famous example of somebody with gigantism is probably Robert Wadlow (1918–1940) who, at 8ft 11in tall (2.71m), was known as the Giant of Illinois and remains the tallest man in recorded history. The actor Richard Kiel (1939–2014), who played the character Jaws in the James Bond films, had the same condition but stood a mere 7ft 1.5in (2.17m) in comparison. Hypo-secretion of GH in childhood results in reduced linear bone growth and soft tissue development. It is one of the many causes of dwarfism (in this case: pituitary dwarfism).

PROLACTIN

Prolactin is a peptide hormone (secreted by the anterior pituitary gland) that stimulates the production of milk by the mammary tissue of the breast. The word mammal describes a type of animal, including humans, that feed their young on milk secreted by the mammary glands. In Chapter 3, we noted that mammary glands are actually a type of modified apocrine or sweat gland. Consequently, they are present in both men and women but typically only function in women. Each mammary gland consists of about 20 lobules situated within the connective tissue and fat of the breast and arranged in a circular fashion around the nipple. Most of the structural changes that are essential for the successful production of milk (lactation) take place during the first four months of pregnancy under the influence of prolactin, progesterone and oestrogen (discussed in Chapter 14). After childbirth has taken place, the secretion of these hormones decreases dramatically as the stimulus for production is removed. However, the suckling action on the nipple during breast feeding stimulates the production of further prolactin by the anterior pituitary gland and lactation commences. At the same time, the posterior pituitary hormone oxytocin triggers contraction of the smooth muscle that surrounds the mammary tissue and is responsible for the release of the milk from the ducts. This is known as the 'let-down' reflex and is explained in more detail in Chapter 3. Occasionally, new-born babies (of either gender) secrete a milky substance from their nipples known as galactorrhea (Greek for 'milk' + 'flow') or, more theatrically, 'witch's milk'. The latter expression stems from European folklore and refers to the belief that witches' cats (and other supernatural beings) stole or fed on this milk. Galactorrhea occurs because some of the mother's hormones are able to cross the placenta and it usually resolves spontaneously within a couple of months as hormone levels decline. No treatment is required unless the area becomes inflamed or infected. Finally, prolactin is inhibited by dopamine which is also known as prolactin-inhibiting hormone (PIH). Dopamine plays an important role in sexual arousal and hyper-secretion of prolactin is thought to contribute to male impotence since it counteracts the effects of dopamine. In women, hyper-secretion of prolactin may result in galactorrhea and/or changes to their menstrual cycle (see Chapter 14).

THYROID-STIMULATING HORMONE AND THE THYROID GLAND

Thyroid-stimulating hormone (TSH) is secreted by the anterior pituitary gland in response to the secretion of thyroid-releasing hormone (TRH) by the hypothalamus (e.g. as a result of exercise, stress and/or reduced plasma glucose levels). As its name suggests, TSH stimulates the thyroid gland to produce and release further hormones: triiodothyronine (T_3) and the much easier to pronounce thyroxine (T_4). The thyroid gland itself is situated just below the larynx (between the carotid arteries) and resembles a butterfly or bowtie in shape (Figure 13.4). T_3 and T_4 are amino acid derivative hormones and are formed when thyroglobulin (a protein) is combined with iodine and the amino acid tyrosine. The body cannot produce iodine itself and must obtain it from a number of dietary sources including dairy products, vegetables (grown in iodine-rich soil), seafood and seaweed (sushi ticks both boxes). Poor dietary intake can result in hypothyroidism (see below) and developmental delay or mental retardation in children whose mothers are iodine deficient during pregnancy. The thyroid gland produces much more T_4 (90%) than T_3 (10%) but the latter is more potent. Both are transported in the blood by the plasma protein thyroxine-binding globulin. In Chapter 4, we noted that T_3 and T_4 are essential for normal development of endochondral and intramembranous bone during childhood and the regulation of bone mineral density in adults. They also increase the rate of oxygen consumption and energy production in most cells of the body. This increases basal metabolic rate (BMR) which generates heat and helps to maintain normal body temperature. We also saw in Chapter 3 that adults are able to secrete additional T_4 (and T_3) for a limited period of time in response to prolonged exposure to cold/hypothermia. Finally, T_3 and T_4 regulate protein, fat and carbohydrate metabolism and are essential for normal cell development and differentiation.

HYPOTHYROIDISM

Hypothyroidism (an underactive thyroid) occurs when the thyroid gland is unable to secrete enough T_3 and T_4 to maintain normal cellular metabolism. The most common cause of hypothyroidism is the autoimmune disease Hashimoto's thyroiditis (first described by the Japanese scientist Hakaru Hashimoto in 1912) where the body's immune system produces

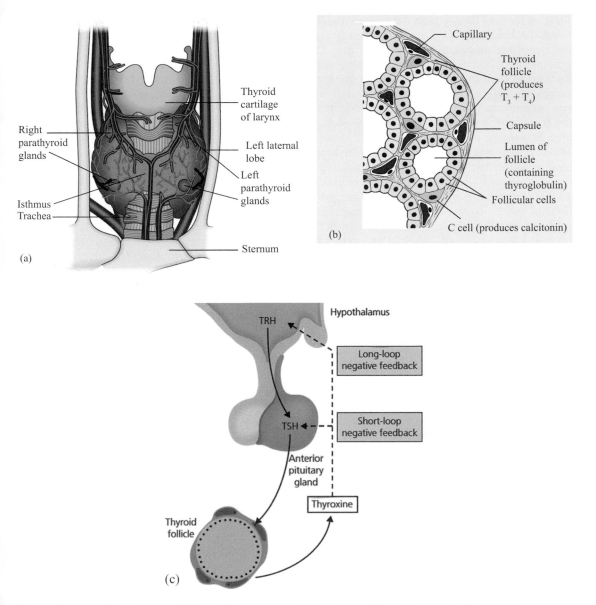

Figure 13.4 (a) Thyroid gland. (b) Thyroid hormone-producing cells. (c) Thyroxine negative feedback loop.

antibodies (immunoglobulins) that attack the thyroid tissue. This can cause enlargement of the thyroid gland (goitre) but eventually the tissue may atrophy and decrease in size. Other causes of hypothyroidism include iodine deficiency, benign tumour of the pituitary gland (resulting in a reduction of TSH), surgical excision of the thyroid gland (thyroidectomy), and as a side effect of some medications (e.g. amioderone used to treat cardiac arrhythmias). The symptoms of hypothyroidism reflect the fact that cellular metabolism is diminished in the absence of T_3 and T_4 and include fatigue, feeling cold, weight gain, constipation, drying of the skin and slow thought processes. Myxoedema is a disease caused by hypothyroidism and has many of the same symptoms. It was whilst researching this disease that the British surgeon Victor Horsley (1857–1916) first identified the link between thyroid deficiency and the symptoms associated with myxoedema. He transplanted thyroid glands from sheep into humans to demonstrate that it was possible to reverse the effects of the disease. Although this was an important breakthrough, the benefits of the transplant were limited to about a week at best. It was one of Horsley's assistants, George Murray, who eventually provided a more long-term solution by straining mashed-up sheep's thyroids, in carbolic acid, to produce an injectable solution he gave the catchy name 'pink thyroid juice'. Today, treatment for hypothyroidism usually involves taking a synthetic (man-made) version of thyroxin as a tablet in order to restore normal hormone levels.

HYPERTHYROIDISM

Hyperthyroidism (an overactive thyroid), on the other hand, occurs when too much T_3 and T_4 are secreted from the thyroid gland resulting in increased cellular activity. Symptoms include restlessness, tachycardia, palpitations, weight loss, diarrhoea, bulging eyes (exophthalmos) and goitre. The most common cause is the autoimmune disease Graves' thyroiditis (first described by the Irish physician Robert James Graves in 1835) where antibodies bind to the cells of the thyroid tissue and mimic the action of thyroid-stimulating hormone (TSH). The antibodies stimulate the growth and function of thyroid follicular epithelium and are known as long-acting thyroid stimulants (LATS). Treatment for hyperthyroidism includes medication to supress the production of thyroxin and the ingestion of radioactive iodine which, when absorbed by the thyroid tissue, causes it to shrink. If a large goitre is present, total or partial thyroidectomy may be necessary to prevent compression of the airway.

CALCITONIN AND PARATHYROID HORMONE

Another hormone produced by the thyroid gland is the peptide hormone calcitonin which helps to maintain and regulate bone mineral density and the concentration of calcium and phosphate in the blood plasma. It is secreted in response to high plasma levels of calcium (Ca^{++}) and encourages the uptake of calcium and phosphate into the bone matrix. Calcitonin also increases calcium excretion in the urine and inhibits the reabsorption of spongy bone by osteoclasts (see Chapter 4). Calcitonin works collaboratively with another peptide hormone called parathyroid hormone (PTH). PTH is produced and secreted by four small parathyroid glands situated on the posterior surface of the thyroid gland. It is secreted in response to low levels of plasma calcium and increases the number and activity of osteoclasts in order to liberate calcium and phosphate from the bone. It also promotes the reabsorption of calcium (and magnesium) from the nephrons of the kidney and converts biologically inert vitamin D_3 into calcitriol (also in the kidney). Consequently, parathyroid hormone is indirectly responsible for the absorption of dietary calcium from the gastrointestinal tract. Both hormones are controlled by negative feedback.

ADRENOCORTICOTROPIC HORMONE

Adrenocorticotropic hormone (ACTH) is cursed with a name as intimidating as any we have encountered so far. However, like so many others, it simply describes what it does.

Adreno + cortico + tropic + hormone = adrenal + cortex + 'turn on' + hormone

Or: 'the hormone that turns on the cortex of the adrenal gland'. The adrenal glands themselves are a pair of pyramid-shaped structures, situated on top of each kidney (ad + renal = on + kidney). They are also known as the suprarenal glands (supra = above) and always remind me of a pair of oversized berets perched on top of each kidney's head (I can only apologise for the anthropomorphism). Like the kidneys, the adrenal glands comprise an inner medullary layer and an outer cortical layer surrounded by a fibrous capsule (Figure 13.5). The endocrine cells of the adrenal medulla are regulated and

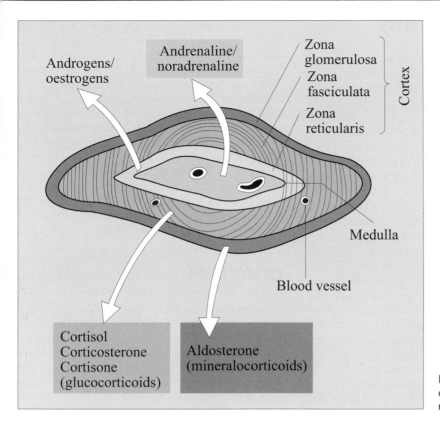

Figure 13.5 Hormones of the adrenal cortex and medulla.

controlled by the autonomic nervous system whilst the adrenal cortex is stimulated by ACTH (secreted into the blood by the anterior pituitary gland following the secretion of corticotropin-releasing hormone by the hypothalamus). ACTH promotes the production and secretion of three groups of fat-based or steroid hormones collectively known as adrenocorticosteroids (adrenal + cortex + steroids). Each of these three groups is manufactured in one of three distinct layers or zones within the adrenal cortex. The outermost layer, situated directly below the capsule, is known as the zona glomerulosa and is responsible for the production of mineralocorticoids. This family of steroid hormones are essential for the regulation of plasma sodium (Na^+) and potassium (K^+) levels, and the reabsorption of sodium (and water) by the kidney in response to low blood pressure. It should come as no surprise then that the most important mineralocorticoid is our 'old friend' aldosterone. In Chapters 8 and 10, we observed how cells in the afferent arteriole

secrete the hormone renin in response to low blood pressure/volume (Figure 8.4). Renin converts the chemical angiotensinogen into angiotensin I, which is then converted into angiotensin II by another enzyme called angiotensin-converting enzyme (ACE). Angiotensin II has two important functions. Firstly, it is a powerful vasoconstrictor which increases systemic blood pressure. Secondly, it stimulates cells in the zona glomerulosa of the adrenal cortex to secrete aldosterone. Aldosterone increases the amount of sodium reabsorbed from the glomerular filtrate by cells in the distal convoluted tubule (DCT) of the nephron. This facilitates the osmotic transport of water from a relatively hypotonic concentration in the DCT to a relatively hypertonic concentration in the renal cells and peritubular capillary blood. In short, aldosterone encourages the reabsorption of salt and water from the kidney into the blood when blood pressure is low. It is inhibited by an increase in blood pressure/volume and an increase in plasma sodium concentrations.

GLUCOCORTICOIDS

The central and largest region of the adrenal cortex is known as the zona fasciculata and is responsible for the production and secretion of steroid hormones known as glucocorticoids (Figure 13.5). The most important and abundant of these is cortisol (hydrocortisone) but small amounts of cortisone and corticosterone are also produced. Cortisol influences the metabolism of most cells in the body and is absolutely essential for the maintenance of healthy activity. Under normal circumstances, cortisol helps to ensure that blood glucose levels remain within the normal range by stimulating liver cells (hepatocytes) to convert amino and lactic acid into glucose (see below). This process is known as gluconeogenesis (glucose + new + creation) and occurs in the liver and kidney when substances other than glycogen or monosaccharides are converted into glucose. Cortisol also plays an important role in damping-down inflammation by reducing the number of available mast cells (which secrete histamine) and inhibiting the production and action of cytokines (see Chapter 6).

In health, cortisol levels are highest first thing in the morning, just after we get out of bed, and decline progressively throughout the day (reaching their lowest level after we fall asleep). However, this pattern can be disrupted by a number of factors including strenuous exercise, infection, physical or emotional stress and trauma (particularly haemorrhage). In these circumstances, the sympathetic nervous system triggers the secretion of corticotropin-releasing hormone (CRH) which stimulates the release of adrenocorticotropic hormone (ACTH) which, in turn, promotes the production of cortisol from the zona fasciculata of the adrenal cortex (Figure 13.6).

CORTISOL

A rise in plasma concentration of cortisol has a number of effects. Firstly, it increases the availability of raw materials for gluconeogenesis by stimulating the breakdown (catabolism) of fats in adipose tissue (into glycerol and fatty acids) and proteins in muscle and connective tissue (into amino acids). Cortisol is also 'glucose

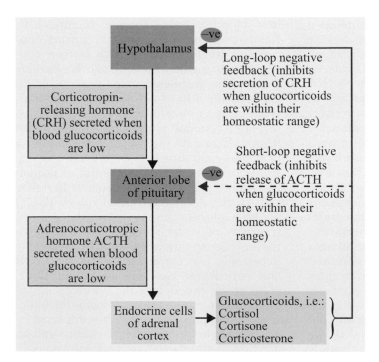

Figure 13.6 Negative feedback loops for secretion of glucocorticoid hormones.

sparing' and, like growth hormone, blocks the uptake of glucose into cells other than those of the central nervous system. In order to ensure that these essential nutrients and raw materials are quickly delivered to where they are required, cortisol also enhances the sensitivity of blood vessels to adrenaline which increases blood pressure (see below). Finally, high levels of cortisol not only damp-down the inflammatory response, they also inhibit immune system activity including T cell proliferation. This explains why synthetic corticosteroids, such as prednisolone, are often used to manage inflammatory conditions such as chronic bronchitis (see Chapter 9) and autoimmune disease such as rheumatoid arthritis (see Chapter 4).

CUSHING'S DISEASE

High cortisol levels, or prolonged use of corticosteroid medication, can lead to a number of undesirable and potentially dangerous side effects and complications. These include elevated blood glucose levels (hyperglycaemia), high blood pressure (hypertension), weight gain, accumulation of fat in the face (moon face) and at the back of the neck (buffalo hump), muscle wasting, poor wound healing and fatigue (to name but a few). A benign tumour called a pituitary adenoma can also produce large amounts of ACTH which stimulates the secretion of cortisol from the adrenal cortex. Crucially, the abnormal pituitary cells are not 'turned off' by negative feedback and plasma cortisol levels continue to rise well above normal. This condition is known as Cushing's disease (first described by the US neurosurgeon Harvey Cushing in 1912) and accounts for about 70% of cases of hypercortisolism not attributed to corticosteroid medication use. Another, much rarer, cause of hypercortisolism is ectopic ACTH syndrome that results when a benign or malignant tumour, situated elsewhere in the body, begins to secrete ACTH. The most common type of ACTH secreting tumours are small cell lung cancers (which account for about 15% of all lung cancers) but tumours originating in the thymus gland and pancreatic islet cells are also capable of producing ACTH. In the

interest of clarity, it is important to note that all of the examples of hypercortisolism mentioned above (including high-dose steroid use) are collectively known as Cushing's syndrome as opposed to Cushing's disease which specifically refers to pituitary adenoma.

ADDISON'S DISEASE

The polar opposite of Cushing's syndrome is Addison's disease (first described by the British physician Thomas Addison in 1855) which occurs when the adrenal cortex begins to fail. The most common cause of Addison's disease, in the UK, is autoimmune adrenalitis (i.e. the adrenal cortex is attacked by antibodies produced by its own immune system) but it can also result from the bacterial infection tuberculosis (TB) and the viral infection AIDS. Symptoms do not usually become apparent until about 90% of the adrenal cortex has been destroyed, at which point cortisol and aldosterone production is significantly reduced. Symptoms include weight loss, weakness, fatigue, hyper-pigmentation of the skin, increased urination, salt cravings, low blood pressure (hypotension), muscle pains, nausea and vomiting. However, because the symptoms typically progress quite slowly, they are often overlooked until a stressful or traumatic event causes them to become worse (e.g. illness or trauma). This is known as an Addisonian crisis and can result in sudden abdominal pain, nausea, vomiting, hypotension, weakness, loss of consciousness and coma. If untreated (with intramuscular or intravenous hydrocortisone) it can prove fatal. Former US president John F. Kennedy (1917–1963) suffered from Addison's disease (amongst other things) and required daily glucocorticoid therapy to avoid the potentially dangerous consequences of adrenal insufficiency.

ANDROGENS

The final (and innermost) region of the adrenal cortex is called the zona reticularis and is responsible for the production and secretion of a number of androgens (Figure 13.5). The Greek word *andro* means 'masculine' and this group of steroid hormones contributes to the development of secondary sexual characteristics in men (e.g. muscle and facial hair growth) as well as male and female libido (sex drive). Like the other hormones produced by the adrenal cortex (mineralocorticoids and glucocorticoids), androgen secretion is stimulated by ACTH. The first stage of puberty is known as adrenarche and represents the maturation of the zona reticularis. This typically occurs between the ages 8 and 10 and results in increased secretion of androgen hormones (cortisol secretion from the zona fasciculata remains unchanged). However, the quantity of androgens produced by the adrenal cortex is very low compared to that produced by the male and female gonads during late puberty and adulthood and their effects are limited (see Chapter 14). The most abundant adrenal androgens (dehydroepiandrosterone and androstenedione) are also relatively weak, despite their macho names, and both are converted into more potent testosterone and oestrogen elsewhere in the body. After the female menopause, when ovarian secretion of oestrogen stops altogether, the only source of oestrogen is that derived from the conversion of adrenal androgens. It is also interesting to note that although men naturally produce small amounts of oestrogen as a result of androgen conversion, this process (aromatisation) can be significantly enhanced by anabolic steroid use (e.g. testosterone injections used by body builders). If this occurs, high oestrogen levels can result in gynecomastia (breast tissue enlargement in men) and other more serious health problems.

ADRENALINE AND NORADRENALINE

The adrenal medulla is situated in the centre of the adrenal gland and comprises specialised chromaffin cells that surround a series of capillaries (Figure 13.5). They are unlike the endocrine cells of the adrenal cortex and are known as neuroendocrine cells since they develop from the same embryonic tissue as sympathetic nerve cells. Consequently, the adrenal medulla is regarded as an extension of the autonomic nervous system and is innervated by the sympathetic nervous system. We noted earlier in the chapter, that when the sympathetic division of the hypothalamus is stimulated it immediately activates neuroendocrine (chromaffin) cells in the adrenal medulla to secrete the catecholamines adrenaline and noradrenaline. Both hormones are amino acid derivatives and are described as sympathomimetic since they mimic (and sustain) the effects of the sympathetic nervous system. For example, they increase cardiac output and blood pressure, they encourage the breakdown of fat (lipolysis) and glycogen (glycogenolysis) to increase blood glucose levels, and they dilate bronchial smooth muscle and the pupils of the eyes. In short, adrenaline and noradrenaline stimulate or enhance anything that is of physiological benefit when we need to run for our lives from the fictitious bear I first mentioned in Chapter 2 (flight-or-fight). There are some differences between the two hormones, however, and adrenaline is secreted in much larger quantities than noradrenaline (a ratio of about 4:1) and has a more potent effect on the heart. In Chapter 7, we noted that during cardio-pulmonary resuscitation (CPR), intravenous adrenaline is used to stimulate myocardiocyte activity and to increase blood flow to the heart and brain. Noradrenaline, on the other hand, has a greater influence on peripheral vasoconstriction which helps to increase blood pressure. Finally, unlike the hormones of the adrenal cortex, neither adrenaline nor noradrenaline are essential for normal everyday activity and both are metabolised and broken down very quickly. Earlier in the chapter we noted that adrenaline has a half-life of about two minutes.

PINEAL GLAND AND MELATONIN

In Chapter 12, we saw that the cone-shaped pineal gland is situated in a region of the brain called the epithalamus (part of the diencephalon). It consists of nervous tissue and specialised secretory cells called pineal-ocytes that synthesise the amino acid derivative hormone melatonin (from another neurotransmitter serotonin). Melatonin helps to regulate the sleep-wake cycle and is secreted and inhibited in response to the strength and duration of daylight, detected by photoreceptors in the retina of the eye. These light-sensitive cells activate retinal neurons that transmit nerve impulses to the suprachiasmatic nucleus (SCN) of the hypothalamus. The SCN is responsible for controlling circadian rhythm (see Chapter 3) and sends information to other hypothalamic nuclei and the pineal gland. In darkness, retinal neurons transmit fewer impulses to the SCN which encourages the pineal gland to synthesise melatonin that makes us feel drowsy. Bright light, on the other hand, results in the transmission of more impulses to the SCN which inhibits melatonin secretion in the pineal gland and makes us feel more alert or awake. This has obvious consequences for those who have visual loss, or regularly work at night, since the transmission of light from the retina to the hypothalamus is diminished. Irregular secretion of melatonin can result in the occurrence of 'free-running' circadian rhythms that make insomnia and sleep disorders more likely. Finally, melatonin is also a powerful antioxidant that helps to protect nervous tissue from damage by free radicals (see Chapter 2).

HORMONES OF THE GASTROINTESTINAL TRACT

The gastrointestinal tract produces a number of hormones that help to control the rate and regularity of digestion. These include gastrin and ghrelin secreted by the stomach (and elsewhere in the case of the latter), and cholecystokinin and secretin synthesised by enterogastric cells in the duodenum. The pancreas also produces five hormones that control and regulate cellular metabolism of glucose (see below). In Chapter 11, we saw that when the stomach is empty it produces the peptide hormone ghrelin that triggers the sensation of hunger by inhibiting receptors in the satiety centre of the hypothalamus. Ghrelin also plays a role in the regulation of blood glucose levels and stimulates areas of the brain associated with reward and addiction. Secretion is inhibited when the stomach is stretched (following a meal) and by the action of another peptide hormone leptin. Leptin is produced by fat cells (adipocytes) and acts upon receptors in the satiety centre of the hypothalamus to suppress appetite (i.e. it performs the opposite function of ghrelin). It also helps to regulate energy expenditure and body temperature over long periods of time.

GASTRIN, CHOLECYSTOKININ AND SECRETIN

The stomach also produces the peptide hormone gastrin in response to distension of the pyloric antrum (see Chapter 11, Figure 11.3). Gastrin stimulates the production of hydrochloric acid and intrinsic factor (necessary for the absorption of vitamin B_{12}) by the parietal cells of the gastric mucosa. It is also responsible for the secretion of pepsinogen (the inactive precursor of the enzyme pepsin) by the chief cells of the stomach and encourages contraction of gastric smooth muscle to aid digestion. We also noted in Chapter 11, that the small intestine produces the peptide hormones cholecystokinin (CCK) and secretin. CCK derives its name from the Greek for 'bile + sac + move' (chole + cysto + kinin) and it stimulates the contraction of the gall bladder and the expulsion of bile. It also increases the production of digestive enzymes by the acinar cells of the pancreas and relaxes the hepatopancreatic sphincter which allows pancreatic juice and bile to enter the duodenum. Secretin, on the other hand, stimulates cells in the liver and pancreas to secrete alkaline bicarbonate into the duodenum that helps to neutralise the potentially damaging effects of acidic chyme on the epithelial cells and brush border of the small intestine. It also inhibits gastric motility and the production of gastric secretions.

INSULIN AND GLUCAGON

In Chapter 11, we saw that the pancreas is situated just behind the stomach (within the loop of the duodenum) and resembles a squashed banana in shape (Figure 11.1). We also noted that the hormone-producing endocrine cells only account for about 1% of the total mass of the pancreas. These are organised into cell clusters known as pancreatic islets or the islets of Langerhans (first identified by the German scientist Paul Langerhans in 1869). A healthy pancreas contains about 2 million pancreatic islets, subdivided into four different types of cell: alpha, beta, delta and F cells. Alpha (α) cells account for about 20% of pancreatic islets and secrete the peptide hormone glucagon in response to low blood glucose levels (hypoglycaemia). Glucagon increases the quantity of glucose in the blood by forcing liver cells (hepatocytes) to release stored glucose, converting glycogen into glucose (glycogenolysis) and producing glucose from lactic acid and non-carbohydrate molecules such as fatty and amino acids (gluconeogenesis). It is estimated that a single molecule of glucagon can stimulate the release of 100 million molecules of glucose into the blood. Beta (β) cells, on the other hand, are much more numerous than alpha cells (about 70% of the total) and secrete the peptide hormone insulin in response to high blood glucose levels (hyperglycaemia). Insulin is often compared to a key that unlocks the cell and allows glucose to enter (to be used for cellular metabolism). This is as good a comparison as any and when insulin binds to receptors on the cell membrane it signals protein carriers to transport glucose through the plasma membrane (a process known as facilitated diffusion). It is estimated that about 35% of glucose absorbed from the gastrointestinal tract is used immediately for cellular metabolism whilst the rest is stored in the liver and skeletal muscle cells as glycogen or converted into fat in the adipose tissue.

AMYLIN, SOMATOSTATIN AND PANCREATIC POLYPEPTIDE

Beta cells also secrete very small quantities of another peptide hormone called amylin (a ratio of about 100:1 with insulin). Amylin slows down gastric emptying, blocks glucagon production and promotes satiety which helps to avoid spikes in blood glucose following a meal. Amylin is a very important hormone therefore but is always overshadowed by its more abundant 'cell-mate' insulin. The delta (δ) cells account for about 5% of the pancreatic islets and secrete the peptide hormone somatostatin. This is identical to growth hormone inhibiting hormone (GHIH) secreted by the hypothalamus and inhibits the secretion of both insulin and glucagon, and slows the absorption of nutrients from the gastrointestinal tract. Finally, the F cells account for the remaining pancreatic islet cells and secrete a hormone known as pancreatic polypeptide. This regulates the production of a number of pancreatic enzymes and inhibits the contraction of the gall bladder and the secretion of somatostatin by delta cells.

DIABETES MELLITUS

In almost every chapter we have noted that glucose is essential for healthy cellular metabolism and if you are thoroughly sick of reading the equation 'glucose + O_2 → energy + CO_2 + H_2O' I have succeeded in reinforcing this point (my work here is almost done). The secretion of insulin and glucagon by the pancreas allows the body to maintain blood glucose levels within a very narrow range (between about 4–6 mmol/l before meals and between about 4–8 mmol/l after meals) and ensures a constant supply of glucose is available for cellular respiration. Diabetes mellitus occurs when pancreatic beta cells produce little or no insulin or when the cells of the body become resistant to its effects. The Greek word *diabetes* means 'siphon' or 'flow through' and refers to the production of large quantities of urine. The Latin word *mellitus* means 'honeyed' or 'sweet' and refers to the presence of glucose in the urine.

TYPE 1 AND TYPE 2 DIABETES MELLITUS

There are two types of diabetes mellitus, unimaginatively, but sensibly, known as type 1 and type 2. Type 1 is an autoimmune disease that typically occurs in childhood or youth following a period of illness or viral infection. The exact cause remains unknown and it affects about 5–10% of those who have the disease. Treatment for type 1 diabetes is insulin-replacement therapy administered by subcutaneous injection several times a day (dependent on regime). The aim of treatment is to mimic normal insulin secretion patterns and stimulate the uptake of glucose into the cells for metabolism and storage. Type 2 diabetes, on the other hand, typically affects those over the age of 40 and is far more common than type 1 (90–95% of cases). It occurs when pancreatic beta cells produce less insulin than normal or when the cells of the body become resistant to its effects due to changes in the cell membrane which obstruct facilitated diffusion. Treatment for type 2 diabetes typically includes dietary control of blood glucose levels and the use of oral hypoglycaemic medications that stimulate the beta cells to produce more insulin or increase insulin sensitivity in peripheral tissue. It is interesting to note that the incidence of type 2 diabetes in children and young people is becoming increasingly common. Although the reasons for this are not fully understood it is thought that obesity, physical inactivity and a diet high in sugar are contributory factors.

HYPERGLYCAEMIA AND KETOACIDOSIS

If type 1 or type 2 diabetes is poorly controlled, it can lead to elevated blood glucose levels (hyperglycaemia) and diabetic ketoacidosis. Hyperglycaemia occurs when glucose cannot be transported into the cells (for the reasons mentioned above) and accumulates in the blood. In Chapter 10, we saw that water-soluble glucose is filtered from the blood into the proximal convoluted tubule (PCT) of the nephron where, in health, it is entirely reabsorbed into the capillary circulation via active transport. However, if plasma glucose levels exceed about 10 mmol/l, the protein carriers (symporters) are unable to work fast enough to reabsorb all of the glucose from the glomerular filtrate and it is lost in the urine (glycosuria). Before the invention of reagent strips (dipsticks) to test for the presence of glucose in the urine, physicians would place a drop on their tongue to see if it tasted sweet! Ketoacidosis refers to the accumulation of ketones in the blood, leading to a reduction in plasma pH (i.e. it becomes more acidic). Ketones are produced when the body breaks down fats and amino acids to synthesise glucose. But why would the body produce more glucose when the blood is already saturated with it, I hear you ask? The answer is that although blood glucose levels are high, there is very little glucose available for cellular metabolism since it is unable to access the cell without insulin. This encourages the cells of the liver (and elsewhere) to undertake glycogenolysis and gluconeogenesis to increase the availability of glucose. However, without insulin, it simply results in the progressive elevation of blood glucose levels and worsening ketoacidosis. If uncorrected, this can result in hyperventilation, hypotension, ketotic breath (smelling of nail varnish remover), ventricular arrhythmias, lethargy, mental confusion, fitting and coma. Treatment involves insulin and fluid replacement with appropriate correction of electrolyte imbalance and metabolic acidosis. The first person with diabetes to receive insulin was a 14 year-old Canadian boy called Leonard Thompson in 1922. The insulin had been harvested from the pancreas of a dog (by Frederick Banting and Charles Best) and proved remarkably effective. Today it is typically manufactured in a laboratory.

HYPOGLYCAEMIA

Low blood sugar levels (hypoglycaemia) most commonly occur when insulin administration is in excess of requirement. However, a variety of factors can contribute to hypoglycaemia including illness and exercise (which increase cellular metabolism of glucose), alcohol consumption, failing to vary insulin injection site and (rarely) insulin-secreting tumours. Symptoms of hypoglycaemia include fatigue, sweating, trembling, headache, heavy breathing, nausea and vomiting, irritability, slurred speech and coma. Many of these symptoms are similar to, and could be mistaken for, alcohol intoxication. This is because neurons are unable to store glucose in the same way as other cells and glucose deprivation results in disturbed neural functioning and can lead to irreversible brain damage. Treatment involves the rapid administration of glucose (dextrose) either orally or intravenously.

HORMONES OF THE KIDNEY

In Chapters 4, 5, 7 and 10, we saw how the kidneys are responsible for the production and secretion of three important hormones. The first is the steroid hormone calcitriol that helps to regulate the absorption of dietary calcium from the gastrointestinal tract. Calcitriol is the active form of vitamin D and is originally derived from calciferol (vitamin D_3) synthesised in the epidermis of the skin following exposure to ultraviolet light. Calciferol is converted into 25-hydroxy vitamin D by the liver before it is carried to the kidneys (bound to globulin) and converted into calcitriol by the cells of the proximal convoluted tubule (PCT). Calcitriol encourages the absorption of calcium (and phosphate) in the small intestine and increases reabsorption of calcium in the nephron. It also stimulates osteoclast activity which releases calcium from the bone in order to increase plasma concentration (in response to parathyroid hormone mentioned above).

ERYTHROPOIETIN AND RENIN

The second hormone synthesised by the kidney (and to a lesser degree the liver) is the peptide hormone erythropoietin (EPO). EPO is secreted in response to low levels of oxygen in the blood (hypoxaemia) and stimulates myeloid stem cells in the bone marrow to produce more erythrocytes (see Chapter 5). This increases the quantity of oxygen in the blood which in turn slows or inhibits EPO production by the kidney (negative feedback). Since erythrocytes only last for about 120 days (before they are recycled by pancreatic and hepatic macrophages), EPO ensures that erythrocyte numbers remain fairly constant and that the oxygen-carrying capacity of blood is always sufficient to meet the metabolic requirements of the body. The final hormone produced by the kidneys is another peptide hormone renin which is secreted by cells in the afferent arteriole in response to low blood pressure. We noted earlier in the chapter, that renin kick-starts the renin-angiotensin-aldosterone system (RAAS) which increases the amount of sodium (Na^+) and water reabsorbed from the nephron into the capillary circulation (see Chapter 8, Figure 8.4). The RAAS is essential, therefore, for the maintenance of normal blood pressure and fluid balance.

HORMONES OF THE HEART AND THYMUS GLAND

In Chapters 8 and 10, we noted that atrial myocardiocytes (muscle + heart + cells) secrete the peptide hormone atrial natriuretic hormone (ANH) in response to rising blood pressure and distension of the atrium. In essence, ANH performs the opposite function to aldosterone which is secreted in response to low blood pressure/volume. ANH relaxes vascular smooth muscle (vasodilation) and helps to reduce the reabsorption of Na^+ in the nephron. This results in increased urine output (diuresis and natriuresis) which reduces circulatory volume and blood pressure. The pyramid-shaped thymus gland is also situated in the mediastinum and partially overlays the heart and aortic arch (see Figure 6.2). It secretes a group of peptide hormones known as thymosins that are essential for the normal development and maturation of lymphocytes. It is also one of the places T cells develop a sense of 'self-tolerance' in order to distinguish between self and foreign cells. The thymus gland is most active during the early years of life since the body is exposed to a constant stream of new microorganisms and pathogens. It must ensure that the T cells mature and are available to participate in the immune response as soon as possible. The thymus continues to enlarge until the child reaches puberty at which point it begins to atrophy (waste away) and eventually only fibrous and fatty tissue remain. It is estimated that the thymus weighs about 15 g at birth, increasing to about 35 g during puberty, before declining to as little as 6 g by the time we reach 70 years old. Calves and lambs' thymus glands are considered something of a delicacy and are known as ris or throat sweetbreads (as opposed to 'heart sweetbreads' which are actually the pancreas of the same animals). If you want to acquaint yourself more closely with cooked glandular tissue, apparently they are very nice lightly dusted in flour or breadcrumbs and pan-fried. Sweetbreads are often mistakenly thought to be another type of glandular tissue – testis (testicles). In culinary terms, calves or bulls testicles are known by a number of colourful nicknames including rocky mountain oysters, prairie oysters, huevos del toros (literally 'bulls eggs' in Spanish), cowboy caviar, dusted nuts and swinging beef (to name but a few). There are also numerous annual festivals throughout Western Canada and the US dedicated to celebrating and eating these glandular delicacies. On which appetising note, I invite you to read the final chapter: the reproductive system.

CHAPTER 13: TEST YOURSELF

Q. There are three main groups of hormones: peptides, amino acid derivatives and lipid derivatives. Briefly explain how they differ from one another.

A. Peptide hormones are made from chains of amino acids and are soluble in water. Amino acid derivatives are derived from two types of amino acids and are mostly soluble in water (thyroid hormones are fat soluble only). Lipid derivative hormones are made from cholesterol or fatty acids and are fat soluble only.

Q. Where are hormones secreted from?

A. Hormones are secreted into the blood by an endocrine gland or by specialised cells situated within an organ (e.g. pancreatic beta cells).

Q. Explain the difference between water-soluble and fat-soluble hormones in relation to speed and duration of action.

A. Water-soluble hormones are unable to penetrate the phospholipid membrane of the cell and must bind to receptors located on its surface. Consequently, they tend to act quickly but have a short duration of action since they are broken down rapidly in the interstitial fluid. Fat-soluble (steroid) hormones are able to pass through the cell membrane and bind with receptors situated on the nuclear membrane. Typically, they are slow to start but tend to have a longer duration of action.

Q. Which two glands (located in the brain) control and regulate most endocrine activity in the human body?

A. The hypothalamus and pituitary gland.

Q. What is the hypophyseal portal system and why is it important?

A. The hypophyseal portal system is a network of blood vessels that connects the hypothalamus to the anterior lobe of the pituitary gland. This allows the hypothalamus to control

(Continued)

(Continued)

the endocrine activity of the anterior pituitary gland by secreting a variety of regulatory hormones known as releasing and inhibiting hormones.

Q. List as many of the seven anterior pituitary hormones as you can.
A. Growth hormone (GH), thyroid-stimulating hormone (TSH), adrenocorticotropic hormone (ACTH), prolactin, melanocyte-stimulating hormone (MSH), follicle-stimulating hormone (FSH) and luteinising hormone (LH).

Q. What are the names of the two hormones secreted by the posterior pituitary gland?
A. Oxytocin and antidiuretic hormone (ADH).

Q. What is most abundant hormone produced by the anterior pituitary gland?
A. Growth hormone.

Q. What does the hormone prolactin do?
A. Prolactin stimulates the production of milk by the mammary tissue of the breast.

Q. Thyroid-stimulating hormone (TSH) stimulates the production of two thyroid hormones: triiodothyronine (T_3) and thyroxine (T_4). What are their principles functions?
A. Both are essential for normal development of bone during childhood and the regulation of bone mineral density in adults. They also increase the rate of oxygen consumption and energy production in most cells of the body.

Q. Which hormone is secreted by the parathyroid gland?
A. Parathyroid hormone.

Q. What is the function of adrenocorticotropic hormone (ACTH)? Remember to break up the word: adreno + cortico + tropic + hormone.
A. It stimulates the adrenal cortex to secrete three groups of steroid hormones (adrenocorticosteroids).

Q. Glucocorticoids are steroid hormones secreted by the adrenal cortex and include cortisol, cortisone and corticosterone. What are the principle functions of these hormones?
A. Glucocorticoids play an important role in damping-down the inflammatory response and can inhibit immune system activity. They also help to ensure that blood glucose levels remain within the normal range.

Q. Adrenaline and noradrenaline are both secreted by cells in the adrenal medulla. What are the principles functions of these hormones during exercise and/or stress?
A. Adrenaline and noradrenaline help to increase cardiac output and blood pressure. They encourage the breakdown of fat (lipolysis) and glycogen (glycogenolysis) to increase blood glucose levels. They also dilate bronchial smooth muscle and the pupils of the eyes.

Q. Melatonin is secreted by the pineal gland of the brain. What is the principle function of this hormone?
A. Melatonin helps to regulate the sleep-wake cycle and is secreted and inhibited in response to the strength and duration of daylight.

Q. Glucagon is secreted from pancreatic alpha cells and insulin is secreted from pancreatic beta cells. Explain how these hormones manage and maintain normal blood glucose levels.
A. Glucagon is secreted in response to low blood glucose levels (hypoglycaemia). It increases the quantity of glucose in the blood by forcing liver cells to release stored glucose,

converting glycogen into glucose, and producing glucose from non-carbohydrate molecules (gluconeogenesis). Insulin is secreted in response to high blood glucose levels (hyperglycaemia). It facilitates the transport of glucose into the cell (where it is used for cellular metabolism) and stores glucose as glycogen in the liver and skeletal muscle.

Q. What is the normal range for blood glucose following a meal?
A. About 4–8 mmol/l.

Q. What is the function of the steroid hormone calcitriol and where is it secreted from?
A. Calcitriol helps to regulate the absorption of dietary calcium from the gastrointestinal tract and is secreted by the kidneys.

Q. What is the name of the group of hormones secreted by the thymus gland and what do they do?
A. The thymus gland secretes thymosins that are essential for the normal development and maturation of T cells.

Contents

CHAPTER 14

REPRODUCTIVE SYSTEM

REPRODUCTION

In humans, reproduction refers to the ability to conceive and produce the next generation of offspring. This usually occurs as a result of sexual intercourse between a man and a woman, although artificial insemination (directly inserting sperm into the woman's womb) and in vitro fertilisation (fertilising the egg in a laboratory before implanting it into the womb) also enables this process to take place without the need for actual sex. The most important attribute or quality of reproduction is the combination and mixing of genetic material from both biological parents to ensure that the child is as genetically diverse as possible. In Chapter 2, we saw that human characteristics are transferred from generation to generation by genes located on 23 pairs of chromosomes (46 in total). In order to ensure

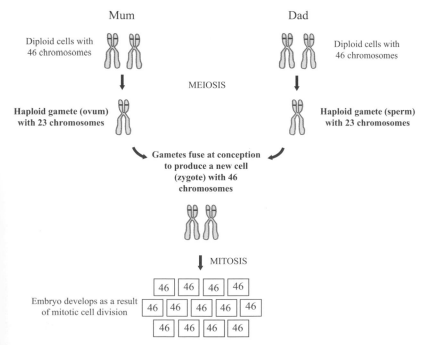

Figure 14.1 Meiosis and mitosis pre- and post-conception.

that the child receives a mix of genetic material from each parent, male and female sex cells (gametes) have 23 unpaired chromosomes. These cells are known as haploid cells and are created during meiotic (or reductive) division of the cell nucleus. The 23 chromosomes in each gamete is not a random selection from the 46 chromosomes of the parent. It consists of one (of each pair) of the 22 autosomes, plus either an X or Y chromosome. X and Y chromosomes are called sex chromosomes since they determine gender (see below). Cells that are produced via mitosis are known as diploid cells and have 46 chromosomes (or 23 pairs). The only haploid cells produced by the human body are male and female gametes: spermatozoa and ova (see below). At fertilisation, they combine to create a new (diploid) cell with a full complement of chromosomes (Figure 14.1). This is why reproduction produces children that resemble their parents but are not identical to them. Each individual (apart from identical twins) has a unique combination of genes (located on their chromosomes) known as a genotype.

ALLELES

Even though we all share the same genes, there are many different forms or variants known as alleles. For example, the gene for eye colour has an allele for brown eyes and an allele for blue eyes. Some alleles are said to be dominant (e.g. brown eyes) and some are recessive (e.g. blue eyes). Since we receive a gene for eye colour from each parent, we may receive two dominant genes (BB), two recessive genes (bb) or one dominant and one recessive gene (Bb). Dominant characteristics such as brown eye colour will be present even if there is only one copy of that gene in the pair (e.g. BB or Bb). Recessive characteristic such as blue eye colour, on the other hand, require both recessive alleles to be present (bb). Characteristics or traits with the same alleles (e.g. BB or bb) are known as homozygous (same + joined) whereas characteristics with different alleles (e.g. Bb) are known as heterozygous (different + joined). Punnet squares are often used to illustrate the likelihood or probability of inheriting particular traits. For example, the probability of having a child with brown eyes is 100% if the father has homozygous alleles for brown eyes (BB) and the mother has homozygous alleles for blue (bb) (Figure 14.2). This explains why some children look more like one parent than the other despite the fact their genotype is 50/50. The observable characteristics we actually exhibit (e.g. height, nose shape, hair colour, eye colour, etc.) are known as our phenotype. That is to say, the children of parents BB and bb will have brown eyes (phenotype) despite the fact they carry the genes for brown and blue eyes (genotype Bb). We will discuss genetic inheritance later in the chapter when we get to fertilisation.

GENETIC DIVERSITY

Genetic diversity is important for the health and well-being of the child and for the health and well-being of the population as a whole. This is because many genetic disorders only occur when both alleles (disease-causing variants) are present on a chromosome and this is much more likely to occur in offspring from close family members. Most cultures and social groups prohibit (or at least strongly discourage) sexual relationships with family members but this hasn't stopped many royal families from giving it a go, so to speak, over the centuries. Perhaps the most famous example of a genetic disorder made worse by generations of royal intermarriage and inbreeding is the so-called Habsburg jaw. Part of the Hapsburg family ruled Spain from 1516 to 1700, and marriages between first cousins, and uncle and

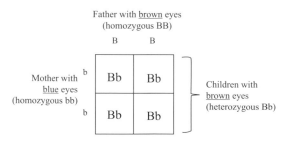

Figure 14.2 Punnet square for eye colour (homozygous parents).

niece, were commonplace. The final 'Spanish' Hapsburg was Charles II who died aged 39 and was considered to be physically and mentally impaired. It is reported that he didn't speak until he was 4 and, even as an adult, it was difficult to understand what he was saying because of his oversized jaw and tongue (which supposedly drooled continuously). The physician who undertook Charles's autopsy, recorded that his heart was the size of a peppercorn, he had a single testicle ('black as coal') and that his head was full of water. Although the accuracy of this report is questionable, it is fair to say that Charles was not a vigorous specimen of manhood and it is generally agreed that the shrinking gene-pool, that resulted from centuries of interbreeding between uncles/nieces and first cousins, directly contributed to his ill-health and early death. The Habsburgs (and many other interbred royal dynasties) provide persuasive evidence that genetic uniformity or 'purity' is both undesirable and dangerous. We'll come back to genes and inherited characteristics later in the chapter but first we need to understand the processes that contribute to the production of male and female sex cells (gametes) in health.

MALE REPRODUCTIVE SYSTEM

In the previous chapter, we saw that the anterior pituitary gland secretes seven peptide hormones including follicle-stimulating hormone (FSH) and luteinising hormone (LH). These two hormones are collectively known as pituitary gonadotropins since they control activity within the male and female gonads (testes and ovaries). Although there are clear similarities in the way in which these hormones influence the male and female reproductive systems (e.g. the maturation of gametes and the production of steroid hormones), there are also important differences. The male reproductive system has two main functions: to produce and transport male gametes (spermatozoa/sperm) and to deposit them within the female reproductive system. It consists of a number of interconnected structures including the testes (singular: testis), epididymides (singular: epididymis),

vasa deferentia (singular: vas deferens), seminal vesicles, prostate gland, bulbourethral glands, urethra and penis (Figure 14.3).

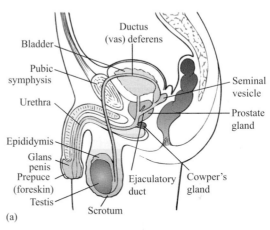

(a)

Structure	Homeostatic function
Testes	Produce sperm and sex hormone
Accessory organs	
Vas deferens, urethra	Transports sperm out of the body
Glands – seminal vesicles, prostate, Cowper's	Contribute the majority of fluid within semen
Scrotum	House the testis outside the pelvic cavity – essential for viable sperm production
Penis	Organ of copulation and excretion

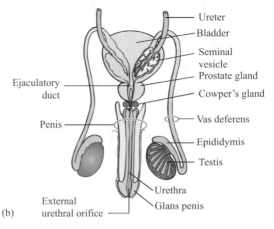

(b)

Figure 14.3 (a) Male reproductive tract, sagittal view. (b) Posterior view.

SCROTUM

The testes (or testicles) are the only organs that are not located within one of the main body cavities. Instead, they are housed within the scrotum or scrotal sac, directly behind the penis and in front of the anus. The scrotum is divided into two compartments (left and right) each of which contains one testis, one epididymis and the testicular-end of each spermatic cord. But why house these sensitive organs in such a vulnerable location – 'dangling' precariously behind the penis? The answer is simple: temperature. We know that core body temperature is maintained at around 37°C in health (see Chapter 3). Sperm production, however, is inhibited at temperatures any higher than about 35°C. Consequently, the testes must be kept at a slight distance from the warmer abdominal cavity if they are to continue to produce high-quality sperm at optimum capacity. This also explains why the scrotum shrinks or retracts when the external temperature falls below gamete producing range (e.g. jumping into a cold swimming pool). The testes and spermatic cords are covered by the cremaster muscle (one each side) which contracts to draw the scrotum and testes upwards towards the warmer abdominal cavity. Similarly, if the external temperature rises, the cremaster muscle relaxes and the testes descend away from the body (e.g. in a hot bath). As men get older, the cremaster muscle declines in strength and elasticity, just like any other muscle, and the testes begin to hang lower than they did in youth. The characteristic wrinkles or rugae of the scrotum are formed by bundles of smooth muscle fibres (dartos muscle) found in the subcutaneous tissue of the scrotum. These increase surface area and also assist the cremaster muscle to elevate the testes if required.

TESTES

Adult testes vary in size and can be measured using an instrument called an orchidometer. This sounds like a terrifying piece of equipment but is in fact a string of 12, numbered, wooden/plastic beads of increasing size from 1 to 25 ml (facetiously known as the endocrine rosary or worry beads). A normal adult testis measures 12–25 ml and weighs 10–15 g (slightly smaller than a calf's testicle/rocky mountain oyster discussed in the previous chapter). It is surrounded by a serous membrane called the tunica vaginalis and a dense capsule of connective tissue called the tunica albuginea. The tunica albuginea also extends inwards and repeatedly divides to form hundreds of small compartments called lobules (Figure 14.4). Each lobule contains between two and three tightly wound vessels known as seminiferous tubules (from the Latin for 'seed carrying'). The outer layer of the seminiferous tubule consists of smooth muscle that is able to contract to move sperm and fluid along the vessel. The inner layer is lined with millions of specialist epithelial cells called sertoli cells that are responsible for sperm production (spermatogenesis). Follicle-stimulating hormone (FSH), secreted by the anterior pituitary gland, encourages primary spermatocytes (diploid cells) to undergo the first division of meiosis to form secondary spermatocytes (haploid cells). The spermatocytes develop into spermatids and eventually become spermatozoa (sperm). Sertoli cells also secrete a hormone called inhibin which exerts negative feedback on the anterior pituitary gland and inhibits secretion of FSH.

TESTOSTERONE

It is estimated that the seminiferous tubules of an average man can produce between 200 and 300 million sperm per day. It takes about 72 days for sperm to develop and fully mature but, in order for this to occur, they must be exposed to a number of hormones. Leydig cells (also known as interstitial cells) are situated in the connective tissue that supports the seminiferous tubules. They are activated by luteinising hormone (LH) and synthesise and secrete testosterone and other androgen hormones required for healthy sperm production. For example, one of the functions of testosterone is the removal of unnecessary cytoplasm and organelles from the spermatids as they develop their characteristic tail and become sperm. The mature sperm are eventually moved through the seminiferous tubule, by peristaltic

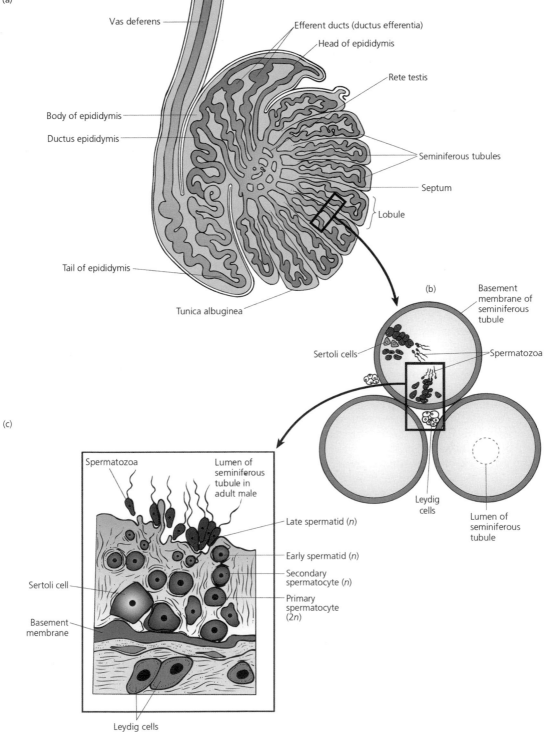

(a)

Vas deferens

Efferent ducts (ductus efferentia)

Head of epididymis

Rete testis

Body of epididymis

Ductus epididymis

Seminiferous tubules

Septum

Lobule

Tail of epididymis

Tunica albuginea

(b) Basement membrane of seminiferous tubule

Sertoli cells

Spermatozoa

Leydig cells

Lumen of seminiferous tubule

(c)

Spermatozoa

Lumen of seminiferous tubule in adult male

Late spermatid (n)

Early spermatid (n)

Secondary spermatocyte (n)

Primary spermatocyte ($2n$)

Sertoli cell

Basement membrane

Leydig cells

Figure 14.4 (a) Seminiferous tubules. (b) Sertoli and leydig cells. (c) Stages of spermatogenesis.

muscular contractions, to the epididymis where they are stored and become mobile within 18–24 hours. Testosterone is also necessary for the development of male, secondary sexual characteristics such as the thickening of the vocal cords, enlargement of the thyroid cartilage (Adam's apple) and growth of body and facial hair. This is best illustrated by the phenomenon of castrato – men who were castrated before they reached puberty in order to preserve their soprano singing voice. The procedure (which persisted into the late 19th century) prevented the secretion of testosterone and therefore the thickening of the vocal cords. At the same time, the man continued to grow in size (and vocal strength) since testosterone also contributes to the gradual 'closure' of growth plates (see Chapter 4).

EPIDIDYMIS

The epididymis is situated on the posterior aspect of each testis and consists of a single, tightly wound tubule or duct that, if uncoiled, would measure 6–7 m in length (Figures 14.3, 14.4). However, in its normal, wound state it is only about 4 cm long which is a tremendous relief from the point of view of testicle size. The epididymis is divided into three sections: head, body and tail. The head is the widest region and receives sperm from the seminiferous tubules of the testes. The body of the epididymis extends along the posterior margin of the testis, and the tail connects to the vas deferens (see below). The epididymis is lined with columnar epithelial cells surrounded by a layer of smooth muscle that slowly propel the sperm though the tubule. The epithelium also secretes nutrients that nourish the sperm, whilst any dead or defective sperm are reabsorbed. Sperm can remain in the epididymis for about a month before they are phagocytosed (devoured) by the epithelial cells and replaced by younger gametes.

SPERM TRANSPORT

A healthy sperm has a head, body and whip-like tail that it uses for propulsion. The head is almost completely filled by the nucleus that contains its 23 chromosomes. However, it also contains a small acrosomal cap or compartment that is filled with enzymes necessary for the sperm to penetrate the outer layer of the female gamete and reach the genetic material. The body or mid-piece of the sperm is packed with mitochondria, positioned in a spiral arrangement around a series of microtubules. The mitochondria produce energy (ATP) that fuels the propelling corkscrew action of the tail and allows the sperm to become mobile. In order to reduce size and weight, sperm lack many of the traditional organelles found in less-specialised cells (e.g. endoplasmic reticulum, golgi apparatus, lysosomes etc.). Sperm can also be stored and remain viable for several months in the next part of male reproductive system: the vas deferens or deferent duct. The vas deferens is a tube that measures about 30 cm in length and extends from the epididymis (in the scrotum) to the seminal vesicles (in the abdominal cavity) via the spermatic cord. The final part of the vas deferens is known as the ampulla (from the Latin for 'small bottle' or 'jar') and attaches to the seminal vesicles to form the ejaculatory duct (Figure 14.3). Like the epididymis, the vas deferens is lined with columnar epithelium but it is also surrounded by three layers of smooth muscle that allow it to contract during orgasm and propel the sperm past the ejaculatory ducts into the urethra.

SEMINAL VESICLES, PROSTATE AND BULBOURETHRAL GLANDS

The seminal vesicles are a pair of finger-like glands situated on the posterior surface of the bladder that produce and secrete seminal fluid containing fructose, amino acids, ascorbic acid (vitamin c), potassium and prostaglandins. This fluid is essential for sperm motility since it is a both a transport medium (i.e. liquid) and provides the raw materials necessary for ATP production by the sperm's mitochondria. Seminal fluid also contains an enzyme called visiculase that is responsible for the clotting reaction that takes place following ejaculation. This helps to ensure that semen is retained within the vagina rather

(a)

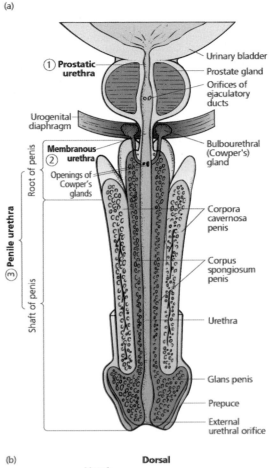

(b)

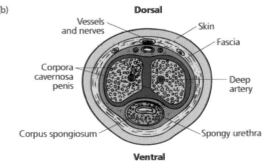

Figure 14.5 (a) Structure of the penis. (b) Transverse view.

It is roughly the same size and appearance as a chestnut and surrounds part of the urethra known as the prostatic urethra. This provides a common pathway for urine (from the bladder) and sperm and seminal fluid (from the vas deferens/seminal vesicles). Although it is possible for men to urinate when the penis is erect (despite the obvious positional difficulties) it is not possible to urinate and ejaculate at the same time. This is because once male orgasm commences, the internal urethral sphincter closes to prevent semen from entering the bladder and urine from exiting. The prostate gland secretes a milky-coloured fluid that gives semen its characteristic appearance. It also contains citric acid (used by sperm to produce ATP) and a number of enzymes (e.g. prostate specific antigen) that help to liquefy the clotted semen and allow sperm to swim freely. Prostatic fluid accounts for about 30% of the total volume of semen ejaculated. Situated directly below the prostate gland are the bulbourethral or Cowper's glands (Figure 14.5). These pea-shaped glands secrete alkaline mucus (known as pre-ejaculate) into the male urethra to protect the sperm from chemical and mechanical damage during/following ejaculation. For example, the alkaline mucus helps to neutralise acidic urine that may still be present in the male urethra and provides a degree of protection from the acidic environment found in the vagina (see below).

PROSTATE ENLARGEMENT

The prostate gland continues to increase in size (hyperplasia) as men get older. It is estimated that about 40% of men in their fifth decade, and about 90% of men in their ninth decade, will experience urinary symptoms as a result of benign prostatic hyperplasia (BPH). For example, an enlarged prostate can compress and distort the prostatic urethra resulting in poor flow, incomplete bladder emptying, urinary frequency and urgency (particularly at night). Prostate cancer, on the other hand, refers to the proliferation (multiplication) of malignant cells within the prostate tissue. These cells can infiltrate adjacent structures/tissue and spread to other parts of the body via the blood or lymph

than just sliding out again (I can't think of a more polite way to describe this). Seminal fluid accounts for about 60% of the total volume of semen at ejaculation (see below). The next part of the male reproductive system is the prostate gland situated directly below the bladder and seminal vesicles (Figure 14.5).

vessels (metastasis). There are a number of investigations and tests that can be performed to indicate a diagnosis of prostate cancer including digital rectal examination (DRE) and prostate specific antigen (PSA) levels in the blood. The former investigation involves manually assessing the size and shape of the prostate gland (with a gloved and lubricated finger) against the anterior wall of the rectum. When I worked in Accident and Emergency, many years ago, I remember that there was a cube-shaped paperweight on the desk in the doctor's office. Each side possessed a small hole into which you could insert your finger and feel a replica of a normal/enlarged/abnormal prostate gland. It was always amusing to walk into the office and find a medical colleague sitting in front of their notes absent-mindedly exploring the 'anus cube' with their finger. The words 'Am I interrupting you, doctor' would always elicit rapid retraction of the finger followed by flustered praise of what an excellent educational tool it was (which, of course, it was).

URETHRA, PENIS AND FORESKIN

The male urethra is approximately 20 cm in length and can be divided into three sections: prostatic urethra, membranous urethra and penile urethra (Figure 14.5). The prostatic urethra is completely enclosed by the prostate gland and measures about 2.5 cm in length. It is the widest section of the male urethra and is attached to the ejaculatory ducts at approximately the mid-point. The membranous urethra is the narrowest and shortest section at about 1.5 cm and is surrounded by a layer of muscle known as the urogenital diaphragm. The penile or spongy urethra extends the length of the penis and typically measures about 16 cm (6.2 in). It is covered by a mass of spongy tissue called the corpus spongiosum (Latin for 'porous body') that prevents the urethra from becoming squeezed or pinched during erection. The penile urethra exits the body at the external urethral opening (meatus) of the glans penis. The word glans means 'acorn' in Latin and is essentially the expanded cap of the corpus spongiosum. We noted in Chapter 3, that the glans is one of the few parts of the body not covered in vellus hair and (in uncircumcised men) it is enclosed by a retractable hood of skin and smooth muscle known as the prepuce or foreskin (Figure 14.5). Going off on a foreskin tangent, it was widely believed in medieval Europe that the only part of Jesus that had not ascended to heaven (following the resurrection) was his foreskin, which had been circumcised when he was 8 days old in accordance with Jewish custom. There are many accounts of holy foreskin relics and their various powers, including the one given to Pope Leo III by King Charlemagne as a Christmas present in 800 (if that wasn't weird enough, Charlemagne claimed it had been given to him by an angel). Unfortunately, church leaders were not able to agree on which of the many foreskin relics had actually belonged to Jesus and, in 1900, the Roman Catholic Church (thoroughly fed up with all the bickering) ruled that, henceforth, anyone who wrote or spoke about this delicate subject would find themselves excommunicated. If only they had listened to the 17th-century scholar Leo Allatius who proposed that none of the relics could be genuine since Jesus' foreskin had independently ascended to heaven where it had been transformed into Saturn's rings (seems obvious now).

ERECTION

Two large masses of erectile tissue known as the corpora cavernosa ('hollow bodies') are situated directly above the penile urethra and corpus spongiosum (Figure 14.5). They extend along the shaft of the penis as far as the glans and are essentially two large cavities (venous sinusoids) surrounded by a strong fibrous capsule. The 'functional state' of the penis (up or down) is governed by smooth muscle tone. That is to say, sympathetic nervous system activity maintains the penis in its flaccid (limp) state, whilst parasympathetic nervous activity brings about erection. For example, following erotic stimulation (or sometimes completely spontaneously) parasympathetic activity triggers the release of nitrous oxide (NO) from nerve endings within the penis. This results in the relaxation of smooth muscle in the penile arteries (vasodilation) and blood flow into the penis increases. The corpus spongiosum and corpora cavernosa quickly become engorged with blood (since venous drainage remains unchanged) and the penis becomes rigid and erect. The erection pathway is naturally inhibited by an enzyme (phosphodiesterase type 5 or PDE-5) that causes constriction of the penile arteries. Viagra (and other PDE-5 inhibitor drugs) temporarily inactivate this enzyme in order to ensure that even small quantities of nitrous oxide are sufficient to achieve and maintain an erection. The most common cause of erectile dysfunction or impotence (inability to achieve/sustain an erection) is narrowing or obstruction of the arteries that supply blood to the penis. In the previous section, we noted that the penile urethra typically measures about 16 cm but, for obvious reasons, there is some variation from individual to individual. However, the average man has a penis-to-body-length ratio of about 1:12. This is fairly respectable amongst primates such as gorillas and chimpanzees but pretty unimpressive in relation to much of the animal kingdom. Surprisingly, the humble barnacle has the largest penis-to-body-length ratio at 40:1 whilst the blue-bill duck, waddles around with a corkscrew penis that can reach the same length as its body (1:1). Leopard slugs have both male and female sex organs (they are hermaphrodite) and are able to reproduce with any willing leopard slug they may encounter on their unhurried travels. When the time is right, they twist their bodies together and dangle upside-down from a long rope of sticky mucus (much more elegant than it sounds). Once the correct position has been accomplished, a blue-tinted penis emerges from the side of each slug's head and wraps around the other to form a translucent 'penis-ball'. Once fertilisation has taken place, the slugs disengage from one another (one often falling from the mucus cord) and continue on their way. Unsurprisingly, many leopard slugs don't bother with sexual intercourse and simply fertilise their own eggs.

SEMEN

The word semen is derived from the Latin for 'seed' and it is a common misconception that it is comprised solely of sperm. Mathematicians amongst you have hopefully totted up the various constituents of semen as follows: seminal fluid = c.60%; prostatic fluid = c.30% and sperm = 5–10% However, despite the fact that sperm only accounts for as little as 5% of the total, there are still an awful lot of them and, it is estimated, that each ml of healthy semen contains about 120 million sperm. Since men typically ejaculate between 2 and 5 mls of semen this works out at 240–600 million sperm per ejaculation. If sperm numbers fall below about 20 million per ml, infertility is likely. This is because sperm 'wastage' within the female reproductive tract is enormous and only about 50 sperm (out of a possible 600 million) are expected to arrive at the correct location for fertilisation to occur. Another factor that contributes to male fertility is the health and vigour of the sperm and it is not uncommon for over 50% of those ejaculated to be either dead-on-arrival or unable to swim properly! For sperm, therefore, ejaculation is something of a suicide mission even when conditions are favourable as we will see later in the chapter.

EJACULATION

Ejaculation is a spinal reflex that occurs in two stages, usually as a result of sexual stimulation but it can occur spontaneously (e.g. a wet dream). The first stage is known as emission and involves the propulsion of sperm and seminal fluid from the ejaculatory ducts into the prostatic urethra where it is combined with milky-coloured prostatic fluid. As noted above, the semen is trapped here and cannot enter the bladder since the internal urethral sphincter is closed. This stage of ejaculation is controlled by sympathetic nerves from T10 to L2 (see Chapter 12). The second stage is known as expulsion and occurs when the bulbospongiosus muscles of the perineum and penis (and to a lesser extent the muscle that surrounds the glandular tissue of the prostate) contract in order to propel the semen through the urethra and out of the penis. The rhythmic contraction of these muscles at orgasm results in the spurting nature of ejaculation and typically lasts between two and five seconds. Once the contractions have ceased, the arterioles in the penis vasoconstrict (narrow) and the penis returns to its flaccid state (regulated by the sympathetic nervous system). This is known as the latent period and the man is unable to achieve another erection for at least several minutes, and possibly several hours, depending on the individual. The expulsion stage of ejaculation is governed by somatic (voluntary) nerves that originate in the sacral spine at S2 to S4.

VASECTOMY

Some men opt to undergo a minor surgical procedure called a vasectomy as a method of permanent contraception (although surgical reversible is possible). This involves tying or sealing the vas deferens to prevent sperm entering the ejaculatory duct. Sperm continue to be produced in the seminal vesicles and are phagocytosed and reabsorbed in the manner described above. One of the questions health professionals are often asked regarding this procedure is whether it is still possible for a man to ejaculate afterwards. As I'm sure you have worked out, the quantity and appearance of the ejaculate will remain largely unchanged since sperm only account for 5–10% of the final product so to speak. Bizarrely, in the early 20th century, the Austrian physiologist Eugen Steinach claimed that it was possible to reverse the ageing process, and increase energy levels, by performing a vasectomy. He believed that tying-off the vas deferens would increase

the quantity of testosterone secreted by sertoli cells. We now know that testosterone secretion is controlled by negative feedback (i.e. increasing levels inhibit further secretion) but it did not stop a large numbers of men from all over the world volunteering for the procedure (known as the 'Steinach operation').

FEMALE REPRODUCTIVE SYSTEM

The female reproductive system consists of the vulva, vagina, uterus, fallopian tubes, fimbriae and ovaries. In terms of its overall role and function, it is much more complex and versatile than the male reproductive system. For example, the female reproductive system generates and transports female gametes (ova); receives and retains male gametes (sperm); provides the correct environment for fertilisation, placentation and gestation and, when necessary, undertakes labour and delivery of the new-born (neonate). When discussing the female reproductive system it is convenient to divide it into two parts: the external genitalia and the internal components. The external genitalia consist of a number of protective and other structures collectively known as the vulva (from the Latin word for 'wrap around' or 'cover'). The first part of the vulva is known as the mons pubis (literally 'pubic mountain') and consists of a fatty mound of tissue that covers the pubic symphysis (Figure 14.6). It separates (inferiorly) into two prominent folds

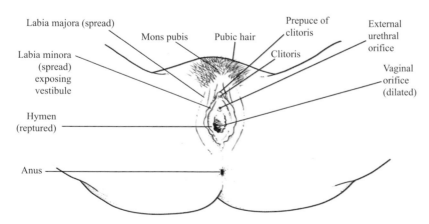

Figure 14.6 Female external genitalia (vulva).

of skin called the labia majora ('large lips') that encircle and partially conceal two smaller folds of skin called the labia minora ('small lips'). Both structures enclose the vaginal and urethral openings and provide some protection from opportunistic infection. During sexual arousal, increased blood to the area causes them to swell and drawback which allows access to the vagina. The upper folds of the labia minora unite to form a hood of skin called the prepuce (equivalent to, but much smaller than, the male foreskin). The prepuce houses a small mound of highly sensitive erectile tissue called the clitoris (Greek for 'little hill'). The visible part of the clitoris is known as the glans ('acorn') and, like the glans penis, it plays an important role in sexual arousal and becomes engorged with blood when stimulated. Situated directly below the clitoris, the labia minora enclose an area called the vestibule (Latin for 'forecourt' or 'entryway') that

contains the external urethral opening and the vaginal opening. Skene's glands (lesser vestibular glands) are situated on either side of the urethral opening and secrete mucus into the vestibule to keep it moist. Bartholin's glands (greater vestibular glands) are situated on either side of the vaginal opening and secrete small amounts of mucus during sexual arousal/intercourse to aid vaginal lubrication.

VAGINA

It is a common and persistent misconception that the word vagina describes the external genitalia when, as we know, this area is celled the vulva. The vagina is an internal structure that extends from the vestibule of the vulva to the cervix (neck) of the uterus (Figure 14.7). The word vagina itself means 'sheath' or

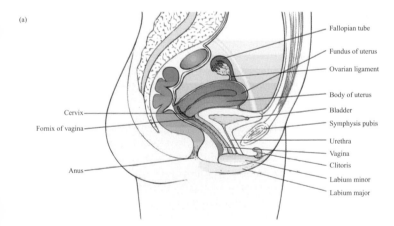

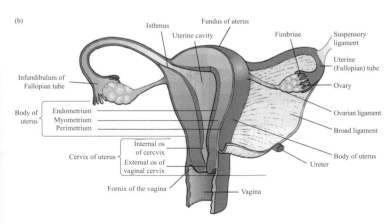

Figure 14.7 (a) Female reproductive tract, sagittal view. (b) Frontal view.

'scabbard' in Latin and it is essentially a fibro-muscular tube. The walls of the vagina consist of three layers of tissue: adventitia, smooth muscle and mucosa. The adventitia consists of an outer layer of connective tissue that anchors the vagina to surrounding organs and structures such as the bladder and rectum. The middle layer of tissue contains two sheets of smooth muscle (circular and longitudinal) that enable to vagina to stretch and dilate during sexual intercourse and childbirth. The inner mucosal layer is lined with stratified, squamous epithelial cells (similar to those found in the mouth) which are able to withstand friction and wear and tear. The mucosa is also folded into pleats (rugae) that increase surface area and provide a corrugated appearance. These allow the vagina to stretch and expand when necessary, and also stimulate the penis during penetration. In Chapter 6, we noted that vaginal secretions have a pH of about 4–5 which helps to inhibit opportunistic bacterial colonisation. We also noted that much of the body is already colonised by 'friendly' bacteria (commensals) and the vagina is no different. The mucosal cells produce and secrete large amount of glycogen which the vaginal bacteria convert into organic acids.

UTERUS

The uterus or womb is a hollow muscular organ that is comparable in size and shape to an upside-down pear (Figure 14.7). Sperm swim though the uterus in order to fertilise the mature female gamete (ovum) in one of the two fallopian tubes. The fertilised egg (zygote) then implants itself into the lining of the womb and develops and grows (gestates) over the course of the following nine months or so (see below). The uterus can be subdivided into three anatomical regions: cervix, body and fundus. The cervix or neck of the uterus opens into the upper (proximal) end of the vagina via a narrow opening or canal called the cervical os (Latin for 'mouth'). The vaginal canal surrounds the cervix and produces a recess known as the fornix (Latin for 'arch' but not to be confused with the limbic fornix described in Chapter 12). The external os is normally

plugged with a barrier of mucus to protect the uterus from colonisation by vaginal bacteria. This also blocks the passage of sperm into the uterus except at the mid-point of the menstrual cycle when it thins to allow access. The large central portion of the uterus is known as the body whilst the domed region between the two fallopian tubes is called the fundus (Latin for 'base' but not to be confused with the fundus of the stomach, bladder or eye). The height of the uterine fundus (in relation to the top of the pubic bone) is used to assess foetal growth and development during pregnancy.

UTERINE TISSUE

The walls of the uterus are comprised of three layers of tissue known as the perimetrium, myometrium and endometrium. The perimetrium (peri + metrium = around + womb) covers most of outer uterine surface and is continuous with the peritoneum discussed in Chapter 11. The myometrium (muscle + uterus) consists of a thick layer of smooth muscle that is able to accommodate the growing foetus during the gestation period. It is also able to contract with sufficient force to push the baby through the vagina during birth. In Chapter 3, we noted that this process is triggered by sustained pressure from the baby's head on the internal surface of the cervix, resulting in secretion of oxytocin from the posterior pituitary gland (the Ferguson reflex). The final layer of the uterus is the endometrium (inner + uterus) that consists of a sheet of columnar epithelium resting on a supporting framework of connective tissue (stroma). The connective tissue is highly vascular and varies in thickness according to the quantity of oestrogen and progesterone secreted during the menstrual cycle (see below).

FALLOPIAN TUBES AND FIMBRIAE

The fallopian or uterine tubes are situated on either side of the uterine fundus and measure about 10 cm in length (Figure 14.7). They are held in place by a pair of suspensory ligaments (above) and the broad ligament (below). The tubes consist of a thin layer of smooth muscle and are lined with ciliated and non-ciliated epithelial cells. The funnel-shaped portion of the fallopian tube is known as the infundibulum (not to be confused with stalk of cells that attach the pituitary gland to the hypothalamus discussed in Chapters 12 and 13). The infundibulum ends in a series of finger-like projections known as fimbriae (Latin for 'fringe') that surround the ovary and 'catch' or direct the female gamete into the fallopian tube following ovulation. The gamete is then transported towards the uterus by a combination of smooth muscle contraction (peristalsis) and the sweeping action of the cilia. The non-ciliated cells also produce and secrete mucus that is ideal for the movement of the gamete (and sperm if present). Fertilisation of the gamete by the sperm must take place in the fallopian tube in order for the newly fertilised cell (zygote) to successfully implant in the uterus (see below). Occasionally the zygote implants into the thin wall of fallopian tube, the ovary or the abdominal cavity itself. This is known as an ectopic pregnancy (from the Greek word *ektopos* for 'out of place') and will typically abort spontaneously since the fertilised egg cannot survive outside the uterus. However, there is a danger that ectopic pregnancy will result in the rupture of the fallopian tube and surgery may be necessary to remove the zygote. If the fallopian tube has ruptured, or is severely damaged, it may need to be removed during surgery to prevent further complications. Women can also opt to have their tubes sealed or obstructed with an implant as a method of contraception since it prevents the egg cell from reaching the sperm/uterus. The principle is similar to the male vasectomy discussed above but is more invasive.

OVARIES

Like the male testes, the ovaries are both gonads and endocrine glands since they produce female gametes and secrete steroid hormones necessary for gamete maturation and development. They are held in place within the pelvic cavity (between the parietal and visceral peritoneum) by a pair of ovarian ligaments, a pair of suspensory ligaments and the broad ligament (Figure 14.7). In size and shape (but not in colour) they resemble a pair of dried apricots and consist of an outer

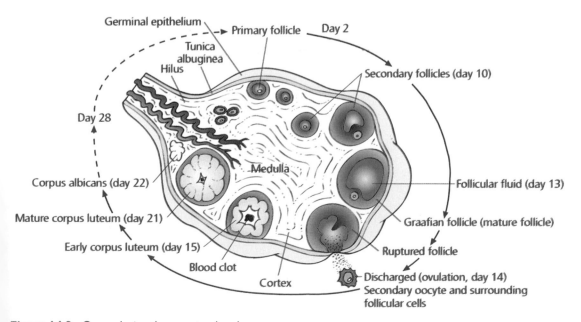

Figure 14.8 Ovary during the menstrual cycle.

cortex and inner medulla surrounded by two further layers of tissue (Figure 14.8). The outermost layer is known as the germinal epithelium and forms a smooth covering of simple epithelium continuous with the peritoneum. The next layer is a dense capsule of connective tissue called the tunica albuginea that surrounds and protects the delicate underlying tissue. The ovarian cortex is also composed of connective tissue (stroma) but, uniquely, it contains a large number of tiny sac-like structures called ovarian follicles (from the Latin word *folliculus* for 'little bag'). Each follicle surrounds and supports a single oocyte (egg cell) that has the potential to develop into a mature ovum (egg). It is estimated that, at birth, the ovarian cortex contains as many as 2 million follicles but by puberty *only* about 40,000 remain. This process is known as atresia and refers to the degeneration and reabsorption of immature ovarian follicles over time (a little like the reabsorption of sperm in the epididymis). Although this seems rather wasteful, less than 500 oocytes will ever be required to mature into ova and be ovulated (between menarche and menopause). Follicular cells also produce and secrete the steroid hormone oestrogen (see below). The final and innermost region of the ovary (the medulla) consists of lose connective tissue and contains a large number of nerves and blood vessels that support the other layers.

said, prospects. The smaller of the two cells is known as the first polar body and is essentially a packet of unwanted nuclear material. The other much larger cell (almost visible to the human eye) is called the secondary oocyte and contains 23 chromosomes, as well as the vast majority of cytoplasm and organelles from the primary oocyte. This is because it must provide all of the organelles, nourishment and genetic programming necessary to support the developing embryo for several days following conception. The role of the sperm it simply to deliver the father's genetic material to the site of fertilisation. The secondary oocyte suspends progression of the cell cycle (meiosis) and is swept into the fallopian tube by the fimbriae (along with the first polar body) at ovulation. If sperm are present and penetrate the secondary oocyte, it completes meiosis II to produce one large fertilised ovum (zygote) and a second, much smaller, polar body that quickly degenerates. The first polar body may also undergo meiosis II at this point resulting in the production of two even smaller polar bodies. However, like the polar body produced by the secondary oocyte following fertilisation, these also degenerate. If sperm is not present in the fallopian tube and fertilisation does not take place, the secondary oocyte suffers the same fate as the primary bodies and eventually degenerates. In order to properly understand this process properly, we need to look at the hormones (pituitary gonadotropins and ovarian steroids) that influence the female reproductive system.

OOGENESIS

The production of female gametes in the ovaries is known as oogenesis (egg + creation) and, like spermatogenesis, it involves meiosis (reductive division of the cell nucleus). From the onset of puberty, a small number of primary oocytes are activated each month by follicle-stimulating hormone (FSH). Of these, typically, only one oocyte will undergo meiosis I and produce two haploid cells (each with 23 chromosomes). Although both daughter cells have the same number of chromosomes, they differ considerably in size and, it has to be

MENSTRUAL CYCLE AND OESTROGEN

The ovarian and uterine cycles are controlled and coordinated by the pituitary gonadotropic hormones: follicle-stimulating hormone (FSH) and luteinising hormone (LH). The two cycles take place concurrently each 28 days or so and are collectively known as the menstrual cycle. For the sake of convenience, the menstrual cycle is subdivided into two halves or phases each lasting approximately 14 days. The first phase is known as the follicular phases and, as its name suggests, involves the development of the primordial follicle containing an oocyte (Figure 14.8). The oocyte matures and increases in size under the influence of follicle-stimulating hormone and luteinising hormone. It is suspended by a stalk of cells within a fluid-filled cavity, a little bit like a lollipop on a small stick. As it grows, it begins to synthesise fats and nutrients to sustain it after ovulation (a packed lunch). It also produces and secretes increasing quantities of the steroid hormone oestrogen. In actual fact, there are three types of oestrogen produced by the body: oestradiol, oestrone and oestriol. Collectively, they exert a number of important effects on the female reproductive system and the body as a whole. For example, oestradiol (the most potent of the three oestrogens) promotes the secretion of large amounts of thin cervical mucus and stimulates the myometrium of the uterus to become more excitable and contractile during the follicular phase of the menstrual cycle. This aids the transit of the sperm towards the fallopian tubes prior to ovulation. It also increases the rate of smooth muscle contraction and cilia activity within the fallopian tube to encourage the transit of the secondary oocyte towards the sperm following ovulation. Finally, the endometrium of the uterus begins to thicken under the influence of oestradiol and develops a rich blood supply in preparation for implantation of the (potentially) fertilised ovum. In terms of general health, oestrogens promote the development of female secondary sexual characteristics including breast tissue. They also lower blood cholesterol, maintain bone density and encourage protein synthesis. This partially explains why women are more likely to suffer from cardiovascular disease and bone demineralisation (osteoporosis) following the menopause (cessation of the menstrual cycle).

OVULATION

Oestrogen levels remain low during the first half of the follicular phase but gradually increase towards the mid-point of the menstrual cycle.

During this stage, oestrogen inhibits the secretion of large amounts of follicle-stimulating hormone (FHS) and luteinising hormone (LH) from the anterior pituitary gland. However, once oestrogen levels reach a threshold value, there is a sudden shift from negative to positive feedback and large amounts of LH (and to a lesser degree FSH) are released. This is known as the LH surge and occurs at about day 12 or 13. LH is responsible for the completion of meiosis I by the primary oocyte and it is quickly transformed into a secondary oocyte (see above). LH also breaks down the stalk of cells that support the oocyte and ovulation occurs when the ballooning wall of the ovary ruptures and the contents of the follicle are expelled into the fallopian tube. In a very small number of ovulations, more than one secondary oocyte is ovulated which can result in the production of non-identical twins (discussed below). Ovulation marks the mid-point of the menstrual cycle and the beginning of the luteal phase. Although secretion of luteinising hormone quickly declines following ovulation, it remains the dominant gonadotropin for most the second half of the menstrual cycle. During the luteal phase, luteinising hormone acts upon the cells of the ruptured follicle and transforms it into a new (temporary) structure called the corpus luteum (Latin for 'yellow body'). The corpus luteum varies in size between 2 cm and 5 cm and synthesises and secretes the steroid hormone progesterone (Figure 14.8). In general terms, therefore, the first half of the menstrual cycle is characterised by the secretion of FSH by the pituitary gland, and oestrogen from the developing follicle; whilst the second half is characterised by the secretion of LH from the pituitary gland, and progesterone from the corpus luteum (Figure 14.9).

PROGESTERONE

Although the corpus luteum produces large quantities of progesterone, it also secretes a small amount of oestrogen since both hormones are necessary for the development and maintenance of the endometrial

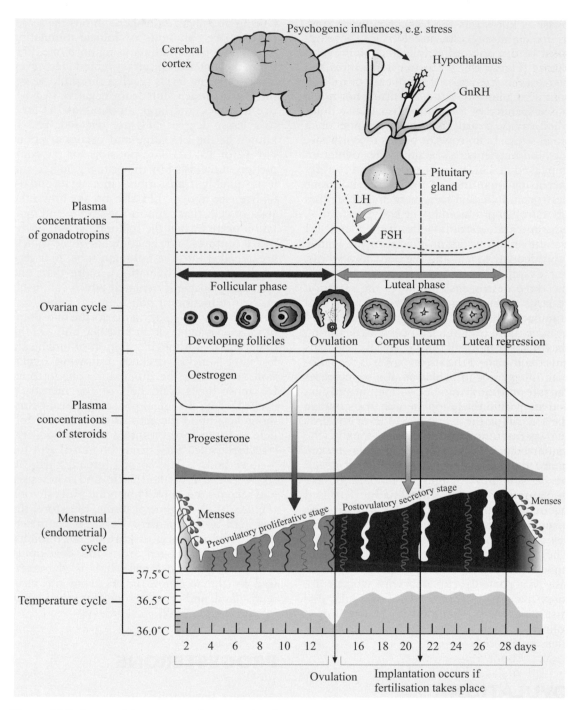

Figure 14.9 Stages of the ovarian and menstrual cycle.

lining of the uterus. However, progesterone is the more influential during the luteal phase and, under its influence, the endometrium becomes thicker and more vascular as it prepares for implantation of a fertilised ovum. At the same time, it inhibits myometrium activity, and thickens and slows production of cervical mucus, to deter further sperm from entering the fallopian tubes (the opposite action to oestrogen). If they haven't got there yet, they've missed the boat, so to speak, for that cycle. Finally, progesterone helps to raise body temperature by about 0.5°C following ovulation and prepares the mammary glands (with oestrogen and prolactin) for milk production following childbirth (see Chapter 13). The fertility awareness method (FAM) of contraception (also known as the rhythm method) takes account of some of these factors to predict when a woman is most fertile (i.e. either side of ovulation since sperm can survive in the female reproductive system for between 48 and 72 hours). Typically, this involves monitoring temperature, examining the consistency/colour of cervical mucus, and comparing the time of ovulation to previous menstrual cycles (calendar method). However, it is recommended that women track at least six cycles before they begin to rely on this method of contraception in order to familiarise themselves fully with the physiological changes that take place. If the secondary oocyte is not fertilised following ovulation, the corpus luteum begins to degenerate and stops producing progesterone after about ten days or so. Eventually, all that remains of the corpus luteum is a fibrous mass of scar tissue known as the corpus albicans (Latin for 'white body'). Without the support of progesterone, the vascular tissue of the endometrium begins to degenerate and eventually detaches, leaving only a thin layer covering the myometrium called the stratum basalis. About 50 ml of menstrual blood, tissue and mucus is lost in this way each month and exits the uterus through the cervix and vagina. This marks the completion of one cycle and beginning of the next.

FERTILISATION

In the event that the secondary oocyte is fertilised in the fallopian tube, it is essential that the vascular lining of the endometrium remains intact and in situ for implantation to occur. Consequently, the newly fertilised ovum begins to secrete a peptide hormone with the impressive name human chorionic gonadotropin (hCG for short). This signals to luteinising hormone receptors in the ovary, to maintain the corpus luteum until the developing placenta can take over progesterone production in about 3 months' time. In Chapter 13, we noted that peptide hormones (such as hCG) are soluble in water which explains how pregnancy tests are able to quickly confirm/exclude conception from a simple urine sample (typically 96% water). Once the sperm has penetrated the secondary oocyte, and meiosis has been completed, the male and female genetic materials fuse together in a process known as amphimixis (from the Greek for 'mixing on both sides'). The zygote (Greek for 'joined') now has the full complement of 46 chromosomes and grows and develops into an embryo by repeated mitotic divisions.

GENDER DETERMINATION

We noted earlier the chapter, that X and Y chromosomes determine the gender of the child. The ovum only carries an X chromosome, whilst sperm can carry either an X or Y chromosome. We also noted that some traits are dominant and some are recessive and, in the case of gender, Y is dominant and X is recessive. That is to say, if an X sperm penetrates the ovum first, the embryo will be female (XX) since recessive characteristics require both alleles to be present. If, on the other hand, a Y sperm penetrates the ovum first, the embryo will be male (XY) since dominant characteristics only require one copy of that allele in the pair. In either case, it is the sperm that determines gender. Using a Punnet

Genetic
contribution of
father (sperm)

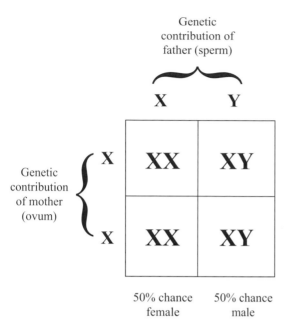

Genetic
contribution
of mother
(ovum)

50% chance
female

50% chance
male

Figure 14.10 Punnett square for male and female gender (XY, XX).

square we can see that the probability of having a male or female child is 50/50 (1:1) since men produce equal numbers of X and Y sperm (Figure 14.10). It is thought that Y sperm swim faster than X sperm but have less endurance (they exhaust themselves). Whilst X sperm start out slower but have greater stamina. Coincidentally, average life expectancy for women also exceeds men (by about two years).

TWINS AND SINGLETONS

Twins can either develop from a single zygote (monozygotic twins) that divides to form two identical embryos; or from two secondary oocytes that are fertilised by separate sperm to form two unique zygotes (dizygotic twins). In the case of the former, the embryos contain exactly the same genetic material since they have developed from the same fertilised ovum. They are always the same gender and may or may not share the same amnion (protective membrane containing amniotic fluid) and placenta. A good example of identical twins

is provided by James and Oliver Phelps who play Fred and George Weasley in the Harry Potter films. In general terms, the later in the pregnancy that the twinning process occurs, the more structures (e.g. placenta) they will share. However, twinning that takes place 12 days or more post-fertilisation, often results in conjoined twins, where the twins are physically joined together and may share the same internal structures (e.g. heart, liver, etc.). Non-identical or dizygotic twins are produced when two secondary oocytes are ovulated by the ovary and are fertilised by separate sperm. Consequently, they are as genetically dissimilar as any other siblings and may be different genders (XX and XY). Notable examples of non-identical twins include Scarlett Johansson and her brother Hunter, and Kiefer Sutherland and his sister Rachel. We noted earlier in the chapter, that typically only one oocyte develops and is ovulated each month. However, some women release multiple eggs in every cycle (hyper-ovulation) and are more likely, therefore, to conceive non-identical or 'fraternal' twins. There is a genetic basis for this trait and it is not uncommon for fraternal twins to run in families. The likelihood of having twins also increases with age and/or if the woman is undergoing fertility treatment. However, most embryos develop alone in the uterus and are known as singletons.

IMPLANTATION

Following fertilisation, the zygote undergoes a process of rapid mitotic divisions known as cleavage. The first cleavage division produces two identical cells called blastomeres that continue to divide to produce four cells, then eight cells and so on. By day 4, the zygote (or pre-embryo) has become a cluster of between 16 and 32 cells forming a ball-shaped structure known as the morula (Latin for 'mulberry'). As the morula progresses along the fallopian tube towards the uterus, it begins to hollow out to produce a fluid-filled space called the blastocoel or blastocyst cavity. This contains a mass of cells known as a blastocyst that will eventually develop into the embryo. At about day 5, the blastocyst frees itself from the layer of cells that surround it (the zona pellucida) and floats freely in the uterus. During the following days, it presses up against the endometrium and begins the process of implantation. Enzymes break down endometrial cells and capillary walls, which allows the blastocyst to penetrate and implant into the endometrium. The blastocyst continues to secrete human chorionic gonadotropin (hCG) to ensure the corpus luteum maintains production of progesterone until the placenta can take over. Implantation is complete by about 12 days after fertilisation and, over the next few weeks, the placenta (Latin for 'flat cake') begins to develop.

PLACENTA

The placenta is a temporary organ that originates from both embryonic and maternal tissue. It allows oxygen and nutrients to pass from the mother to the embryo/foetus without their blood meeting. This is important since it prevents a potential transfusion reaction from occurring (see Chapter 5). The placenta also allows waste products from the developing child, such as carbon dioxide, to pass back along the umbilical cord to the mother's blood supply, and provides protection against bacterial infection. However, it does not protect the developing child from a number of viruses, and rubella (German measles), for example, can cause a variety of birth defects and/or miscarriage. Other potentially harmful substances that are able to cross the placenta include alcohol, nicotine and a variety of drugs and medications. The placenta is fully formed by the end of the third month of gestation and detaches from the uterus following the birth of the child at about nine months (hence it is often referred to as 'the afterbirth'). As this book draws to a close, I can't resist providing a final comment on the trend for eating the placenta after birth or having it ground into powder and encased in a capsule as a 'placenta pill' (people really do this). A quick search on the Internet revealed recipes for placenta lasagne, placenta smoothie and placenta pâté – bon appetit.

CHAPTER 14: TEST YOURSELF

Q. How many chromosomes are found in a human haploid and diploid cell?
A. A haploid cell has 23 chromosomes and a diploid cell has 46.

Q. Provide two examples of haploid cells.
A. Spermatozoa and ova.

Q. What is meant by the terms gene and allele?
A. A gene is a unit of genetic information (e.g. eye colour) that occupies a specific location on a chromosome. The different variants of a gene (e.g. brown, blue, green eye colour) are known as alleles.

Q. What is meant by dominant and recessive characteristics?
A. Dominant characteristics, such as brown eye colour, will be present even if there is only one copy of that gene in the pair (BB, Bb). Recessive characteristics, such as blue eye colour, require both alleles to be present (bb).

Q. What is meant by the terms homozygous and heterozygous?
A. Characteristics or traits with the same alleles (e.g. BB or bb) are known as homozygous and those with different alleles (e.g. Bb) are known as heterozygous.

Q. Use the Punnett square to work out the probability of having a child with blue eyes (bb) when both parents have brown eyes (Bb and Bb)

	B	b
B		
b		

A. 1 in 4 chance of having a child with blue eyes.

	B	b
B	BB	Bb
b	Bb	bb

Q. Why are the testicles housed within the scrotum and not inside the abdominal cavity?
A. Sperm production is inhibited at temperatures higher than about 35°C.

Q. Which anterior pituitary hormones stimulate the sertoli and leydig cells of the seminiferous tubules (in the testes) and what do they produce?
A. Follicle-stimulating hormone (FSH) stimulates the sertoli cells to produce sperm (spermatogenesis). Luteinising hormone (LH) stimulates the leydig cells to produce testosterone.

Q. What is found in the head of a sperm?
A. The head of the sperm is almost completely filled by the nucleus that contains its 23 chromosomes.

Q. Briefly explain the principle functions of seminal fluid.
A. Seminal fluid provides nutrients necessary for energy production by the sperm's mitochondria and contains an enzyme that triggers a clotting reaction following ejaculation. It is also the (liquid) medium of transport for sperm.

Q. How does the vulva differ from the vagina?
A. The vulva consists of a number of structures that make up the female external genitalia (e.g. labia majora, labia minora, etc.) whereas the vagina is an internal structure (fibro-muscular tube) that extends from the vulva to the neck of the uterus.

Q. Briefly describe the three layers of tissue (outer to inner) that constitute the uterus.
A. The perimetrium covers most of the outer surface of the uterus and is continuous with the peritoneum. It surrounds a thick layer of smooth muscle called the myometrium. The innermost layer, the endometrium, is highly vascular and varies in thickness during the menstrual cycle.

Q. What is the function of the fimbriae and fallopian tubes?
A. The fimbriae surround the ovary and direct the egg into the fallopian tube following ovulation. The egg is transported towards the uterus by the sweeping action of cilia and smooth muscle contraction (peristalsis) in the fallopian tube.

Q. Where in the female reproductive tract must fertilisation take place if implantation is to be successful?
A. The fallopian tubes.

Q. What is meant by the term oocyte?
A. An oocyte is an egg cell that has the potential to develop into a mature ovum.

Q. Describe the principle functions of oestrogen during the first half (follicular phase) of the menstrual cycle.

A. Oestrogen promotes the secretion of cervical mucus and stimulates the myometrium to become more contractile. This aids the transit of the sperm towards the fallopian tubes prior to ovulation. Oestrogen also increases the rate of smooth muscle contraction and cilia activity within the fallopian tube to encourage the transit of the egg towards the sperm. Finally, oestrogen encourages the endometrium to thicken and develop a rich blood supply in preparation for (potential) implantation.

Q. Which hormone stimulates oestrogen production in the ovary during the follicular phase of the menstrual cycle?

A. Follicle-stimulating hormone (FSH).

Q. Which hormone stimulates ovulation and the production of progesterone by the corpus luteum?

A. Luteinising hormone (LH).

Q. Describe the principle functions of progesterone during the second half (luteal phase) of the menstrual cycle.

A. Progesterone encourages the endometrium to become thicker and more vascular as it prepares for (potential) implantation. It also inhibits myometrium activity and slows the production of cervical mucus to deter further sperm from entering the fallopian tubes.

Q. What happens to the endometrium when progesterone is no longer produced by the corpus luteum/corpus albicans?

A. Without progesterone, the vascular tissue of the endometrium begins to degenerate and eventually detaches. About 50 ml of menstrual blood, tissue and mucus is lost.

Q. Which hormone is produced by the fertilised ovum (zygote) and what does it do?

A. The fertilised ovum secretes human chorionic gonadotropin (hCG) which signals to luteinising hormone (LH) receptors in the ovary to maintain the corpus luteum until the placenta can take over progesterone production in about three months' time.

GLOSSARY

Acetylcholine: neurotransmitter that exerts an inhibitory effect on cardiac tissue and regulates motor control of skeletal muscle

Action potential: electrical impulse generated by the transient movement of sodium ions across the axon membrane of a neuron away from the cell body

Adenosine triphosphate (ATP): compound consisting of an adenosine molecule bonded to three high-energy phosphate groups (provides chemical energy when phosphate linkage is broken)

Adipocyte: fat cell

Adipose: fat tissue

Adrenal gland: endocrine gland situated on top of the kidney that secretes catecholamines and a variety of steroid hormones

Adrenaline: amino acid derivative hormone secreted by the adrenal gland that stimulates sympathetic nervous system response

Adrenocorticosteroids: group of lipid derivative hormones secreted by the adrenal cortex

Adrenocorticotropic hormone: peptide hormone secreted by the anterior pituitary gland that stimulates the cortex of the adrenal gland

Adventitia: connective tissue covering the outermost wall of an organ, vessel or other structure

Afferent: conducting inwards

Agglutination: clumping of material when held together by antibodies (e.g. following haemolysis)

Agranulocyte: white blood cell (lymphocyte) that contains no granules in its cytoplasm (e.g. B cell and T cell)

Albumin: most abundant plasma protein responsible for maintaining plasma osmotic pressure

Aldosterone: steroid hormone secreted by the adrenal cortex that helps to regulate blood pressure through the reabsorption of sodium and water in the distal convoluted tubule of the nephron

Allele: different form or variant of the same gene (e.g. brown and blue eye colour)

Alveoli: tiny air sacs within the lungs where exchange of oxygen and carbon dioxide occurs

Amino acid: component molecules (building blocks) of proteins

Amnion: thin membrane that surrounds and protects the embryo and contains amniotic fluid

Amphipathic: molecule having hydrophilic and hydrophobic regions

Amygdala: part of the limbic system associated with the storage/retrieval of emotional memories and the expression of anger

Amylase: carbohydrate digesting enzyme

Amylin: peptide hormone secreted by the beta cells of the pancreas that slows down gastric emptying and promotes satiety

Anabolism: process by which simple substances are used to manufacture complex substances (often requires energy to be expended)

Androgen: steroid hormone that promotes the development of male sex characteristics (e.g. testosterone)

Androstenedione: steroid hormone precursor of testosterone and oestrogen secreted by the adrenal cortex

Angiotensin I: precursor to angiotensin II activated by angiotensin-converting enzyme

Angiotensin II: hormone that increases peripheral vascular resistance and stimulates aldosterone secretion from the adrenal cortex

Anion: negatively charged atom that has gained one or more electron

Anterior: front

Antibody: see immunoglobulin

Anti-D: immunoglobulin administered to Rhesus negative women before/after the birth of a Rhesus positive child in order to prevent haemolytic disease of the foetus/neonate

Antidiuretic hormone (ADH): peptide hormone secreted by the posterior pituitary gland to increase permeability of the collecting duct of the nephron and encourage reabsorption of water into the circulatory system

Antigen: substance or marker recognised by the immune system that triggers the formation of an antibody (immunoglobulin)

Aorta: largest artery in the body (transports oxygenated blood from the left ventricle)

Aortic semilunar valve: valve separating the aorta from the left ventricle

Apnoea: temporary cessation of breathing

Apocrine gland: gland found in the skin, breast, ear and eyelid

Apoptosis: programmed cell death

Apyrexia: body temperature below normal range

Arachnoid mater: middle membrane of the meninges

Areola: circular area (commonly used to describe the area surrounding the nipple of the breast)

Arrector pili: small muscles attached to hair follicles that allow them to stand upright

Arrhythmia: irregularity in the force or rhythm of the heartbeat

Arteriole: small artery

Artery: vessel that transports blood away from the heart

Astrocyte: the most abundant glial cell of the central nervous system that provides physical support to neurons and capillaries

Asystole: absence of systolic activity in the heart resulting in no cardiac output

Ataxia: inability to coordinate muscle movement

Atom: smallest particle of an element which can exist as a stable entity (comprised of protons, neutrons, electrons)

ATP: see adenosine triphosphate

Atrial natriuretic hormone: peptide hormone secreted by the atrial myocardiocytes that reduces the reabsorption of sodium in the renal tubules

Atrioventricular (AV) node: small node of specialised cardiac muscle situated in the wall of the right atrium that receives electrical impulses from the sinoatrial node and transmits them to the bundle of His

Atrium: one of the two upper chambers of the heart which receives blood from the superior/ inferior vena cava (right) and pulmonary veins (left)

Auerbach's plexus: network of autonomic nerves situated between the circular and longitudinal muscles of the gastrointestinal tract

Automaticity: the ability of myocardial cells to spontaneously produce an action potential without stimulation from the central nervous system

Autonomic nervous system: regulates key involuntary homeostatic functions (e.g. heart rate and respiratory rate) via two complementary divisions: the sympathetic nervous system and the parasympathetic nervous system

Axolemma: plasma membrane surrounding the axon of a neuron

Axon: long process of a neuron that conducts electrical messages away from the cell body

B cell: lymphocyte that produces and secretes antibodies (immunoglobulins) in response to a particular antigen

Bartholin's glands: situated on either side of the vaginal opening they secrete mucus to aid vaginal lubrication

Basal metabolic rate: the rate at which the body uses energy (and generates heat) at complete rest

Basophil: leukocyte that plays an important role in the inflammatory response (secretes histamine)

Bicuspid valve: heart valve (with two cusps) situated between the left atrium and left ventricle (also known as the left atrioventricular valve and the mitral valve)

Bilirubin: yellow pigment produced in the liver as a result of the breakdown of haemoglobin

2,3-biphosphoglycerate: compound produced by erythrocytes during glycolysis that binds reversibly with haemoglobin

Blastocele: fluid-filled cavity containing a blastocyst within the morula (pre-embryo)

Blastocyst: cluster of cells from which the embryo develops following implantation

Blastomeres: cells produced by mitotic division of the zygote after fertilisation

Body Mass Index: numerical value calculated from a person's height and weight that is used to classify relative weight in adults (e.g. underweight, overweight, obese, etc.)

Bowman's capsule: see glomerular capsule

BPG: see 2,3-biphosphoglycerate

Brainstem: most inferior part of the brain consisting (in ascending order) of the medulla oblongata, pons and midbrain

Broca's area: situated on the left cerebral hemisphere it plays an important role in the production of spoken and written language

Bronchioles: small airways extending from the bronchi to the alveoli (subdivide into terminal and respiratory divisions)

Bronchus: airway that branches off the trachea (left primary bronchus and right primary bronchus)

Brush border: collective name for the microvilli-covered surface of epithelial cells found in the small intestine and nephron

Buffer: chemical or substance that controls the hydrogen ion concentration in a solution (pH)

Bulbourethral glands: pea-shaped glands situated directly below the prostate gland that secrete alkaline mucus into the male urethra

Bulk transport: process where cells release or absorb material or fluid through their outer membrane

Bundle of His: bundle of nerve cells situated in the ventricular septum that provide electrical conduction to the ventricles via the right and left bundle branches

Bursa: sac-like structure filled with synovial fluid that provides a cushion between the skin and the bone at a number of joints

Calciferol: vitamin D_3 synthesised in skin exposed to ultraviolet light

Calcitonin: peptide hormone secreted by the thyroid gland that encourages osteoblast activity in response to high calcium levels in the blood

Calcitriol: hormonally active form of vitamin D secreted by the kidney (promotes absorption of calcium from the gastrointestinal tract)

Calyx: cup-like structure of the renal pelvis surrounding one or more renal papillae

Cancellous bone: see spongy bone

Capillary: narrow blood vessel that consists of a single layer of endothelium and connects arterioles to venules

Capsid: protein shell that protects the genetic material of a virus

Carbaminohaemoglobin: combination of haemoglobin with carbon dioxide

Carboxyhaemoglobin: combination of haemoglobin with carbon monoxide

Cardiac sphincter: ring of muscle situated between the oesophagus and stomach

Cardiovascular centre: situated in the medulla oblongata, it regulates heart rate and blood pressure (consists of cardiac control centre and vasomotor centre)

Carotid artery: situated on either side of the neck/thyroid gland, transports blood to the head and brain

Cartilage: flexible connective tissue found in various forms throughout the body (e.g. hyaline, elastic, fibrocartilage)

Catabolism: process by which complex molecules are broken down into simple ones (often resulting in the release of energy)

Catecholamines: group of amino acid derived hormones including adrenaline, noradrenaline and dopamine

Cation: positively charged atom that has lost one or more electron

Cauda equina: collection of spinal nerves that fan-out through the lumber, sacral and coccygeal vertebrae following the termination of the spinal cord at lumber vertebra 1

Cell membrane: insoluble phospholipid bi-layer that regulates the transport of substances in and out of the cell

Centipoise (cP): measurement of viscosity

Central nervous system: brain and spinal cord

Cerebellar peduncles: connect the cerebellum to the brainstem

Cerebellum: part of the brain situated behind the pons that coordinates voluntary movement and balance

Cerebrospinal fluid: plasma-like fluid secreted by the choroid plexus that circulates through the ventricles into the subdural and subarachnoid spaces in order to maintain uniform pressure within the brain and spinal cord

Cerebrum: largest part of the brain divided into left and right hemispheres each comprising four lobes (frontal, parietal, occipital and temporal). Coordinates activities involved in memory, intelligence, personality, sensory perception and motor control

Cervical: relating to the neck

Cervix: neck of the uterus situated at the proximal end of the vagina

Chemoreceptor: chemical receptor situated in the medulla (central) or carotid arteries/aortic arch (peripheral)

Chemotaxis: movement or orientation of a cell in response to chemical signals

Chief cells (gastric): secrete pepsinogen into the stomach

Cholecystokinin: peptide hormone that stimulates the contraction of the gall bladder and the secretion of digestive enzymes by the pancreas

Chondrocyte: cartilage cell

Choroid plexus: network of blood vessels that project into the ventricles of the brain and secrete cerebrospinal fluid

Chromaffin cells: neuro-endocrine cells situated in the adrenal medulla that secrete adrenaline and noradrenaline

Chromosome: linear, thread-like collection of genes that carries heredity information in the form of DNA

Chyle: lymph containing dietary fat

Chyme: partially digested, acidic stomach contents that passes into the duodenum through the pyloric sphincter

Chymotrypsin: protein-digesting enzyme

Chymotrypsinogen: inactive form of chymotrypsin secreted by pancreatic acinar cells

Cilia: tiny hair-like processes projecting from epithelial cells

Cingulate gyrus: part of the limbic system that helps to regulate acute pain and emotion

Coagulation: transformation of blood from a liquid to a solid state (via the clotting cascade)

Cobalamin: see vitamin B_{12}

Codon: sequence of three consecutive nucleotides

Collagen: protein constituent of connective tissue such as bone, cartilage and tendon

Collecting duct: final part of a nephron that collects early urine from the distal convoluted tubule and transports it towards the renal pelvis

Colon: large intestine (consists of: ascending, transverse, descending and sigmoid colon)

Colostrum: breast milk secreted in the first week of lactation

Columnar cell: epithelial cell shaped like a column

Commensal: organism participating in a symbiotic relationship

Compact bone: dense, rigid outer layer of bone formed from osteons (cortical bone)

Complement system: small proteins found in the blood that stimulate histamine release and promote chemotaxis and phagocytosis

Compound: chemical substance that contains more than one type of atom (e.g. H_2O)

Corpus: Latin for 'body' or 'mass'

Corpus albicans: mass of fibrous scar tissue produced when the corpus luteum degenerates

Corpus callosum: bundle of nerve fibres situated beneath the cerebrum that connects the right and left hemispheres

Corpus cavernosum: one of two masses of erectile tissue situated within the penis directly above the urethra and corpus spongiosum

Corpus luteum: progesterone and oestrogen secreting structure that develops in the ovary following ovulation

Corpus spongiosum: erectile tissue that surrounds the male urethra

Cortex: outer region or layer of an organ, tissue or structure

Cortical bone: see compact bone

Corticotropin: see adrenocorticotropic hormone

Corticotropin-releasing hormone: peptide hormone secreted by the hypothalamus that facilitates the release of adrenocorticotropic hormone by the anterior pituitary gland

Cortisol: steroid hormone (glucocorticoid) secreted by the adrenal cortex essential for normal regulation of plasma glucose and inhibition of inflammation

Co-transporter: see symporter

Covalent bond: formed by the sharing of one or more electrons between atoms

Cowper's glands: see bulbourethral glands

Creatinine: waste compound produced by muscle metabolism

Cuboidal cell: epithelial cell shaped like a cube

Cutaneous: relating to the skin

Cyst: membranous sac containing liquid or semisolid material

Cytokine: generic term for a number of small proteins that have an effect on cell interactions including attraction and activation of phagocytes and natural killer cells

Cytoplasm: fluid component of the cell (includes cytosol)

Cytosol: fluid component of cytoplasm

Dehydroepiandrosterone: steroid hormone precursor of testosterone and oestrogen secreted by the adrenal cortex

Dendrite: short branch-like extension from the cell body of a neuron that receive (and transmit) signals from other neurons or tissue

Deoxyribonucleic acid: double-stranded nucleic acid molecule arranged as a double helix

Dermatophytes: fungi that cause skin, hair and nail infections

Dermis: layer of skin between the epidermis and subcutaneous fat containing a number of appendages including hair follicles, nerve endings, sweat and sebaceous glands

Dermotome: area of skin innervated by a single nerve from a single nerve root of the spinal cord

Diaphysis: shaft of a long bone

Diastole: relaxation of the heart muscle to allow the chambers to fill with blood before systole

Diencephalon: part of the brain containing the thalamus, hypothalamus and epithalamus

Diffusion: movement of a substance from a high concentration to a low concentration

Diploid: a cell that contains a complete set of chromosomes (46 in humans)

Distal: situated away from the point of origin or attachment (e.g. the wrist is distal to the shoulder)

Distal convoluted tubule: section of the renal tubule situated between the loop of Henle and collecting duct

Diuresis: increased or excessive urine production

Diuretic: substance or drug that increases urine production and output

DNA: see deoxyribonucleic acid

Dopamine: hormone and neurotransmitter that helps to regulate movement/motor control, motivation, arousal and reward (also known as prolactin-inhibiting hormone)

Duodenum: first and shortest section of the small intestine

Dura mater: outermost and thickest membrane of the meninges

Dural venous sinuses: large collecting veins situated between the folds of the dura mater

Efferent: conducting outwards

Effusion: accumulation or escape of fluid

Ejection fraction: percentage of blood pumped from a filled ventricle following one heartbeat (55–70% is considered normal)

Elastin: protein constituent of connective tissue which provides elastic recoil

Electrolyte: substance that will dissociate into ions in solution and acquire the capacity to conduct electricity

Electron: negatively charged subatomic particle found in the outer shell of an atom

Element: chemical substance whose atoms are all of the same type (e.g. O_2)

Embryo: fertilised egg in its early stages of development (especially before it has reached a recognisable form)

End-diastolic volume (EDV): volume of blood in the ventricle at the end of diastole (filling)

End systolic volume (ESV): volume of blood in a ventricle at the end of systole/contraction

Endo: prefix meaning within

Endocardium: inner surface of the heart (layer of squamous epithelium that line the chambers/myocardium)

Endochondral: occurring within cartilage (e.g. endochondral ossification)

Endocrine: relating to glands or specialised cells that secrete hormones into the blood

Endocytosis: bulk transport into the cell (e.g. phagocytosis, pinocytosis)

Endometrium: inner lining of the uterus consisting of epithelial and connective tissue

Endoplasmic reticulum: membrane network within the cytoplasm (rough and smooth) involved in the synthesis and transport of proteins, hormones and other substances

Endosteum: thin vascular membrane that lines the inner surface of long bones

Endothelium: layer of cells lining the closed internal spaces of the body

Entero: Prefix referring to the intestine

Enterocyte: simple columnar epithelial cells situated in the small and large intestine

Enteroendocrine cell: specialised hormone-secreting cells situated in the stomach, intestine and pancreas

Enterokinase: enzyme produced in the duodenum that converts inactive trypsinogen into active trypsin

Enteropepsidase: see enterokinase

Enzyme: protein catalyst that can influence the rate of a biological reaction

Eosinophil: phagocytic white blood cell (granulocyte) responsible for the destruction of parasitic organisms

Ependymal cell: glial cell of the central nervous system that line the ventricles and secrete cerebrospinal fluid

Epicardium: inner layer of the pericardium (visceral pericardium)

Epidermis: outermost layer of the skin

Epididymis: coiled duct situated on the posterior surface of the testis that store sperm

Epiglottis: flap of elastic cartilage that covers the entrance to the larynx

Epiphysis: end (distal) part of a long bone

Epithalamus: part of the diencephalon that houses the pineal gland

Epithelium: layer of cells that covers the outside surfaces of the body including the mucous membranes that communicate with the outside of the body

Erythrocyte: red blood cell

Erythropoiesis: process that produces erythrocytes

Erythropoietin: hormone secreted by the kidneys that stimulates erythropoiesis in response to hypoxaemia

Ethmoid bone: separates the nasal cavity from the brain and olfactory bulbs

Eustachian tube: narrow passage that connects the middle ear to the nasopharynx

Exo: prefix meaning outside or external

Exocrine gland: secrete their products via a duct or directly onto the surface of the skin

Exocytosis: bulk transport out of the cell

Extracellular: outside the cell

Extrusion: process where a cell exports large particles through its cell membrane into the extracellular compartment (exocytosis)

Fallopian tubes: pair of narrow tubes connecting the ovaries to the uterus

Fascia: layer of connective tissue that surrounds muscles, blood vessels and nerves

Fascicle: bundle or cluster

Fibrillation: uncoordinated muscular twitching or 'fluttering'

Fibrin: insoluble protein fibres formed from fibrinogen during coagulation

Fibrinogen: soluble plasma protein and clotting factor (I) produced by the liver

Fibrinolysis: fibrin splitting

Fibroblast: cell that secretes collagen proteins (important for bone formation and wound healing)

Fimbriae: finger-like projections that surround the ovary at the end of each fallopian tube

First polar body: small haploid cell produced by primary oocyte following meiosis I

Follicle: small body cavity or sac

Follicle-stimulating hormone: peptide hormone secreted by the anterior pituitary gland that stimulates the production of gametes in the male and female gonads

Fontanelle: soft membranous gap between the partially formed cranial bones of a foetus/baby

Foramen: opening or hole in the bone through which nerves and blood vessels pass

Foramen magnum: large opening at the base of the skull (occipital bone)

Fornix (brain): arch-shaped bundle of axons that connect the hippocampus to the hypothalamus

Fornix (cervix): recess formed where the proximal vagina surrounds the neck of the cervix

Fructose: monosaccharide found in plants and fruit

G cell (gastric): secretes gastrin into the stomach

Galactose: monosaccharide found in milk and milk products

Gametes: male or female reproductive cells (spermatozoa or ova)

Ganglion: cluster or group of neurons situated in the peripheral nervous system

Gastrin: peptide hormone secreted by gastric G cells that stimulates the production of hydrochloric acid and pepsinogen and regulates the rate of gastric emptying

Gene: sequence of nucleotides in DNA or RNA situated on a chromosome (functional unit of inheritance controlling the transmission/expression of one or more traits)

Genotype: total combination of genes inherited by an individual from both parents (genetic makeup)

Germinal cell: cell from which other cells are derived

Gestation: period of foetal development in the uterus from conception to birth

Ghrelin: peptide hormone produced by the stomach that stimulates the sensation of hunger

Gland: group of cells or organ that produce a secretion or hormone (e.g. exocrine or endocrine)

Glial cell: non-excitable nerve cells that perform maintenance functions for neurons

Globulin: plasma protein important for transportation of small ions, hormones and other compounds and, in the case of gamma globulins, the destruction of pathogens (see immunoglobulin)

Glomerular capsule: cup-like double membrane surrounding the glomerulus of a nephron (also known as the Bowman's capsule)

Glomerulus: ball-shaped structure composed of capillary blood vessels involved in the filtration of the blood

Glottis: opening at the upper part of the larynx that houses the vocal folds (cords)

Glucagon: peptide hormone secreted by the alpha cells of the pancreas that increase blood glucose levels

Glucocorticoids: steroid hormones secreted by the adrenal cortex essential for normal regulation of plasma glucose and inhibition of inflammation

Gluconeogenesis: synthesis of glucose from fats and amino acids by the liver and kidneys

Glycogen: polysaccharide that is the main form of stored glucose in the liver and muscle

Glycogenolysis: breakdown of glycogen into glucose

Glycolysis: sugar splitting (phase of cellular respiration)

Goblet cell: columnar epithelial cells that secrete mucus

Golgi body: series of flattened intracellular membranous sacs involved in packaging proteins and other substances for secretion

Gonads: male or female reproductive organs (testes or ovaries) that produce gametes

Granulocyte: leukocyte that contains granules in its cytoplasm e.g. neutrophil, basophil, eosinophil

Growth hormone: peptide hormone secreted by the anterior pituitary gland that promotes growth and repair

Growth hormone: inhibiting hormone peptide hormone secreted by the hypothalamus that inhibits the release of growth hormone, thyroid-stimulating hormone, cholecystokinin and insulin

Growth hormone releasing hormone: peptide hormone secreted by the hypothalamus that facilitates the release of growth hormone

Growth plate: see physis

Gyrus: folded surface of the cerebrum

Haematocrit: ratio of the volume of red blood cells to the total volume of blood (packed cell volume)

Haemoglobin: oxygen-carrying protein and pigment of red blood cells

Haemolysis: the rupture or splitting open of red blood cells

Haemopoiesis: formation and development of blood cells and platelets in the red bone marrow

Haemostasis: homeostatic process that stops bleeding (see clotting cascade)

Haploid: cell that contains half the number of chromosomes of somatic cell (23 in humans – see also gamete)

Haustra: pouches found in the large intestine/colon produced by contraction of the teniae coli

Haversian canals: network of ducts in cortical bone (contain nerves and blood vessels)

Hepatocyte: liver cell

Hepatopancreatic ampulla: union of the common bile duct and pancreatic duct

Hepatopancreatic sphincter: controls the flow of digestive juices into the duodenum from the common bile duct and pancreatic duct (through the hepatopancreatic ampulla)

Heterozygous: characteristic or trait (e.g. eye colour) represented by two different alleles (e.g. Bb)

Hippocampus: part of the limbic system associated with memory and spatial navigation

Histamine: vasoactive chemical produced by basophils and mast cells

Homeostasis: maintenance of stable internal environment

Homozygous: characteristic or trait (e.g. eye colour) represented by two copies of the same alleles (e.g. BB or bb)

Hormone: chemical messenger that modifies/influences cellular activity within a target cell

Human chorionic gonadotropin: peptide hormone secreted by the fertilised ovum (zygote) that signals to the corpus luteum to continue producing progesterone

Hydrolysis: chemical reaction in which water reacts with a compound to produce other compounds (involves splitting a bond)

Hydroxylapatite: mineral and main inorganic constituent of bone and tooth enamel

Hyperaemia: excess accumulation of blood in the tissue/s

Hypercapnia: high concentration of carbon dioxide in the blood

Hypercortisolism: high concentration of cortisol in the blood

Hyperglycaemia: high concentration of glucose in the blood

Hyperkalaemia: high concentration of potassium in the blood

Hypernatremia: high concentration of sodium in the blood

Hypertension: high blood pressure

Hypertrophy: growth or enlargement of tissue/organ resulting from an increase in the size of its cells

Hypoglycaemia: low concentration of glucose in the blood

Hypokalaemia: low concentration of potassium in the blood

Hyponatremia: low concentration of sodium ions in the blood

Hypophyseal portal system: network of blood vessels that connects the hypothalamus to the anterior pituitary gland

Hypotension: low blood pressure

Hypothalamus: area of the diencephalon situated below the thalamus that regulates a large number of endocrine and autonomic activities

Hypothermia: low core temperature (below 35°C)

Hypovolaemia: low volume of circulating blood

Hypoxaemia: low levels of oxygen in the blood (particularly arterial blood)

Hypoxia: inadequate oxygen supply to the cells and tissues of the body

Hypoxic drive: respiratory drive mediated by low levels of oxygen in the arterial blood (typically less than 60 mmHg)

Ileocaecal valve: sphincter that separates the small and large intestines

Ileum: third and final section of the small intestine situated between the jejunum and ileocaecal valve

Ilium: largest and most superior bone of the pelvis

Immunoglobulin (Ig): Y-shaped proteins produced by B cells which attach to foreign substances and assist in destroying them (also known as antibodies). There are five classes: IgA, IgG, IgM, IgD and IgE

Inferior: situated toward the feet (e.g. the stomach is inferior to the heart)

Infundibulum: funnel-shaped structure (e.g. stalk of cells that attach the pituitary gland to the hypothalamus)

Inguinal: situated in the groin

Inhibin: peptide hormone secreted by the sertoli cells of the testes that inhibits secretion of follicle-stimulating hormone

Innervation: to supply an organ/part of the body with nerves (neurons)

Insulin: peptide hormone secreted by the beta cells of the pancreas that lowers blood glucose levels

Insulinlike growth factors: peptide hormones that stimulate growth

Interferon: small proteins (cytokines) released by lymphocytes in response to viruses (and other pathogens) that interfere with replication

Interstitial: small, narrow spaces between cells or tissue

Intracellular: inside the cell

Intramembranous: occurring within a membrane (e.g. intramembranous ossification)

Ion: electrically charged atom (group of atoms) formed by the loss or gain of one or more electrons

Ionic bond: formed between two atoms when an electron is transferred or donated from one to the other

Ischaemia: insufficient blood supply to an organ or part of the body

Jejunum: second and middle section of the small intestine situated between the duodenum and ileum

Keratin: tough, water-resistant protein found in hair, nails and epidermal cells (secreted by keratinocytes)

Keratinocyte: keratin-producing cell

Ketoacidosis: complication of hyperglycaemia that occurs when large amounts of ketones accumulate in the blood and lower plasma pH (<7.35)

Ketone: compound produced when fats and amino acids are broken down for energy (e.g. acetone)

Kinins: broad group of small proteins (polypeptides) that stimulate vasodilation during the inflammatory response

Krause's end bulbs: nerve ending found in the dermis, sensitive to cold

Kupffer cell: fixed macrophage in the liver that destroys worn-out red blood cells, bacteria and foreign proteins

Lacteal: small lymphatic vessel that absorbs dietary fat (as chyle) in the small intestine

Lacuna: cavity (especially in bone)

Lamella: thin layer of tissue (especially in bone)

Langerhans cell: cell found in the epidermis that recognise and attack pathogens

Lateral geniculate nucleus: situated in the thalamus, it relays visual information from the optic nerve to the primary visual cortex of the cerebrum

Leptin: peptide hormone produced by fat cells that triggers the sensation of satiety and regulates energy expenditure

Leukocyte: white blood cell

Leukotrienes: group of hormones/inflammatory mediators derived from arachidonic acid

Leydig cells: situated in the connective tissue that supports the seminiferous tubules, they secrete testosterone

Limbic system: group of interconnected structures situated in the brain that help to regulate emotion, memory and the perception of smell

Lipase: fat digesting hormone

Loop of Henle: U-shaped section of the renal tubule situated between the proximal and distal convoluted tubules – site of sodium and water reabsorption

Luteinising hormone: peptide hormone secreted by the anterior pituitary gland that is responsible for ovulation in women and the production of testosterone in men

Lymph: clear fluid that contains and carries white blood cells (mostly lymphocytes and macrophages)

Lymph nodes: numerous bean-shaped masses of tissue situated along the course of lymphatic vessels

Lymphocyte: type of white blood cell derived from lymphoid stem cells (includes B cells, T cells and natural killer cells)

Lyse: separate or split

Lysozyme: enzyme that destroys cell walls of certain bacteria (found in exocrine sweat, nasal secretions, saliva and tears)

Macrophage: large phagocytic white blood cell

Mammillary bodies: part of the limbic system associated with the recollection of specific events, experiences and emotions

Mean arterial pressure (MAP): average arterial pressure during single cardiac cycle (MAP >60 mmHg is necessary to perfuse major organs)

Meatus: opening (usually external) or passage

Mediastinum: central compartment of the thoracic cavity that contains the heart

Medulla: inner region or layer of an organ, tissue or structure

Medulla oblongata: most inferior part of the brainstem containing the cardiovascular and respiratory centres

Megakaryocyte: large, nucleated, bone-marrow cell responsible for the production of thrombocytes (platelets)

Meiosis: process of cell division that reduces the number of chromosomes in reproductive cells from diploid to haploid (23 in humans)

Meissner's corpuscle: nerve ending found in the dermis, sensitive to light touch

Melanin: brown/black pigment secreted by epidermal melanocytes

Melanocyte: epidermal cell which secretes melanin

Melatonin: hormone secreted by the pineal gland that helps to regulate the sleep-wake cycle

Meninges: three fibrous membranes (dura mater, arachnoid mater, pia mater) that surround and protect the brain and spinal cord

Meniscus: crescent-shaped cartilage pad that absorbs weight in the knee joint

Merkel cell: situated in the epidermis, sensitive to localised pressure

Mesentery: double layer of the peritoneum that supports the jejunum and ileum (and other structures within the abdominal cavity)

Messenger RNA (mRNA): RNA molecule that transports genetic information from the cell nucleus to the ribosomes and serves as a template for protein synthesis

Microglia: small glial cells of the central nervous system that function primarily as phagocytic immune cells

Microvilli: microscopic finger-like projections present on the surface of some epithelial cells

Midbrain: most superior part of brainstem that contains the substantia nigra and centres that process visual and auditory information

Mineralocorticoids: steroid hormones secreted by the adrenal cortex essential for the regulation of plasma sodium and potassium

Miosis: excessive constriction of the pupil

Mitochondria: intracellular organelle responsible for production of ATP (cellular energy) during cellular respiration

Mitosis: process of cell division where two identical daughter cells are produced (see: diploid)

Mitral valve: see bicuspid valve

Molecule: two or more atoms that form chemical bonds with each other (can be the same or different types of atom)

Monocyte: large white blood cells that differentiate into macrophages

Monomer: molecule that can combine with others to form a polymer

Monosaccharide: any sugar that cannot be broken down into a simpler form by hydrolysis (e.g. glucose)

Morula: pre-embryo made up of a mass of blastomeres

Mydriasis: excessive dilation of the pupil

Myelin: fatty insulating material found around the axon of most neurons

Myocardiocyte: cardiac muscle cell (also known as cardiomyocyte)

Myocardium: cardiac muscle

Myoglobin: oxygen transporting protein (pigment) of muscle

Myometrium: middle, smooth muscle layer of the uterus

Myotome: group of muscles that a single spinal nerve root innervates

Natriuresis: excretion of sodium in the urine

Natural killer (NK) cell: granular lymphocyte that triggers apoptosis in cancer and virus-infected cells

Neonate: new-born

Neoplasm: new growth

Nephron: functional unit of the kidney capable of producing urine (approx. 1 million per kidney)

Neuroglia: see glial cells

Neuromelanin: dark pigment found in the substantia nigra structurally related to melanin

Neuron: nerve cell capable of generating a nerve impulse (action potential)

Neuropathy: damage or disease to nerve leading to numbness or weakness

Neurotransmitter: chemical messenger secreted into a synapse from a synaptic vesicle

Neutron: subatomic particle found in the nucleus of an atom which has no electrical charge

Neutropenia: abnormally low numbers of neutrophils

Neutrophil: abundant phagocytic white blood cell (granulocyte)

Nociceptor: nerve ending that responds to noxious stimuli (pain receptor)

Node of Ranvier: small interruptions in the myelin sheath of an axon that assist rapid transmission of a nerve impulse along its length

Noradrenaline: amino acid derivative hormone secreted by the adrenal gland that stimulates sympathetic nervous system response

Nucleotide: one of a group of molecules that form the building blocks of DNA and RNA (adenine, cytosine, guanine, and thymine for DNA/adenine, cytosine, guanine, uracil for RNA)

Nucleus (atom): core of an atom containing varying numbers of protons and neutrons

Nucleus (cell): core of an animal cell containing genetic material (DNA) wound into chromosomes

Nucleus (CNS): cluster or group of neurons situated in the central nervous system

Oestrogen: female sex hormone secreted by the ovary and corpus luteum during the reproductive cycle

Olfactory bulbs: part of the limbic system that transmits sensory information regarding odours detected in the nasal cavity

Oligodendrocyte: glial cell of the central nervous system that manufactures myelin

Oliguria: decreased urine output

Oocyte: immature female gamete (egg cell)

Oogenesis: growth and maturation of a female gamete in the ovary

Os: opening in the cervix of the uterus

Osmolality: measure of how much of one substance has been dissolved in another substance (osmol/L)

Osmoreceptors: sensory nerve cells situated in the hypothalamus that detect changes in osmotic pressure in the plasma and trigger/inhibit the secretion of antidiuretic hormone

Osmosis: movement of water from high to low concentration across a semi-permeable membrane

Ossification: process of bone formation

Osteoblast: cell that creates new bone (osteoid)

Osteoclast: cell that reabsorbs bone during remodelling or repair

Osteocyte: bone cell

Osteoid: organic substance secreted by osteoblasts prior to mineralisation of bone matrix

Osteon: basic structural unit of compact bone

Ovarian follicle: sac-like structure found in the ovarian cortex that surrounds and supports an oocyte (egg cell)

Ovulation: release of the female gamete (secondary oocyte) from the ovary

Ovum: female gamete following ovulation

Oxyhaemoglobin: combination of haemoglobin with oxygen

Oxytocin: peptide hormone secreted by the posterior pituitary gland that causes muscular contraction of the uterus during labour and stimulates the release of milk from mammary glands

Pacinian corpuscle: nerve ending found in the dermis, sensitive to rapid vibration and pressure

Parasympathetic nerv. system: division of the autonomic nervous system responsible for 'resting and digesting' activities

Parathyroid glands: four small glands embedded in the posterior surface of the thyroid gland

Parathyroid hormone: peptide hormone secreted by the parathyroid glands that encourage osteoclast activity in response to low calcium levels in the blood

Parenchyma: main functional element/s of an organ

Parietal cells (gastric): secrete hydrochloric acid and intrinsic factor into the stomach

Parietal pericardium: outer layer of the pericardium which surrounds the heart and secretes pericardial fluid

Parietal pleura: serous membrane that lines the chest walls and thoracic diaphragm

Paroxysmal: sudden attack, recurrence or intensification of symptoms/disease

Partial pressure: the pressure that any one gas would exert on the walls of a container if it were the only gas present

Pepsin: protein-digesting enzyme

Pepsinogen: inactive form of pepsin secreted by gastric chief cells

Peptide: molecule consisting of two or more amino acids

Pericardium: double membranous sac (consisting of the parietal and visceral pericardium) that surrounds the heart muscle (myocardium)

Perichondrium: layer of fibrous connective tissue that covers the surface of cartilage

Perimetrium: fibrous outer layer of the uterus

Perineum: area between the anus and the scrotum (in men) and vulva (in women)

Periosteum: vascular membrane covering the surface of bones (except at the joints)

Peripheral nervous system: part of the nervous system that is outside the central nervous system and communicates messages to and from it

Peristalsis: involuntary constriction and relaxation of smooth muscle in a tube or canal to push the contents forward

Peritoneum: serous membrane that lines the walls of the abdominal cavity

Peritubular capillaries: network of tiny blood vessels that surround the nephron allowing reabsorption and secretion to take place

Peyer's patch: lymphoid tissue situated in the walls of the small intestine

Phagocyte: type of cell that engulfs or absorbs material

Phagocytosis: ingestion of material into the cell through the plasma membrane (cell-eating)

Phenotype: observable genetic characteristics or traits exhibited by an individual (e.g. eye colour)

Physis: the region in a long bone between the epiphysis and diaphysis where growth in length occurs (also called growth plate)

Pia mater: innermost and thinnest of the meninges

Pineal gland: situated in the epithalamus it secretes the hormone melatonin

Pinocytosis: the ingestion of fluid into the cell through the plasma membrane (cell-drinking)

Pituitary gland: small multi-lobed gland attached to the hypothalamus by the infundibulum that secretes a large number of hormones

Plasma: colourless fluid (part of blood, lymph or cytoplasm)

Plasmin: fibrin-digesting enzyme (activated by tissue plasminogen activator/tPA)

Platelet: see thrombocyte

Plexus: network of nerves or blood vessels

Pneumocyte: one of the cells lining the alveoli of the lungs (type I and II)

Podocyte: cells found in the glomerular capsule that wrap around the capillaries of the glomerulus and provide a barrier through which blood is filtered

Polypeptide: chain of amino acids

Pons: middle section of the brainstem that contains the pontine respiratory centres

Posterior: back or dorsal aspect (of the body)

Preload: force exerted by the blood on the walls of the ventricle before contraction occurs

Prolactin: peptide hormone secreted by the anterior pituitary gland that stimulates the production of milk by the mammary glands

Prostaglandins: group of hormones derived from arachidonic acid that coordinate local cellular activities and influence enzymatic processes

Prostate gland: chestnut-shaped gland situated around the neck of the male bladder that secretes prostatic fluid

Prostate specific antigen (PSA): enzyme secreted by the prostate gland and found in high concentrations in the blood of men with prostate cancer

Prostatic fluid: milky-coloured fluid secreted by the prostate gland that contains citric acid and prostate specific antigen (PSA)

Protein: molecule composed of polymers of amino acids joined together by peptide bonds

Proton: positively charged subatomic particle found in the nucleus of an atom

Proximal: situated towards or nearest to the point of origin or attachment (e.g. the shoulder is proximal to the wrist)

Proximal convoluted tubule: first section of the renal tubule between the glomerular capsule and loop of Henle (site of glucose, sodium and water reabsorption)

Pulmonary artery: transports deoxygenated blood from the right ventricle to the lungs/ pulmonary capillaries

Pulmonary semilunar valve: valve separating the pulmonary artery from the right ventricle

Pulmonary vein: transports oxygenated blood from the lungs/pulmonary capillaries to the left atrium

Pulse pressure (PP): the variation in blood pressure (in an artery) during the cardiac cycle (i.e. systolic – diastolic = PP). It represents the force that the heart generates each time it contracts (measured in mmHg)

Purkinje fibres: network of filaments situated beneath the endocardium of the ventricular walls that distribute the nerve impulse into the cardiac muscle

Pyloric sphincter: ring of muscle situated between the stomach and duodenum

Pyrexia: raised core temperature above the normal range that is not due to exercise or other environmental factors

Pyrogen: chemical that triggers an elevated temperature or fever

Renal corpuscle: structure that consists of the afferent arteriole, efferent arteriole, glomerulus and Bowman's (glomerular) capsule

Renin: peptide hormone secreted by the kidney in response to low blood pressure which transforms angiotensinogen in angiotensin I

Reticular formation: network of interconnected neurons which extend through the brainstem and help to regulate the sleep-wake cycle

Ribosome: intracellular organelle that synthesises proteins from amino acids using a ribonucleic acid (RNA) template

Ruffini's corpuscle: nerve ending found in the dermis, sensitive to vibration, stretching of skin and heat

Rugae: folds or wrinkles that allow expansion and retraction to occur

Schwann cell: glial cell (e.g. in the stomach) of the peripheral nervous system that manufactures myelin

Sebaceous gland: small gland situated in the dermis that secretes sebum

Sebum: oily/waxy substance secreted by sebaceous gland to lubricate and waterproof hair and skin

Second polar body: small haploid cell produced by secondary oocyte following meiosis II

Secondary oocyte: large haploid cell produced by primary oocyte following meiosis I that develops into an ovum if fertilised by sperm

Secretin: peptide hormone that inhibits gastric motility and stimulates the secretion of bicarbonate from the pancreas

Seminal fluid: fluid secreted by seminal vesicles that is essential for sperm motility and nutrition

Seminal vesicle: paired gland on either side of the male bladder that produces and secretes seminal fluid

Seminiferous tubules: tightly wound vessels situated in the testes that are responsible for sperm and testosterone production

Septum: wall or partition dividing a body space or cavity

Serotonin: neurotransmitter that regulates mood, social behaviour, appetite and digestion

Sertoli cells: epithelial cells situated in the seminiferous tubules responsible for sperm production and maturation

Sharpey's fibres: bundles of strong collagenous fibres that connect periosteum to bone and unite the cranial sutures

Sinoatrial (SA) node: small mass of specialised cells situated in the right atrium (close to the entrance of the superior vena cava) that generate electrical impulses and set the pace for ventricular contraction

Sinus: cavity within a bone or other tissue

Sinusoid: venous cavity through which blood passes

Skene's gland: situated on either side of the female urethral opening, they secrete mucus into the vestibule of the vulva

Somatic: relating to the body

Somatic nervous system: part of the peripheral nervous system associated with skeletal muscle and voluntary control of movement

Somatostatin: see growth hormone inhibiting hormone

Somatotropin: see growth hormone

Spermatogenesis: production of sperm by the sertoli cells in the testes

Spermatozoa: male sex cell or gamete produced by sertoli cells in the testes

Sphincter: ring of muscle that (when open) provides access to an opening or tube

Sphincter of Oddi: see hepatopancreatic sphincter

Spongy bone: inner layer of bone formed from lattice-like network of trabeculae (cancellous or trabecular bone)

Squamous cell: epithelial cell shaped like a fish-scale (flat)

Steroid: lipid derivative hormone that is soluble in fat

Stoma: mouth-like opening (often created surgically)

Stratum corneum: outermost (horned) layer of keratinised squamous epithelium

Stroke volume: amount of blood (in ml) pumped from the ventricle in one contraction

Stroma: supportive framework of an organ (or other structure) usually composed of connective tissue

Subarachnoid space: space or cavity between the arachnoid mater and pia mater that is filled with cerebrospinal fluid

Subdural space: narrow (potential) space between the dura mater and arachnoid mater lubricated by a thin film of fluid

Substantia nigra: pigmented area of the midbrain that secretes dopamine

Sulcus: trench or furrow on the surface of the brain caused by folding of the cerebrum

Superior: situated towards the head (e.g. the heart is superior to the stomach)

Superior sagittal sinus: largest of the dural venous sinuses (absorbs cerebrospinal fluid into the venous blood)

Suprachiasmatic nucleus: area of the hypothalamus responsible for regulation of circadian rhythms

Sympathetic nervous system: division of the autonomic nervous system responsible for 'flight-or-fight' response

Symporter: protein that is involved in the movement of two different molecules/ions across a cell membrane in the same direction (co-transporter)

Synapse: minute junction between the synaptic terminal of a neuron and a dendrite/tissue

Synaptic terminal: club-shaped process by which an axon makes synaptic contact with another neuron or tissue

Synaptic vesicle: small membranous sac situated within synaptic terminals that store and secrete neurotransmitters into a synapse

Systole: contraction of the heart muscle to push blood through the aorta and pulmonary artery

T cell: group of white blood cells (lymphocytes) that coordinate the activity of the immune response and recognise, remember and destroy foreign cells (e.g. helper T, cytotoxic T, regulatory T and memory T)

Telodendria: distal branches of an axon which end at synaptic terminals

Teniae coli: longitudinal bands of smooth muscle on the outer surface of the colon

Terminal bouton: see synaptic terminal

Testosterone: steroid hormone secreted by the leydig cells of the testes

Tetanus: prolonged contraction of skeletal muscle (typically associated with the condition of the same name caused by bacterial infection)

Thalamus: egg-shaped structure situated in the diencephalon that relays ascending sensory information to the cerebrum and limbic system

Thermoreceptor: nerve ending that responds to change in temperature

Thrombocyte: clotting cell (platelet)

Thrombokinase: enzyme that converts prothrombin into thrombin at the beginning of the common clotting cascade

Thymosin: hormone secreted by the thymus gland required for T cells to mature and become immunocompetent

Thymus: gland situated behind the sternum that secretes thymosin and is the site of T cell maturation

Thyroid gland: situated in the neck it secretes the hormones triiodothyronine (T_3), thyroxine (T_4) and calcitonin

Thyroid-releasing hormone: peptide hormone secreted by the hypothalamus that triggers the release of thyroid-stimulating hormone

Thyroid-stimulating hormone: peptide hormone secreted by the anterior pituitary gland that stimulates the thyroid gland to secrete triiodothyronine (T_3) and thyroxine (T_4)

Thyroxine (T_4): amino acid derivative hormone secreted by the thyroid gland which regulates cell metabolism

Total peripheral resistance: total resistance to the flow of blood that is contributed by the peripheral (small vessel) circulation

Trabeculae: micro-architecture of spongy/cancellous bone (Latin 'little beam')

Transcription: process by which genetic information is copied from DNA to mRNA

Transfer RNA (tRNA): RNA molecules that transport amino acids to ribosomes for protein synthesis

Translation: process by which proteins are manufactured in the ribosomes by decoding mRNA

Tricuspid valve: heart valve (with three cusps) situated between the right atrium and right ventricle (also known as right atrioventricular valve)

Triglyceride: three molecules of fatty acid combined with a molecule of glycerol

Triiodothyronine (T$_3$): amino acid derivative hormone secreted by the thyroid gland which regulates cell metabolism

Trypsin: protein-digesting enzyme

Trypsinogen: inactive form of trypsin secreted by pancreatic acinar cells

Tunica adventitia: fibrous outer coat of arteries and veins composed of connective tissue

Tunica albuginea: dense capsule of connective tissue that surrounds the male testes and female ovaries

Tunica externa: see tunica adventitia

Tunica intima: inner layer of arteries and veins consisting of a single layer of endothelial cells

Tunica media: the middle layer of arteries and veins composed of smooth muscle and elastic fibres

Tunica vaginalis: serous membrane that surrounds the testes

Tunica vasculosa: delicate network of capillaries that line the tunica albuginea

Ureter: one of two thin muscular tubes that drain urine from the kidneys to the urinary bladder

Urethra: duct that conveys urine out of the body from the urinary bladder

Uterus: hollow muscular organ of the female reproductive tract (womb)

Vacuole: small cavity in the cytoplasm of a cell (bound by a single membrane) often containing fluid, food or metabolic waste

Vagus nerve: pair of cranial nerves responsible for parasympathetic control of the heart and many other internal organs

Valence: number of electrons in an atom's outer shell available for bonding

Vas deferens: muscular tube that transports sperm from the epididymis to the seminal vesicles and male urethra

Vasa recta (renis): series of straight capillaries in the renal medulla parallel to the loop of Henle

Vascular: relating to a vessel or vessels (e.g. carrying blood or lymph)

Vasoconstriction: narrowing of blood vessel wall

Vasodilation: widening of blood vessel wall

Vein: vessel that transports blood towards the heart

Vena cava: one of two large veins that return deoxygenated blood to the right atrium from the chest/neck (superior) or the abdomen (inferior)

Ventricle (brain): one of four communicating cavities in the brain filled with cerebrospinal fluid

Ventricle (heart): one of two lower chambers of the heart that receive blood from the atria and pump it into the pulmonary artery (right) and aorta (left)

Ventricular septum: central partition of the heart that divides the right and left ventricles

Venule: small vein

Vernix: waxy substance coating the skin of new-born babies

Vesicle: membranous fluid-filled pouch or cyst

Villus: small finger-like projection of the mucous membrane found in the small intestine and elsewhere

Visceral pericardium: inner layer of the pericardium which surrounds the heart and secretes pericardial fluid

Visceral pleura: serous membrane that covers the surface of the lungs and dips into the fissures

Volkmann's canals: perpendicular ducts in cortical bone that connect Haversian canals to one another

Vulva: external female genitalia (e.g. labia majora, labia minora, clitoris, vestibule, etc.)

Wernicke's area: situated on the left hemisphere it is involved in language comprehension

Zona fasciculus: central region of the adrenal cortex that secretes cortisol

Zona glomerulosa: outer region of the adrenal cortex that secretes aldosterone

Zona pellucida: thick layer of cells that surrounds the oocyte/ovum/blastocyst

Zona reticularis: inner region of the adrenal cortex that secretes small quantities of androgens

Zygote: cell formed immediately after conception (fertilised ovum with 46 chromosomes)

Zymogen: inactive enzyme precursor (e.g. pepsinogen)

INDEX

Note to index: pages given in italics refer to figures and pages given in bold refer to tables.